"ESSENTIALS OF LITHOTRIPSY"
'LithoTripsy Must Knows'

Prof. Dr. Anil K. Sahni
M.S, F.I.C.S, Advanced D.H.A
Surgeon, Medical Teacher
Urologist, Endoscopist
Lithotripsy Specialist

Life Member:
Austrian Medical Society
The Associaion Of Surgeons Of India
Delhi Urological Society
Association Of Minimal Access Surgeons Of India
Indian Association Of Gastro-Intestinal Endo-Surgeons

Address: A-1 / F-1 Block-A Dilshad Garden Delhi-110095 India.
Mobile : 09873083100
E-mail : dranil_sahni@yahoo.co.in
dranil_sahni@hotmail.com
dranilksahni@gmail.com

Copyright © 2015 Anil K. Sahni
All rights reserved.

ISBN: 1495491927
ISBN 13: 9781495491924

"PREFACE"

Last 2-3 Decades, Clinical Practice Witnessed Drastic Changes,
Due To Advent Availability Of Newer Technologies, Appliances
With Their SucessFul Applicabilities.
CareFul Observations Noticed An Evident Significant Shift In The
"Managemet Of Stone Disease" From Classical 'Open Stone Surgery'
Procedures To 'LithoTripsy' & Endoscopic Removal Of Stones:'PCNL',
Video Uretero-Renoscopy(URS) With Lithoclast,Cysto-Lithoclast Etc.
& More Recently Sucessfully Prcaticed Laproscopic Manovures
Like Lap. UreteroLithotomy.

Amongst Various Differently Practiced Recent Methodologies For
'Urolithiasis'. 'LithoTripsy' Has Established ItSelf As An Acceptable,
Authenticated Treatment Modality.
By Applying Discretely Focussed Extrinsic Shock Waves, Stones Are
Broken Into Minute Particles, That Are Passed Out With Urine Leaving
'Stone Free Patient', With The Advantages Of Simple, Safe, Secure,
Easily Performed, Non-Invasive Procedure, Avoiding Hazards Of
Anaesthesia & Surgical Trauma & Hence Minimal Ambulation.

Being Performed As 'OPD' Procedure, Patient Discharged Same Day,
Resumes Day To Day Routine Work Duties By Next Day,Thus Saving
Huge Infra-Structure,ManPower Resources & Working Hours,
As Compared To,Classical 'Open Stone Surgery' Procedures,
Endoscopic & Laproscopic Manovures For Stones Removal.
By Successful Technical Applicabilities & Ensured Minimal Errors,
Even In The Horizons Of Difficult Anatomical Locations, Secured 'Stone
Remnants Free' Patients, Provide No 'Nidus' For Future Stone Formation,
Resultant Minimally Reduced Recurrences,Subjected To Intensive
Recurrence Control Supportive Treatment Regimes,
Lead To Maximal Result OutComes

Especially In Geographical Regions, With High Prevalence Of
'Stone Diseases' & Hence Increased Susceptibility For Multiple Life
Time Recurrences, Of Differing Sites & Sizes Of Stone Formation,
The Imperative Need Of An Treatment Modality,
As Safely Advisable 'Stone Disease Management' Methodology,
Avoiding 'Repeated' Classical Open Surgeries',PCNLs,
LaproScopic Procedures Etc,
The Extended Scope Of The Established Procedure 'ESWL',
Secures An Authenticated Treatment Modality Status.

To Ascertain The Needed Demands Of Target Audience Including UnderGraduate, PostGraduate, Speciality Medical Students, Gen.Surgeons & Other Clinicians,
Dealing Abundance Of Stone Disease Patients, From CrystallUria To Differing Wide Variety Of Manifestations, In Close Co-operation With Attending Technical & Para-Medical Staff,
The Cautiously Prepared Available Comprehensive 'Text',
'LithoTripsy Study Material' Includes AllMost All Basic Fundamental Aspects Of The Procedure; Relevant Historical LandMarks, Involved Bio-Mechanics,Appliances, Procedural Details, Indications, ContraIndications, Complications,
Various Supportive Measures Regimes To Prevent Recurrences
& Additional Innovative Information Emphasizing For Facilitation Of The UnderStanding For Procedure Methodology - When Performed For Paediatric, Geriatric, Age Groups & Other Anatomical Compromised Stone Situation Circumstances;Lower Pole Stones, Lower Ureteric(VUJ) Stones Etc By-

i. Relevant X-Ray Films.
ii. Illustrative Diagrams Depicting 'Bio-Mechanics Aspects',
   Various Different 'Anatomical ParaMetres Determinants' Of Result Outcome, For Proper UnderStanding Of Complex Fundamentals.
iii. Recent Update Authenticated Work Study, Reports,References By Peer & Pioneers Of Respective Field, Has Been Methodically Concised, To Provide A Concise Systematic Reading UnderStanding, Regarding Various Aspects Of Different Involved Concepts With Further Reading Options.

Role Of Lithotripsy In "Biliary Stone Diseases"
& Scope For Other Indications,
Relevant Aspects Of 'Intra-Corporeal Litho-Tripsy',
With Recent SuccessFully Practiced Role Of 'Lasers' In 'Stone Disease' & Evolving Technique Methodology Of 'Extra –Corporeal Shock Wave LithoTripsy' Applicabilities, Have Been Summarized In Different Chapters.

In 'Discussion' & 'Conclusion' Parts Of The 'Text", All Relevant Key Points For Success In Achieving Maximal Result OutCome Of About >95% Success Rates, Along With Emphasis Upon Different Aspects Of 'Comprehensive Stone Management Strategies' Are Included.

Prof.Dr.Anil K. Sahni
M.S, F.I.C.S, Advanced D.H.A
Surgeon
MedicalTeacher

"SCIENTIFIC STUDY PRESENTATIONS APPRAISALS"

- "Extracorporeal Shock Wave Lithotripsy (ESWL), And Its Role In Urolithiasis, With Emphasis On Lower Pole, Inferior Calyx Kidney Stones, Lower Ureteric, VUJ Stones, And Gall Stone Diseases".
  62 AnnualConference,The Association Of Surgeons Of India, ASICON 2002, Science City, Kolkata,India,December'2002.

**Was Selected Amongst Several Papers On "Lithotripsy",
By The Scientific Paper Computer Code For Sectional Scientific Session- Urology, "New Technology In The Urological Field",
"The Association Of Genitourinary Surgeons Of India",
& Is The First Paper On Lithotripsy Presented, At National Level.**

- "ESWL(Modified Technique): Role in Inferior Calyx, Lower Pole Kidney Stones,Lower Ureteric, VUJ Stones, & Choledocho-Lithiasis".

Presentations During Various Different 'Academic Lecture Series', CME, CPD, LLL Programmes, At Local, State, National & International Levels.

Appraised For Availability Of Comprehensive Concise 'Study Material', With Evidence Based Support, For The SucessFul Treatment Modality, Applicabilities In 'Stone Disease ManageMent'.

"Abstract"

Objectives: Urolithiasis (Urinary Tract Calculi) Is A Common Clinical Problem Demanding Treatment, With Varying Incidence,Prevalence, Geographical Distribution Etc.
This Study Includes More Than 300 Patients Of Renal And Ureteric Calculi That Were Completely Removed By Extracorporeal Shock Wave Lithotripsy (ESWL).
Unless Associated Nonsupportive AnatomicalLandmarks Determinants Or Other Anatomical Abnormalities Within The Kidney, Such As Outflow Obstruction, E.G., Pelvi-Ureteric Junction Obstruction, Leading To Future Stones Formation By Promoting Stasis, Indicating Surgical Extraction Of Stone And Simultaneous Correction Of Defect,
Open Surgical Stone Extraction Procedures Are Considered Of Decreasing Interest, With The Advent Of Recent Successful Endourology & Laparoscopic Procedural Techniques.

Materials and Methods: More Than 300 Patients Of Variable Renal And Ureteric Calculi, Including Gall Stone Disease(Choledocholithiasis) Etc., Were Included In The Study Recording Successful Management With ESWL .
About 20 Slides Of X-Rays Abd. KUB Of About Seven Patients Demonstrating Gradual Removal Of Renal And Ureteric Calculi Were Included.
Adequately Powered And Frequency (Time Spaced), Shock Delivery With Discrete Coherence Upon Stone Throughout The Procedure Remains Key To Success.
Minutely Shattered Stone Particles Pass With Urine Spontaneously, Avoiding Obstructive Complications And Thus, Minimizing Need Of Double J Stent Insertion And/Or Other Complications Incidence.
Supportive Measures Such As Metabolic Evaluation, Stone Analysis, Diet Regulation, Various Regimes Of Medical Treatment Including Forced Diuresis, Proper In Regards To Dosage Duration And Supportive Compliance For Stones Up To 8 Mm And Residual Stone Fragments Utilized, Specially For Recurrence Management.
Specialized Procedural Emphasis Upon The ESWL Role In Lowerpole Inferior Calyx Renal Stone, Lower Ureteric, Vesico-Ureteric Junction Stones, And Gall Stone Disease:Solitary Gallstones,Choledocholithiasis, Pancreatic Calculi, With Or Without Contrast Delineation Included.

Results: More Than 300 Patients Of Renal And Ureteric Calculi Were Completely Removed By ESWL, Maintaining An Average Of About Two Sittings And More Than 95% Success Rate, While Single Sitting Clearance Achieved In About ≥50% Cases.

Conclusions: For All Practical Purposes, Renal And Ureteric Calculi Can Be Treated With ESWL With Almost Cent Percent (Complete) Success,Up To A Solitary Stone Size Of 45 Mm, With/Without Supportive Measures, Excluding Various Limiting Conditions.

Key words: ESWL**1)**, OSS(Open Surgical Stone Extraction) **2)**,
Lower Pole Renal Stones(LPS) **3)**,
Lower Ureteric, Vesico-Ureteric Junction(VUJ) Stones **4)**,
Choledocholithiasis **5)**, Diameter Of Infundibulum(IW) **6)**,
Infundibulopelvic Length(IL) **7)**, Lower Infundibulopelvic Angle(LIP) **8)**,
Spatial Distribution Of Calyces **9)**.

Foreward

It Has Given Me Great Pleasure To Peruse Dr.Sahni's Manual And It Has Been A Learning And Refresher Experience Too.

This Book Is A Detailed Account Of Not Only Lithotripsy But Stone Disease, Its Pathophysiology, Symptoms, Management And Their Complications.
The Chapters On Lithotripsy Traces The Various Generations Of Lithotripters To The Present. This Complex Methodology Has Been Simplified And Made Easy To Understand.

Renal Anatomy, Physiology Has Been Well Outlined. All Causes Of Stone Disease Have Been Dealt With And So Have TheirManagement, Including Non-Surgical.

It Also Includes Chapters On Indications, The Procedure Itself, Limitations And Side –Effects.

To Make It Complete, Stone Disease At Non Renal Sites Have Also Been Included.

This Is A Complete Book On Lithotripsy And Should A Compulsory Accompaniment Of All Medical Personnel

Dr. Sitangshu Basu
M.B.B.S., M.S., F.R.C.S.(UK)
Sr. Consultant Surgeon & Specialist Male Infertility

Max Superspeciality Hospital, Shalimar Bagh, Delhi- 110019,India.

FormerlySenior Consultant & Head Department Of Surgery And Urology

Jaipur Golden Hospital, Delhi.India.

'CONTENTS'

CHAPTERS	PAGE No.s
(1.) INTRODUCTION	1- 27

   (i.) Definition
   (ii.) Historical Aspects
   (iii.) Bio-Mechanics
   (iv.) Lithotriptors

(2.) ESWL:UROLITHIASIS   28 - 171

   (i) Urinary Stones: General Considerations
   (ii.) Procedural Details
   (iii.) Indications, ContaIndications Anatomical Determinants
   (iv.) Complications
   (v.) Emphasis Management Stones
   (vi.) Supportive Measures
      (A) Medical Therapy
      (B) Forced Diuresis
      (C) Stone Analysis
      (D) Dietary Regulations
      (E) Metabolic Evaluation
      (F) Treatment Of Cause

(3.) i. IntraCorporeal Lithotripsy   172 - 183
     ii. Role Of 'Lasers'

(4.) i. **ESWL: BILIARY STONE DISEASE**   184 - 233
     ii. **ESWL: OTHER INDICATIONS**
     III. **EXTRA-CORPOREAL TISSUE LITHOTRIPSY**

(5.) i. DISCUSSION   234-240
     ii. CONCLUSION

ACKNOWLEDGEMENTS   241-241
ABOUT THE AUTHOR   242-243

CHAPTER(1.)
INTRODUCTION

The Term 'Lithotripsy', Refers To A Medical Procedure,
Involving The Physical Destruction Of Hardened Masses Like Kidney Stones, Bezoars Or Gallstones.
Although Commonly Implied For 'Extracorporeal Shock Wave LithoTripsy (ESWL), The Various Different Implications Of Litho-Tripsy,
Have Been Discussed In The Subsequent Chapters.

(1.)(I.)DEFINITION

The Word 'Lithotripsy', Originated From Two Greek Words,
Litho - Meaning Stone, And Trip - Meaning To Break,
The First Known Use, Dates Back To 1834.
Medical Definition Of *LITHOTRIPSY*: The Breaking Of A Calculus
(As By Shock Waves Or Crushing With A Surgical Instrument)
In The Urinary System Into Pieces Small Enough To Be Voided Or Washed Out—Called Also ***Litholapaxy, Lithotrity.***

Successfully Acceptable Management Modality Of Urolithiasis,
With Extendable Scope For Other Stone Diseases.
Extra Corporeal Shock Wave Lithotripsy (ESWL),
Being Convenient Noninvasive, Safely Performed OPD Procedure,
Comprising Fragmentation Of Stone Into Minute Particles,
By Shock Waves.
Fragmented Stone Particles Are Passed With The Passage Of Urine,
In Due Course Of Time, Resulting In A Stone-Free Patient.
Usually, The Patient Undergoes The Procedure In The Morning,
Discharged In The After-Noon, And Can Go To Day-To-Day Work
By The Next Day With Advice For Follow-Up.
Since The Shock Waves Are Generated, Using A High-Voltage Spark
Or An Electromagnetic Impulse Outside Patient's Body,
The Procedure Is Termed Extracorporeal Shock Wave Lithotripsy(ESWL).

(1.)(II.)HISTORICAL ASPECTS

Urolithiasis Management Has Undergone Drastic Changes
Since Early 1980s, With Popularization Of Endourology,
ESWL, And PCNL Techniques.
High-Energy Shock Waves Have Been Recognized For Many Years,
Beginning 1969, Dornier (German Ministry Of Defense) Reported
Studies Of Shock Wave Effects On Tissue.
However, The Production And Distribution, Dornier HM3 Lithotripter
Availability, Began Late In 1983,
Whereas US Food And Drug Administration Approval For ESWL
Obtained In 1984.
Since Then, Numerous Companies Came With Different Models, Using
Various Technical Know-How And Varying Efficacies, Lithotripters.

Anil K. Sahni

Historical Landmarks

'Crushing The Stone': The first Minimally Invasive Surgery,
For Thousands Of Years Before The 19th Century,
'Cutting For The Stone' Or Lithotomy Through A Perineal Incision
Was The Ultimate Available Treatment.
A Gruesome Procedure, Performed Without Anaesthesia. Resultant Frightful Morbidity (3) Months Or Longer Recovery Periods, Erectile Dysfunction, Incontinence Or Persistent Draining Sinuses In Several Patients) And Mortality Rates Of At Least One Of Every Four Or five Deaths, Usually From Bleeding Or Sepsis.
Understandably, The Conveyed Message Was To Postpone Any Operation Until The Continued Pain Was Worse Than The Operation Itself.

At The Start Of The Modern European Period,
With The Growth And Progress Of The Science Of Chemistry In The 18th Century, Encouraged The Thought For Dissolving Bladder Stones. Various Medications, Chemicals And Noxious Concoctions Were Tried And Commercialized, Without Success, But It Undoubtedly Led The Thinking Towards Direct Means To Destroy Stones Within The Bladder i.e Intravesical Destruction Of Bladder Calculi,
By **The Modern Lithotrites.**

However, During The Byzantine Era, Dating Back To The 9th Century,
The Egyptians Used To Dilate Urethra To Facilitate The Passage Of Small Stones, Possibly By Some Form Of Lithotripsy Using A Catheter. But The Closely Guarded Secrets Of Surgical Techniques & Derived Information From Historical And Not Medical Sources ,Render Authentication Difficult.
In The Early 19th Century, As An Alternative To The Morbid And Frequently Fatal Perineal Lithotomy, Lithotripsy Emerged In Stages,

  I.   Learning To Pass A Straight Hollow Sound,
  II. Drilling Stones To Break Them By Crushing ,
  III. Followed By Evacuation Of Fragments,
  IV. Finally By Lithotrite Integration With The Cystoscope,
       Permitting Direct Vision Surgery.

Baron Charles Louis Stanislas Heurteloup (1793–1864),
Both A Lithotrite Inventor & Operator, Operating For Up To 2 Hrs Without HarmFul Effects And Achievied Removal Of All Of The Stone, As Compared To Short Time Working Sessions ,
Requiring Repeated Sessions As During Lithotripsy.

Bigelow Named The New Operation As **'Litholapaxy'**.
However, The Secret Of His Success Was Probably **The Use Of Anaesthesia, Discovered In 1846.**

Essentials Of Litho-Tripsy

In 1824 Civiale, Used Lithotrite To Perform The first Successful Lithotrity (Lithotresis) To Crush Bladder Stones.
Herr Civiale, Leroy Gruithuisen., Franz Von Gruithuisen (A Bavarian Physician) (1774–1852) - Procedural Success Of Passing A Straight Tube Into A Bladder.
Heurteloup, 1832- Introduction Of Percuteur, Or Curved Crusher With Hammer.
By 1833, The Developed Basic Principle For The Operation Of Lithotrites Remain Changed,

Until The first Quarter Of The 20th Century-
1877, Max Nitze Invention Of first Practical Cystoscope, Made Better With **Edison's Lamp In 1886**, And For The first Time, Urologists Could Visualize The Procedures Being Performed, Inside The Bladder.

In 1908, The final Phase Of Development To Modern Lithotrite-
Integrating The Cystoscope With The Lithotrite Completed,
Hugh H. Young Of Baltimore, By Using Bigelow's Lithotrite As A Model, Introduced A Lithotrite In Which The Stone Could Be Viewed & Grasped,

The first Lithotriptoscope, Enabling The. Engage, Crush Or Destroy Stones Completely And Safely Under Visualization,
Using Mechanical Or Newer Sources Of Energy.
An Example Is Electrohydraulic Lithotripsy, A More Sophisticated But Not Dissimilar Percussion Method As The Hammer.
The Modern Lithotrites, Several Models Developed in Susequent Years.

Famous people who were kidney stone formers include-Napoleon I, Epicurus, Napoleon III, Peter the Great, Louis XIV, George IV, Oliver Cromwell, Lyndon B. Johnson, Benjamin Franklin, Michel de Montaigne, Francis Bacon, Isaac Newton, Samuel Pepys, William Harvey, Herman Boerhaave, and Antonio Scarpa.

References

Andreassen KH, Dahl C, Andersen JT, Rasmussen MS, Jacobsen JD, Mogensen P. Extracorporeal shock wave lithotripsy as first line monotherapy of solitary calyceal calculi. Scand J Urol Nephrol 1997;31:245-8.

Renner CH, Rassweiler J. Treatment of renal stones by extracorporeal shock wave lithotripsy Nephron 1999;81:71-81.

Anil K. Sahni

Aulus Cornelius Celsus (1831). "Book VII, Chapter XXVI: Of the operation necessary in a suppression of urine, and lithotomy". In Collier, GF. *A translation of the eight books of Aul. Corn. Celsus on medicine* (2nd ed.). London: Simpkin and Marshall. pp. 306–14.

Shah, J; Whitfield, HN (2002). "Urolithiasis through the ages". *British Journal of Urology International* **89** (8): 801–10. doi:10.1046/j.1464-410X.2002.02769.x.PMID 11972501.

Ellis, H (1969). *A History of Bladder Stone*. Oxford, England: Blackwell Scientific Publications. ISBN 978-0-632-06140-2.

Bigelow, HJ (1878). *Litholapaxy or rapid lithotrity with evacuation*. Boston: A. Williams and Company. p. 29.

Desnos, E. C. (1972). The History of Urology up to the latter half of the Nineteenth Century, *In the History of Urology*, Ed. Murphy, LJT, Springfield & Illinois: Charles, C. Thomas, pp. 5-186.

Adams, F. (1846). In the seven books of Paulus Aegineta, Trans. Adams, F., Vol 2, London: The Syndenham Society, pp. 356-363.

Aegineta, P. (1846). *The seven books of Paulus Aegineta*, Trans. Adams F., Vol. 2, London: The Sydenham Society, pp. 354-362.

Albucasis (1973). *Albucasis on surgery and instruments: A definitive edition of the Arabic text with English translation and commentary*, Eds: Spink, M.S. and Lewis, I.L, London: Publications of the Wellcome Institute of the History of Medicine, pp. 414-417

Al-Razi (1961). *Kitabul Hawi Fi Al-Tibb* (Rhazes Liber Continens), Vol. 10, First Edition, Ed. The Bureau, Osmania Oriental Publications, Osmania University, Hyderabad, pp. 110-153.

Andreas a Cruce (1785). In: *A system of surgery*, by Alexander Bell, Second Edition, Edinburgh, C. Elliot publisher.

Charaka (1961). In *Kitabul Hawi Fi Al-Tibb* (Rhazes Liber Continens), Vol. 10, Ed. The Bureau, First Edition, Osmania Oriental Publications, Osmania University, Hyderabad, p. 131.

Cumston, C. G. (1968). *An Introduction to the History of Medicine from the Time of Pharaohs to the End of the XVII Century*. London: Dawsons of Pall Mall, pp. 23-26, 185-212.

Desnos, E. C. (1972). The History of Urology up to the latter half of the Nineteenth Century, *In the History of Urology*, Ed. Murphy, LJT, Springfield & Illinois: Charles, C. Thomas, pp. 5-186.

Dickinson, E.H. (1975). *The Medicine of the Ancients*. Liverpool: Adam Holden.

Dimopoulos, C., Gialas, A., Likourinas, M., Androutsos, G., & Kostakopoulus, A.(1980). Hippocrates: Founder and Pioneer of Urology. *British Journal of Urology*, 52: 73-74.

Essentials Of Litho-Tripsy

1(III) BIO-MECHANICS
Lithotriptor Appliances: Technical Aspects

Extracorporeal Shock Wave Lithotripsy (ESWL), A Well-Established And Most Commonly Performed Procedure For UroLithiasis, With Generally Ensured High Success Rates & Low Adverse Effects.

All Lithotripsy Machines (LithoTriptors) Have 4 Basic Components Essentially:
(1) **A Shockwave Generator;** Source Of Shock Waves
(2) **A Focusing System;** Focussing Devices
(3) **A Coupling Mechanism;** Including Coupling Medium
(4) **Localization Systems;** An Imaging/Localization Unit
   Accurate Device For Stone Targeting
   (Radio-Diagnostic-Ultrasonography, X-Ray/CT Scan Monitors).

(1) SHOCK WAVE GENERATOR
(Source Of Shock Waves)

Depending Upon The **Methodology For Generation Of Shock Waves**, There Are **(3) Primary Types Of Shock Waves Generators**:

(I) Electrohydraulic Shock Wave Lithotripsy (Spark Gap):

The Original Methodology Of Shockwave Generation (Used In The Dornier Hm3), Was Electrohydraulic Based Upon **'Spark-Gap Technology'**.
On The Passage Of High-Voltage Electrical Current Across A 'Spark-Gap Electrode' (About 1 Mm Apart), Located Within A Water-Filled Container (Hemi-Ellipsoid Reflector), The Resultant Underwater High-Voltage Spark Discharge Causes Explosive Vaporization At Electrode Tips, The Discharge Of Energy Produces A Vaporization Bubble, Which Expands And Immediately Collapses, Thus Generating A **High-Energy Spherically Expanding Pressure Waves**, Separated From Patients Body By An Insulated Membrane.

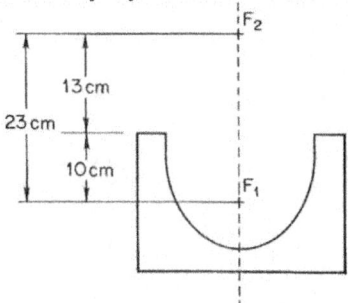

Ellipsoid Reflector In The Original HM3 Dornier LithoTriptor
The Distance Between The Second Focal Point & The Top Fixed At 13 cms, The Limitation Exists For Several LithoTriptors.
Source- JenKins AD, GillenWater JY 1988 Controversies On The Management Of Urinary Stones S Karger AG, Basel p.129

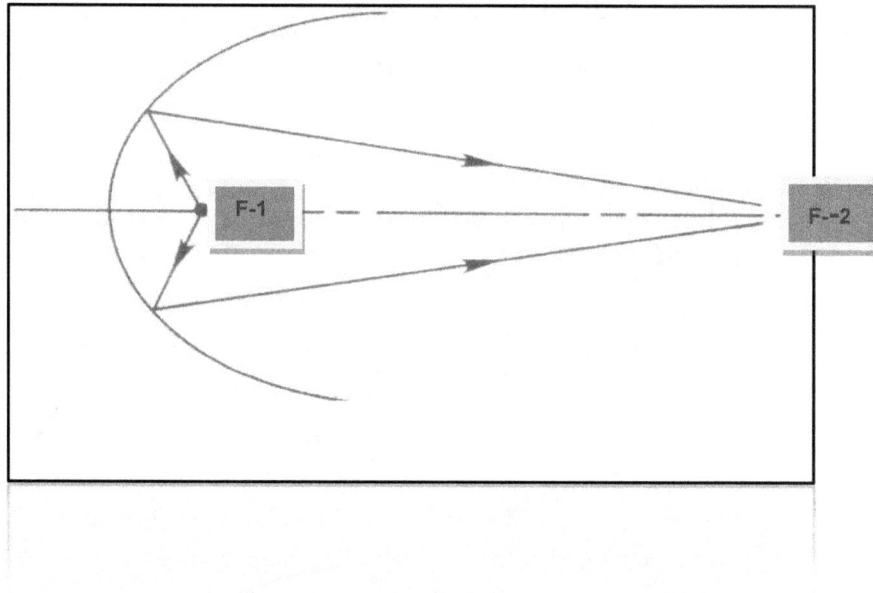

**Electrohydraulic Shock Wave Lithotriptor,
With Rotational Ellipsoid Reflector(Basic Design)**
Shock Waves Produced At F1, With Under Water Spark Discharge,
Focussed Laser Pulse Or Micro-Explosion
<u>Source</u>- JenKins AD 1987 1990 Urology Annual Appleton And Lange, East NorWalk CT, pp.266-273)

With Clear Advantage Of Effectiveness,
Disadvantages Include Substantial Pressure Fluctuations From Shock To Shock And Relatively Short Electrode Life.

(II)<u>Electromagnetic Generator:</u> A High Voltage Is Applied To An Electromagnetic Coil, This Coil, Either Directly Or Via A Secondary Coil, Induces High-Frequency Vibration In An Adjacent Metallic Membrane. This Vibration Is Then Transferred To A Wave-Propagating Medium (Water In Differing Containers),
Resultant Strong Magnetic Field Electromagnetic Force,
Termed 'Magnetic Pressure' Produce **Under Water Pressure ShockWaves, Either Plane Or Cylindrical Variety.**
Plane Waves Focused By **An Acoustic Lens**,
While Cylindrical Shock Waves Reflected By **A Parabolic Reflector**, Are Transformed Into Spherical Waves, Made Target Specific Coherence & Utilized For Stone Fragmentation.

Essentials Of Litho-Tripsy

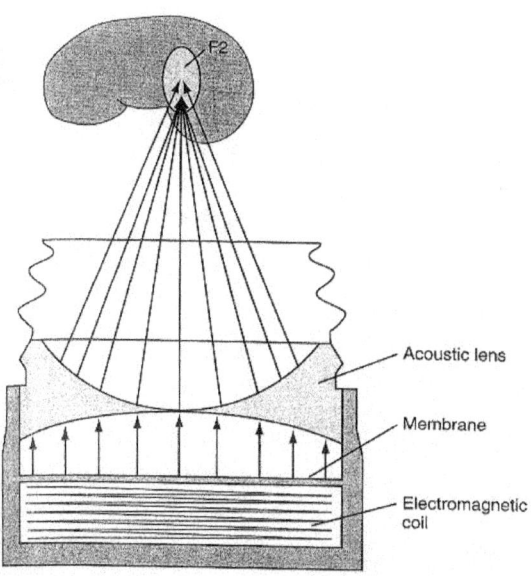

Schematic View-ElectroMagnetic Shock Wave Generator Using An Acoustic Lens For Focussing Shock Waves

Shock Waves Are Generated By ElectroMagnetic Coil
Source – CampBells Urology

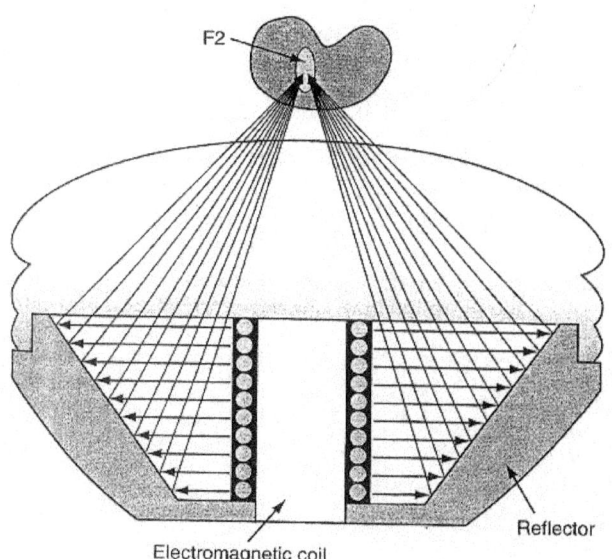

Schematic View-ElectroMagnetic Shock Wave Generator Using A ParaBoloic Reflector For Focussing Shock Waves

Shock Waves Are Generated By ElectroMagnetic Coil.

Source – CampBells Urology

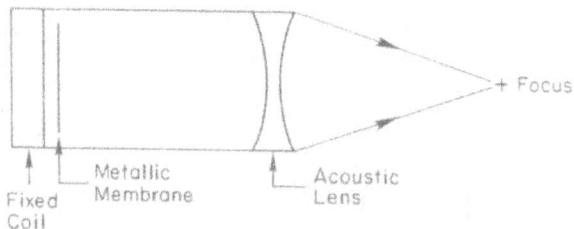

EisenMengerCoil Used In SieMens LithoStar Schematic illustration
ElectroMagnetic Principle With Different Geometric Configuration Used In STORZ Modulith LithoTriptor
Source- JenKins AD 1987 1990 Urology Annual Appleton And Lange, East NorWalk CT, pp.266-273)

Advantages Over The Electrohydraulic Generator:
(1) Due To No "Variable" In The Design, e.g Under Water Spark Discharge, Electromagnetic Generators Are More Controllable And Repeatable.
(2) Energy Entrance Involving A Large Body Surface Area, Through Patients, Rendering EMG Less Painful.

Disadvantages Due To A Small Focal Region Of High Energy Resulting In An Increased 'Subcapsular & Peri-Nephric Hematoma' Formation Incidences Rates In Modified/Unmodified E.M.Gs

III)Piezoelectric Generator: Production Of Electricity Via Application Of Mechanical Stress, The Piezoelectric Effect, First Demonstrated By Curie Brothers In 1880. Gabriel Lippman In The Following Year, Theorized The Reversibility Of This Effect,That Was Later Confirmed By The Curie Brothers. The Piezoelectric Generator Takes Advantage Of This Effect.

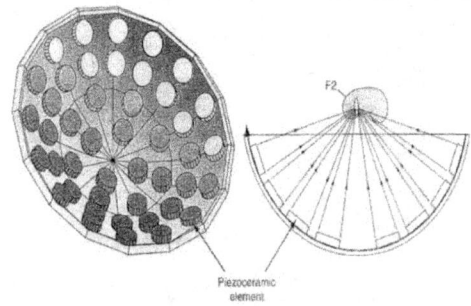

Piezoelectric Shock Wave Generator
Numerous Polarized PolyCrystalline Ceramic Elements Are Positioned On The Inside Of A Spherical Dish.
Source-CampBell's Urology

Essentials Of Litho-Tripsy

Thus Based Upon Piezoelectric Effect Phenomenon,
Utilization Of Polarized Polycrystalline Ceramic Elements, Set In A
Water-Filled Container, Stimulated Via High-Frequency Electrical Pulses.
The Alternating Stress/Strain Changes In The Material Create Ultrasonic
Vibrations, Resulting In The Production Of **Plane Shock Waves With
Direct Convergence Shock Fronts**, Are Used For Stone Fragmentation.

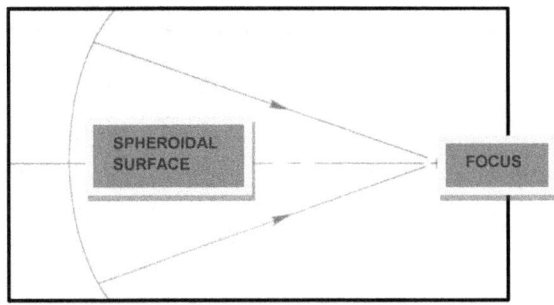

PiezoElectric Lithotriptor,
Numerous Small PiezoElectric Crystals Mounted The Spheroidal Surface,
Or One Large PiezoElectric Crystal Mounted On The Spheroidal Plate At
Central Axis.
Source- JenKins AD 1987 1990 Urology Annual Appleton And Lange, East
NorWalk CT, pp.266-273)

Advantages Include Accuracy, Durability, And Less Painful
Anesthetic Free Treatment Due To Low Energy Density At
Skin Entry Points.
Disadvantages Being Less Efficacy Due To
Insufficient Power Delivery For Stone Fragmentation.

**Others Including Micro-Explosive Generators: Using Lead Azide
Pellets & Laser Beam Multistage Light Gas Guns**
Could Not Gain Mainstream Acceptance.

Intra-Corporeal Appliances: Produced Shock Waves Are Utilized Within
Patients' Body Directly To Stones,
Available As 'Flexible' & 'Rigid' Instrumentations.
SomeTimes Combination Of Ballistic & USG Devices Are In Use.

(Please Note, IntraCorporeal Devices Chapter)

(2) FOCUSING SYSTEMS
(Focussing Devices)

To Direct The Generator-Produced Shockwaves At A Focal Volume In A Synchronous Fashion, The Focusing System Is Used.

An Ellipse Being The Basic Geometric Principle Used In Most Lithotriptors. Shockwaves Are Created At One **Focal Point (F1)** And Converge At The Second **Focal Point (F2).**

The Target Zone Or Blast Path, Is The 3-Dimensional Area At F2, Where The Shockwaves Are Made Coherent And Fragmentation Occurs.

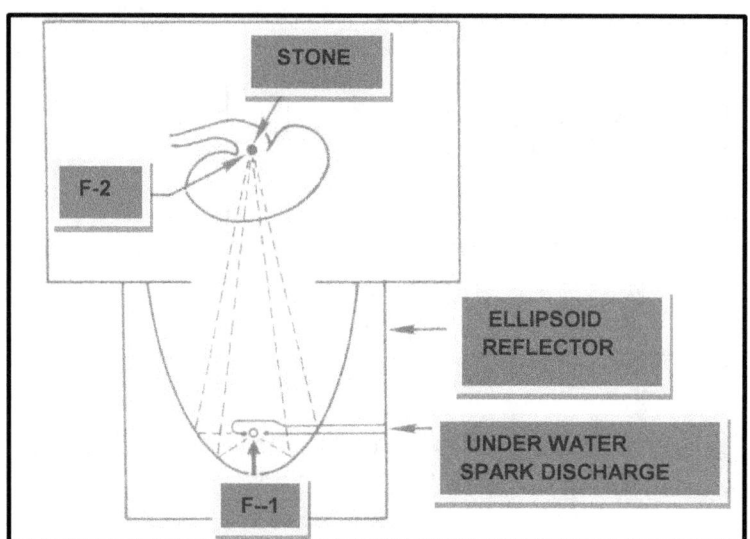

Dornier's ElectroHydraulic LithoTriptor
Spherical Shock Waves Produced At F_1 By Under Water Electrode Discharge. With Patient's Stone Placed At F2, The Spherical Shock Waves Are Focussed At F_2 By Ellipsoid Reflector.
Source- Chaussy & Fuchs 1987b

**Depending On The Shockwave Generator Used,
Focusing Systems Differ:**
Electrohydraulic Systems; Used The Principle Of The **Ellipse** - A Metal Ellipsoid Directs The Energy Created From The Spark-Gap Electrode.
Electromagnetic Systems; The Shockwaves Are Focused With Either, An Acoustic Lens (Siemens System) Or
A Cylindrical Reflector (Storz System).
Piezoelectric Systems; Ceramic Crystals Arranged Within A
Hemispherical Dish Direct The Produced Energy Toward A Focal Point.

Essentials Of Litho-Tripsy

(3) COUPLING MECHANISMS

**During Propagation And Transmission Of A Wave,
Energy Loss At Interfaces With Differing Densities Occurs.
To Minimize The Dissipation Of Energy Of A Shockwave As
It Traverses The Skin Surface, As Such,
A Coupling System Is Needed.
Water Being The Usual Coupling Medium Used**, DueTo A Density Similar To That Of Soft Tissue And Its Readily Availablity.

In **First-Generation Lithotriptors (Dornier Hm3)**,
The Patient Used To Be Placed In A Water Bath.
However, With **Second- And Third-Generation Lithotriptors**,
To Provide Air-Free Contact With The Patient's Skin, Small Water-Filled Drums Or Cushions With A Silicone Membrane Are Used Instead Of Large Water Baths.
The Innovation Facilitates The EfficaciousTreatment Of Calculi In The Kidney Or The Ureter, Often With Less Anesthesia
Than That Required With The First-Generation Devices.

(4) LOCALIZATION SYSTEMS

(An Imaging/Localization Unit; Accurate Device For Stone Targeting
 (Radio-Diagnostic-Ultrasonography, X-Ray/CT Scan Monitors).

The Aims Of Imaging Systems Use ;
1. To Localize The Stone.
2. To Direct The Shockwaves OnTo The Calculus Maximally,
   So AsTo Achieve Better Results.
3. By Tracking The Progress Of Treatment, All Throughout
   'Litho-Tripsy Sitting' And Making Necessary Alterations As
   Needed By The Stone Fragments Status.

The (2) Methods Fluoroscopy And Ultrasonography,
Were Commonly Used To Localize Stones.
Fluoroscopy, Involves Ionizing Radiation To Visualize Calculi & Has Familiarity To Most Urologists. As Such, For Detecting And Tracking Calcified And Otherwise Radio-Opaque Stones,
Both In The Kidney And The Ureter.
Fluoroscopy Is Excellent.
But The **Disadvantage** Of Usually **Poor Localization Of Radiolucent Stones (Eg, Uric Acid Stones)**, Needs Compensation By Introducing **Intravenous Contrast Radiology** Or More Commonly, Retrograde Pyelography i.e Cannulation Of The Ureter With A Catheter And Retrograde Instillation Of Contrast, Can Be Performed.

Ultrasonographic Localization Renders **Visualization Of Both Radiopaque And Radiolucent Renal Stones**,
But The **Real-Time Monitoring Of Lithotripsy**.
Due To Much Less Expensive Cost Than Radiographic Systems, Most Second-Generation Lithotriptors Utilize This Imaging Modality.
Ultrasonography With The Advantage Of Ionizing Radiation Exposure Prevention, Has The Technically Inability To Visualize Ureteral Calculi, Particularly Smaller Stones, & In Interposed Air-Filled Intestinal Loops Situations, Difficulty For Accurate Localization.

Stones Can Either Be Localized With **Ultrasound** Or X-Ray.
The Main Benefits Of **Ultrasound** Are Real Time Monitoring Of The Disintegration Process And The Absence Of Ionizing Radiation.
Fluoroscopy Imaging Usually Is Very Fast And Precise. It Visualizes Areas That Are Not Seen With Ultrasound.
Dornier Lithotripters Are Designed For Dual-Mode Imaging Offering The Choice To Apply Both Imaging Modalities Simultaneously.

The Availability Of CT Scan Continuous Monitoring; By
Available C-Arm & Or Integrated C-Arm Units,
Has A Definite Useful Role In Contributing To The Overall Better Efficay Of III Generation Litho-Triptors.

Bio-Physics:Extra-Corporeal Shock Waves

In The Early 80s, Extra-Corporeal Shock-Wave Lithotripsy (ESWL) Was Introduced In Clinical Practice.
It Is A Minimally Invasive Method , Comprising The Destruction Of Stones (Kidney, Biliary) By The Action Of Multiple Shock Waves (Strong Impulses Of Acoustic Pressure).The Resultant Debris (Fragmented Stone Particles) Are Removed From The Body Via Natural Efferent Passages.

Extra-Corporeal Shock Waves Produced By A Source, Outside The Patient Body, Are Propagated Inside The Body Focused On Stone.
Externally Generated Relatively Weak Nonintrusive Waves, Transmitted Through The Body, Building Sufficient Strength At The Target Site To Break Stone, Is Achieved By Uniqueness Of This Device.

Rapid Energy Deposition Into Fluid Leads To Shock Wave Production Invariably. This Is Described As Surfaces, Dividing Material Ahead, Not Yet Affected By The Disturbance At The Source From Material Behind, Which Has Been Compressed As A Consequence Of The Energy Input (**Sturtevant, 1996**).

Essentials Of Litho-Tripsy

With The Behavioral Characteristic Of Propagation Of Non-Linear Waves Moving Faster Than The Speed Of Sound, Shock Waves' Speed Is In Direct Proportion To The Shock Strength.

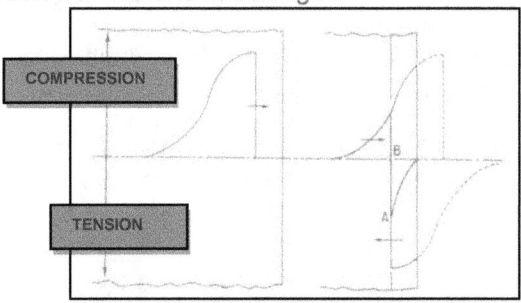

Lithotripsy;Time-Course Of A Shock Wave
Formation Of A Tensile Shock Wave Following Reflection Of A Compressive Shock Wave At An Acoustic InterFace.
Source-Rinehart J 1967 International Symposium On Stress Wave Propagation In Materials. JohnWiley And Sons INC.newYork.pp.247-269

A Rapid Onset Of Pressure Gradient Arises On An Interface Of Two Media, As A Result Of Difference In Acoustic Impedances.
If The Pressure Force Exceeds The Mechanical Resistance Of A Stone, Its Progressive Fragmentation Occurs (Pressures Of About 10^8 Pa Is Necessary).
Many Shock Waves (50 To 4000,On Average 1000) Needs.Application (Synchronous With Heart Beats), For Complete Fragmentation Of Stone.

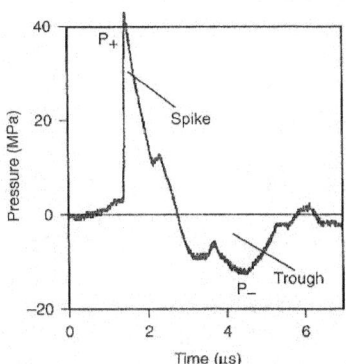

PolyVinylidene DiFluoride Membrane Hydrophone Measured Typical Pressure Pulse At The LitoTriptor Focus(F2).

The Initial Steep Positive Pressure Front Of About 40MPa,
Followed By Negative Pressure Of 10 MPa,
With Entire Pulse Duration Of 4 μsec.
Source- Cole Man AJ, Sauders JE, Preston RC, et al. Pressure Wave Forms Generated By A Dornier ExtraCorporeal Shock Wave LithoTriptor.UltraSound Med Biol 1987;13:651-7.

PATHOPHYSIOLOGY
STONE FRAGMENTATION BIOMECHANICS
By Different LithoTripsy Appliances Has Been Categorized As-

1. Electrohydraulic Lithotripsy: Cavitation Bubble Formation Mechanism.
2. Laser Lithotripsy: Plasma Bubble Formation,
                    Shock Wave Mechanism,
3. Ultrasonic Lithotripsy: By Ultrasound Vibrations
4. Ballistic Lithotripsy: Projectile Movemen Jackhammer Effect

The Potential Mechanisms For 'ESWL' Stone Breakage: Can Be Explained By-

Typical Pressure Pulse
Tensile Pressure (Positive And Negative Phase)
Reversed Pressure Theories;
(1) Compression Fracture
(2) Spallation
(3) Acoustic Cavitations And Bubble Formation
(4) Dynamic Fracture Fatigue

Cumulative Damage Accumulation During Course-Of Treatment Lead To Eventual Stone Destruction.

The Exact Mechanisms By Which Shock Waves Can Damage Stones And Tissue Are Still Not Fully Understood, Although It Is Likely That Direct Stresses And Cavitation Are Dominant In Stone Fragmentation, And That Cavitation Is Dominant In Tissue Injury.

Most Lithotriptors Produce A Similar Type Of Shock Wave, Which Consists Of-
A Leading Positive Pressure Shock Front (Compressive Wave) Lasting About 1 Ms Followed By
A Negative Pressure Trough (Tensile Wave), Which Lasts About 3 Ms.

There Is A Large Range In The Amplitude Of
The Shock Waves Used, With Peak Positive Pressures Of 30 To 110 Mpa Depending On The Type Of Shock Source And The Power Setting.

The Intense Compressive Wave Induces Mechanical Forces Inside The Stone That May Lead To Fragmentation, Most Likely By A Spall Mechanism.
The Tensile Component Of The Shock Wave Is Lower Amplitude (About -8 To -15 Mpa). This Negative Pressure Drives Cavitation Bubble Activity That Is Critical To Stone Comminution, But Also Causes Vascular Trauma To The Kidney.

Essentials Of Litho-Tripsy

Numerous Mechanisms Have Been Proposed To Explain How Shock Waves Break Urinary Stones.
No Single Mechanism Gives An Adequate Explanation, And
It Appears That **Multiple Mechanisms** Involving Cavitation And Spallation Are At Play. For Tissue Injury
On The Other Hand It Appears That Cavitation, And Shock Wave/Bubble Interaction, Are The Most Likely Cause Of Trauma.

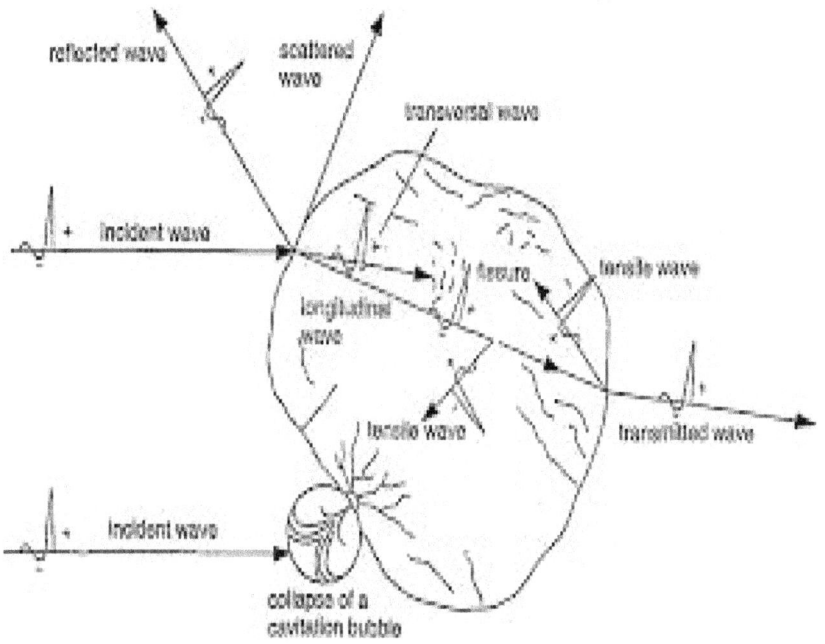

Summary-Bio-Mechanics Of Various Mechanical Forces Generated By ESW LithoTriptor Cause Stone Fragmentation

Source-
The Physics of Shock Wave LithotripsyRobin O. Cleveland, PhD
James A. McAteer, PhD Acknowledgements-Grants From The National Institutes Of Health (NIH DK43881, DK55674) And The Whitaker Foundation (RG-01-0084).

Stone Fragmentation Ocurs When The Shockwaves Forces Overcomes The Tensile Strength Of The Stone. Not Completely Understood, Fragmentation Is Considered To Occur Through A Combination Of Methods, Including Compressive And Tensile Forces, Erosion, Shearing, Spalling, And Cavitation. Amongst These Different Forces, Compressive And Tensile Forces Generation And Cavitation Are Thought To Be The Most Important.

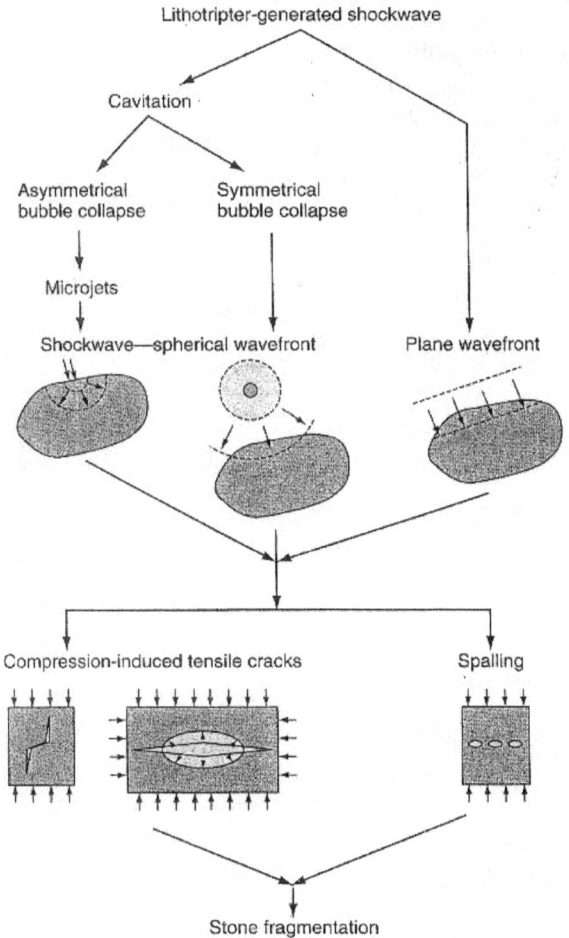

Summary-Bio-Mechanics Of Various Mechanical Forces Generated By ESW LithoTriptor Cause Stone Fragmentation
Source- Dr.Bradley Sturtevant (CampBell UroLogy)

Shockwave Propagation Through A Medium (Water), Causes Very Little Energy Loses, Until While Crosses Into A Medium With A Different Density. If The Medium Is Denser, **'Compressive Forces'** Are Produced On The New Medium. Similarly,
If The New Medium Is Less Dense, **'Tensile Stress'** Is Produced On The First Medium Upon Hitting The Anterior Surface Of A Stone,
The Change In Density Creates **Compressive Forces**, Causing Fragmentation. As The Wave Proceeds Through The Stone To The Posterior Surface, The Change From High To Low Density Reflects Part Of The Shockwave's Energy, Producing **Tensile Forces**, Which Again Disrupt And Fragment The Stone.

Essentials Of Litho-Tripsy

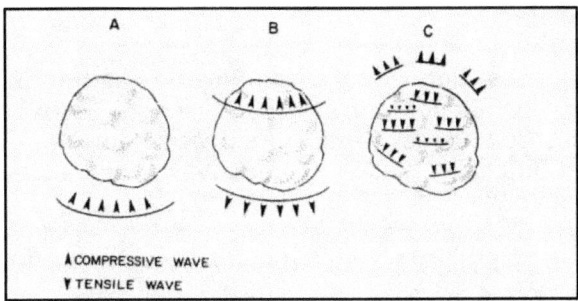

Shock Waves Induced Spalling On The Front & Back Surfaces Of A Representative Stone
Source - Chaussy & Fuchs 1987b

In Cavitation, Shockwave Energy Applied At A Focal Point Leads To Failure Of The Liquid With Generation Of Water-Vapor Bubbles. These Gaseous Bubbles Collapse Explosively, Creating Microjets That Fracture And Erode The Calculus.
The Process **Can Be Monitored With Real-Time Ultrasonography** During TheTreatment And Appears As Swirling Fragments And Liquid In The Focal Zone.

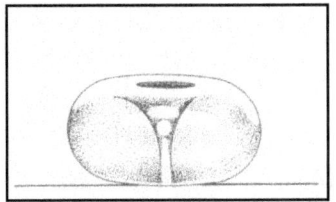

With Visible Cavitation Jet Travelling Through The Centre, Cavitation Bubble Resting On A Surface.
The Liquid Micro-Jet Force Capable Of Deforming Metals & May Be Partially Responsible For Stone Destruction And Tissue Injury
Source – Dr.Larry Crum 1988

Thus, **Stone Fragmentation** Is Primarily Caused By,
High Local Tensile And Shear Waves Created By The Focused Shock Waves Hitting The Stone.
Spherical Shock Wave Fronts Contribute To
Compression-Induced Tensile Cracks Or Spalling
At The Posterior Stone Surface.
Cavitation Is Also Important For Stone Comminution.
The Rapid Collapse Of Cavitation Bubbles On The Surface Of The Stone Or In Liquid-Filled Cracks Within The Stone Produces Shock Waves, Causing Microfractures In The Stone.

ESWL Success, Dependent Upon Several Factors Such As- Stone Location, Stone Composition, Stone Size, Patient's Body Characteristics And Risk Factors, Pain Management, Treatment Strategies, And The Shock Wave Parameters.
The Effectiveness Of The Shock Wave Is Also Related To The Absence Of Anatomical Structures Within The Shock Wave Path And The Accuracy With Which The Stone Is Located And Aligned In The Therapy Focus Of The Shock Wave Source.

Effective Disintegration Energy

Stone Fragmentation Is Firmly Correlated With The Shock Wave Energy Delivered Into The Focal Zone.
Shock Wave Pulse Acoustic Energy Is Determined Within An Area Having A Diameter That Corresponding To The Average Urinary Stones Size.
Effective Energy Contributing To Stone Disintegration, Is Generally Defined As Energy Delivered To An Area Of 12 Mm Diameter In The Focal Plane(12-Mm Area Corresponds To Most Stones Indicated For ESWL Monotherapy).
With Precisely Targeted Stone Delivery, Most Of The Effective Energy Is Utilized For Fragmentation, Except The Portion Not Directly Hitting The Stone ,That Is Absorbed By Surrounding Tissue .
For Larger Stones Fragmentation, Full Effective Energy Application To Stone Is Needed.
Safe Energy Dose (Number Of Shock Waves & Times Dependent Effective Energy) Selection To Disintegrate The Stone,Is Important.

Energy Dose $E_{tot}(12mm) = N * E_{eff}(12mm)$
N - Is Number Of Applied Shocks
$E_{eff}(12mm)$ - Is The Disintegration Energy(Acoustic Energy Per Shock Wave Delivered To An Area Of 12 Mm Diameter In The Focal Plane).

Treatment Success In Terms Of Fragmentation And Side Effects Is Determined ByThe Applied Energy Dose.
Thus, The Success Of ESWL Treatments At Different Intensity Levels Seems To Remain The Same, When The Number Of Shots Is In The Range Receiving Equivalent Energy Dose.
The Energy Dose For Kidney Stones Typically Is In The Range Of 100 To 200 J Per Treatment.

Pulse Repetition Frequency (PRF):
Cavitation Bubbles In The Shock Wave Path Exert A Noticeable Effect On Fragmentation Efficacy, By Shock Wave Attenuation & Resultant

Essentials Of Litho-Tripsy

Fragmentation Efficacy Reduction.
In Vitro Performed Studies Suggest That The PRF Influences Fragmentation Efficacy Due To **Cavitation Effects**.
At Higher PRFs, Shock Waves Become Less Effective.
For This Reason PRF Should Be Kept As Low As Possible.

The Shock Waves Of Energy 1.2-40 Mj Have Energy Density Of 0.14 – 1.8 Mj/Mm^2 In Focus. This Energy Is Sufficient To Penetrate To Max. 60mm In Depth. The Frequency Can Be Changed From 1 To 4 Hz. The Focal Pressure Is 10 – 100-Times Lower That That Produced By A Lithotripter.

1.iv. LITHO-TRIPTER(LITHO-TRIPTOR)

DEFINITION: Lithotripter /**Litho·Trip·Ter/(Lith´O-Trip"Ter)**;
An Instrument For Crushing Calculi In Lithotripsy.
The Term '**Litho –Tripter (Litho-Triptor)**',Is Commonly Used For Appliance Device To Perform Lithotripsy,
Especially **A Noninvasive Device** That Pulverizes Stones By Focusing Shock Waves On A Patient Through Insulated Membrane Or Patient Immersed In A Water Bath(As In Early Models).
HowEver, The Variant Expressions Of Litho-Tripter *Include*
'Lithontriptor', From *Lithontriptic* Breaking Up Bladder Stones, Modification Of **Greek (*Pharmaka Tōn*) *Lithōn Thryptika*** (Drugs) Capable Of Pulverizing Stones,WithThe First Known Use Recorded, In Year 1825.

"**Lithotripsy**", From The Greek Word Meaning "Stone Crushing," Drastically Changed The Uro-Lithiasis Management,With Its Extending Scope In Gall Stone Diseases & Others.
Ultra-Sonic, Electro-Hydraulic And Laser Lithotripters Have Been Adapted For Use With Nephroscopes (Percutaneous Nephrostolithotomy, Or PNL), Ureteroscopes (Transureteral Ureteroscopic Lithotripsy, Or TUL) To Pulverize Urinary Stones,
While, Varieties Of Gastro-Endoscopes For Hepato-Biliary,Pancreatic Stone Diseaes & 'HIFU' Being Amongst Most Recent Available Appliances.

Evolution Of Shockwave Lithotriptors

<u>The Dornier HM3</u>; The First 'Shockwave Lithotriptor' Introduced In The United States, Was Originally Designed To Test Supersonic Aircraft Parts. HM3 Design Based On **'Electrohydraulic Shockwave Generator'** Principles, With **Patient Immersed In A Water**, The Shockwaves Are Focused Via An **Ellipsoid Metal Water-Filled Tub**, For Localization & Placement Of The Calculi, In The Target Zone.
Despite Being Somewhat Dated, It Is **Still One Of The Most Effective Lithotriptors** And RetainsThe **Standard For Comparing The Efficacy Of Other Available Appliances.**

<u>Second-Generation Lithotriptors</u>; The Energy Source Being **Piezoelectric Or Electromagnetic Generators**, Coupled With The Appropriate Focusing Device, These Litho-Triptors Commonly Have A Smaller 'Focal Zone'.
The Coupling Device Being A Silicone-Encased Water Cushion That Coapts To The Patient, Providing Simplified 'Positioning Of Patient' For Procedure.
A Smaller Focal Zone Rendering The Advantages Of Analgesia & Minimal Surrounding Tissue Damage , But At The Cost Of Stone Movement In And Out Of The Focal Zone, During Respiratory Excursion, Thus Compromising Fragmentation Rates.

Essentials Of Litho-Tripsy

The Newest-Generation Lithotriptors; Were Designed To Offer Greater Portability And Adaptability With The **Advantage To Alternate Between Imaging Modalities (Both Fluoroscopy And Ultrasonography Available)**, Compensating The Deficiencies Of Either System.

Most Current Lithotriptors; Utilizing **Electromagnetic Generators** And Their **Focusing Units** Have The Capablity Of Delivering Shockwaves Similar In Intensity To HM3, To A Smaller Focal Zone.
Although The Theoretical Advantage Of Minimized Sourounding Tissue Damage & Stone Movement Away From Target Zone Factor, Compensated By Improved Localization Techniques And Anesthetic Manipulation , Yet OverAll Higher Failure Rates, Incomplete Treatment, And The Needs For Retreatment, Are Reported, With II & III Generation Litho-Triptors.

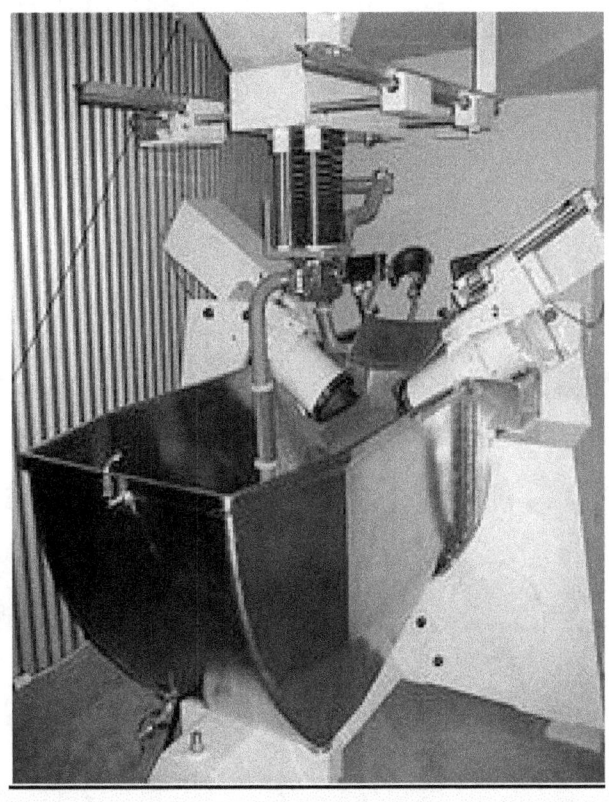

THE DORNIER HUMAN MODEL 1 (HM1) PROTOTYPE LITHOTRIPTER (DEUTSCHE MUSEUM AT BONN).

'LITHOTRIPTER' MACHINES: AVAILABLE VARIETIES

RELEVANT DETAILS:
- Radiolucent Table Holds Up To 186 Kgs (410 Lbs)
- Zero Bladder Cut-Off And Large Travel Ranges Allow The Display Of The Entire Urinary Tract
- Exchangeable, Radiolucent Mid-Sections
- Flexible Table Has X, Y, Z And Trendelenburg Movement With An Isocentric And Non-Isocentric Tilt Feature

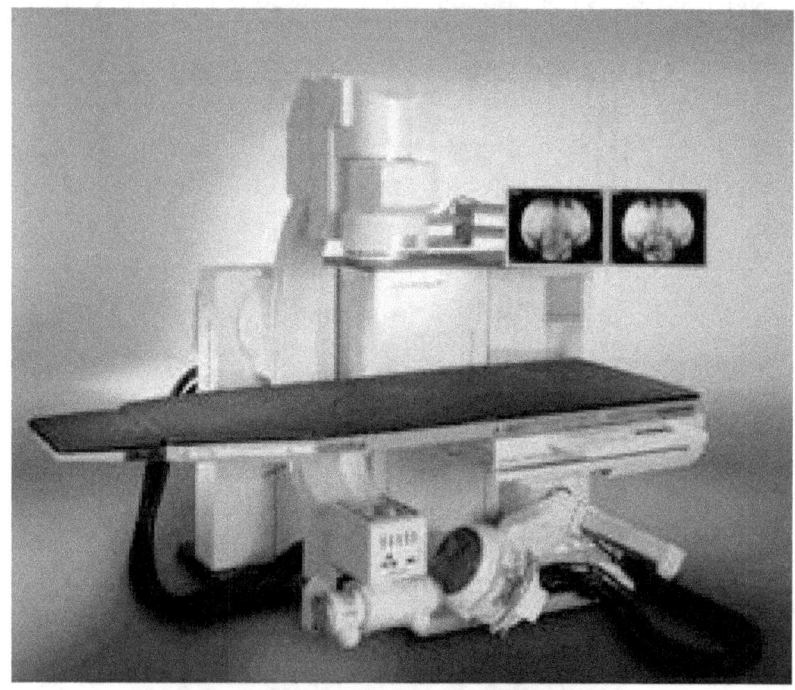

Dornier Lithotripter S II
- **Premium multi-functional lithotripter**
- **Comprehensive patient data management with DICOM 3.0 interface**
- **Integrated urological workstation ideally suited for both ESWL and endourology**
- **Computer controlled automatic positioning**
- **Stationary design**

Essentials Of Litho-Tripsy

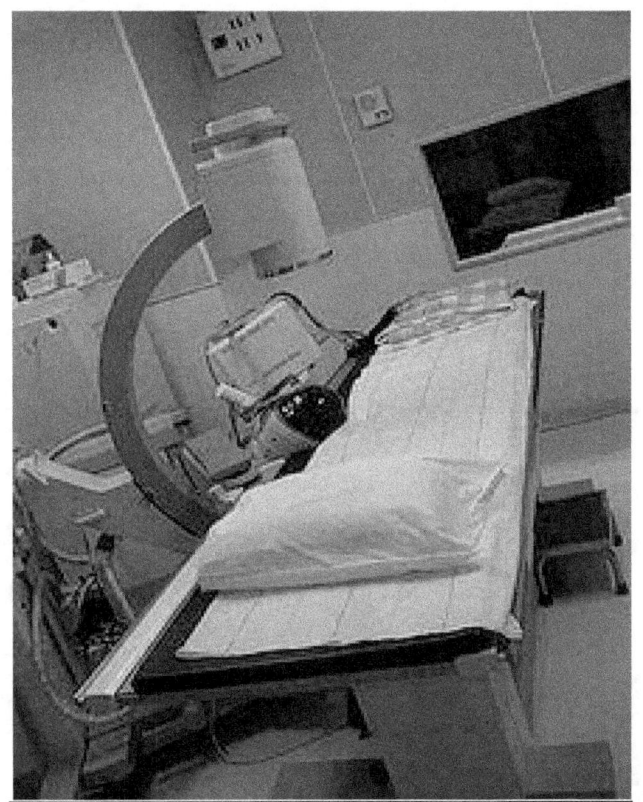

AN ESWL MACHINE (LITHOTRIPTER) INSIDE AN OPERATING ROOM.

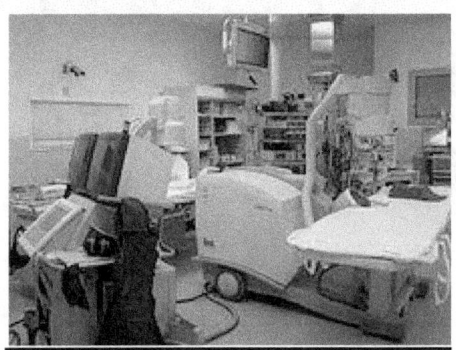

A **Lithotriptor Machine** Is Seen In An **Operating Room**; Other Equipment Is Seen In The Background, Including An **Anesthesia Machine** And A **Mobile Fluoroscopic System** (Or "C-Arm").

STONE-LITH (PCK) LITHOTRIPTER

(1.) Patient Table: Vertical, Horizontal (Up-Side Down, Toward, And Away From Machine), Hydraulic Function

(2.) Ellipsoid, Electrodes, Connecting Tube, Insulated Membrane

(3) C-Arm Unit, Integrated U-Arm

(4.) Monitoring Unit; Operating Unit With Remote Control Devices

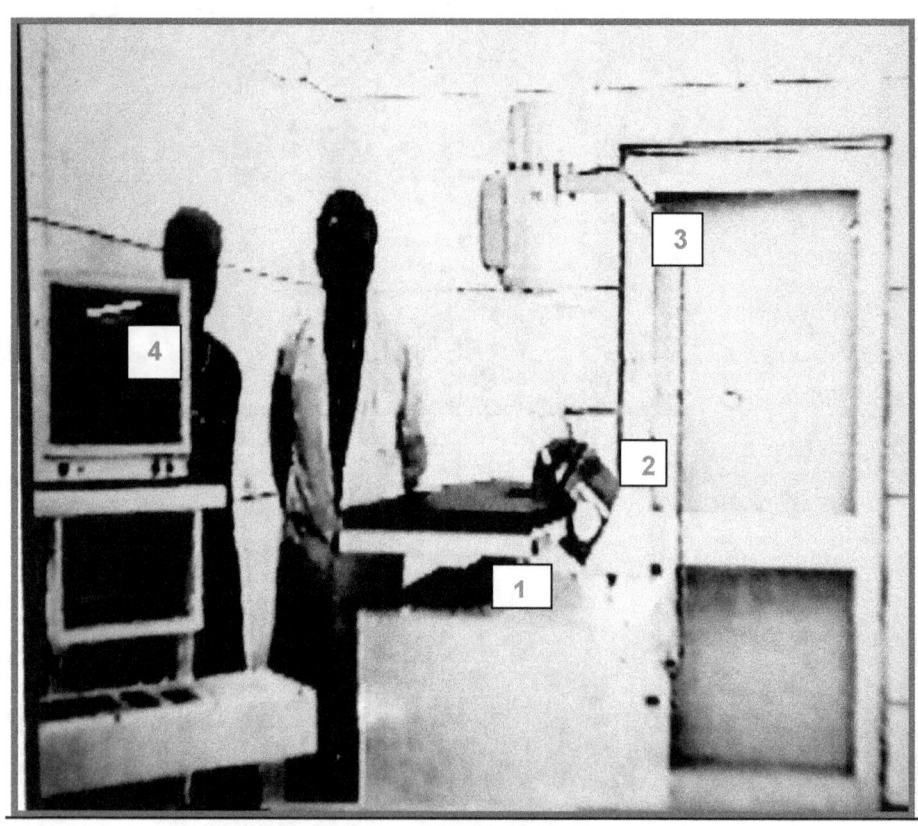

Stone-Lith (PCK) Litho-Triptor

Essentials Of Litho-Tripsy

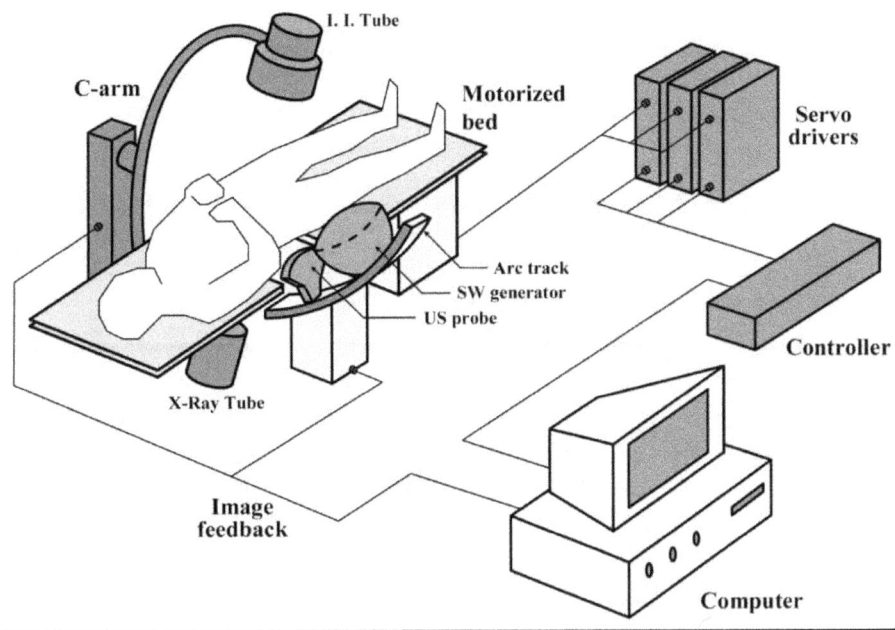

Sensors | Free Full-Text | Design Of The Dual Stone Locating System On An Extracorporeal Shock Wave Lithotriptor
www.Mdpi.Com1024 × 718Search By Image

LITHOTRIPTER COMPARISONS

The Success Of ESWL Has Resulted In Its Rapid Acceptance World Wide (Power.1987:Bloom et al.1991) & Has Also Stimulated Interest In The Development Of AlterNative ExtraCorporeal LithoTripsy Devices By Numerous Manufatures.

Despite Large No. Of Publications Regarding LithoTripsy In Urologic Literature(Mid-1980s), No Appropriately Designed Comparative Trials On Lithotriptors AvailAble, Due To No Agreed-On Standards Amongst Manufacturers, Regarding Quantification Of Power & Efficiency Of LithoTriptor.

Available Various Studies Involving Several Aspects For Lithotripter Comparisons Remained Non-Authentic Due To Lack Of Awareness Regarding Several DeterMinant Factors(LingeMan et al.1994).

Despite The Proliferation Of LithoTriptors & The Variety Of Solutions Devised For Stone Targeting & ShockWave Delivery, No Other LithoTriptor System System Has Convincingly Equalled Or SurPassed The Results Produced By UnModified Dornier HM3 Device.

Despite Claims To The Contrary,Unmodified HM 3 Dornier Lithotripter Remains The Gold Standard For ESWL,
Others Availabillities Included For Comparative Trials,Being Large Variety Productions From Different Manufacturers,Besides Siemens Lithostar, EDAP LT.01 And Sonolith 2000,Sonolith 3000 Versions.

Based Upon **ClayMan & Associates(1989)** Suggestions For Comparing Results Of SWL & PNL Or Comparing Different LithoTriptors, The **Different ParaMetres** Combined Into **"EffectiveNess Ouotient"** For Better Expression Of TreatMent Result & Also Various Comparative Analysis For Appliances & TreatMent Modalities.

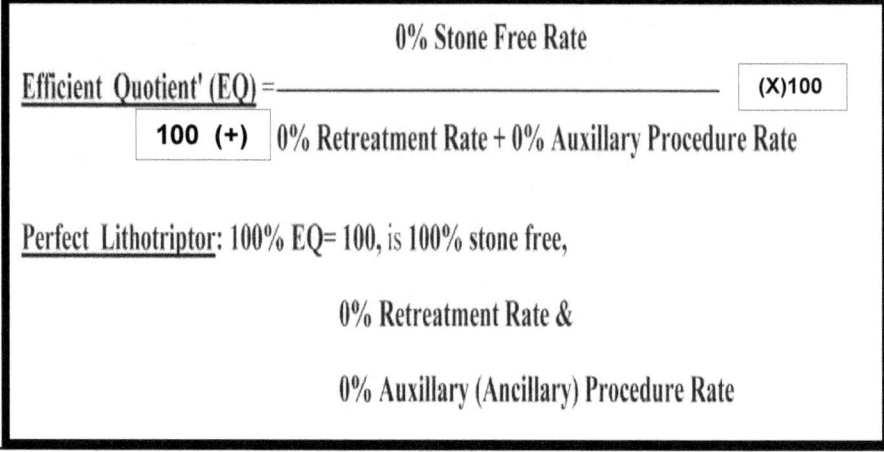

Lithotriptor Efficient Quotient

References

Andreassen KH, Dahl C, Andersen JT, Rasmussen MS, Jacobsen JD,Mogensen P. Extracorporeal shock wave lithotripsy as first line monotherapy of solitary calyceal calculi. Scand J Urol Nephrol 1997;31:245-8.

Renner CH, Rassweiler J. Treatment of renal stones by extracorporeal shock wave lithotripsy Nephron 1999;81:71-81.

Orestona F, Caronia N, Gallo G, et al. Functional aspects of the kidney after shock wave lithotripsy. In: Lingeman JE, Newman DM, editors.Shock wave lithotripsy 2: Urinary and biliary lithotripsy. New York:Plenum Press; 1989. p. 15-7.

Bierkens AF, Hendrikx AJ, de Kort VJ, de Reyke T, Bruynen CA, Bouve ER, et al. Efficacy of second generation lithotripters: A multicenter comparative study of 2206 extra corporeal shock wave lithotripsy treatment with the Siemens Lithostar, Dornier HM4, Wolf Piezolith 2300, Direx Tripter X-1, and Breakstone Lithotripters. J Urol 1992;148:1052-6.

Essentials Of Litho-Tripsy

Strutevant B. The shock wave physics of Lithotripsy. In: Smith AD,Badian DH, Clayman RV, editors. Smith's Text

Sheir KZ, El-Diasty TA, Ismail AM. Evaluation of a synchronous twin-pulse technique for shock wave lithotripsy: the first prospective clinical study. *BJU Int*. Feb 2005;95(3):389-93. [Medline].

Sheir KZ, Elhalwagy SM, Abo-Elghar ME, Ismail AM, Elsawy E, El-Diasty TA. Evaluation of a synchronous twin-pulse technique for shock wave lithotripsy: a prospective randomized study of effectiveness and safety in comparison to standard single-pulse technique. *BJU Int*. Jun 2008;101(11):1420-6. [Medline].

Zehnder P, Roth B, Birkhäuser F, Schneider S, Schmutz R, Thalmann GN, et al. A Prospective Randomised Trial Comparing the Modified HM3 with the MODULITH(®) SLX-F2 Lithotripter. *Eur Urol*. Apr 2011;59(4):637-44. [Medline].

Aulus Cornelius Celsus (1831). "Book VII, Chapter XXVI: Of the operation necessary in a suppression of urine, and lithotomy". In Collier, GF. *A translation of the eight books of Aul. Corn. Celsus on medicine* (2nd ed.). London: Simpkin and Marshall. pp. 306–14.

(2.) ESWL:UROLITHIASIS
(2.)(i)Urinary System Surgical Anatomy Surgical Pathology & Physiolgy

TWO KIDNEYS
A Pair Of Purplish-Brown Organs Located Below The Ribs Towards The Middle Of The Back(Flanks).
Being **Retroperitoneal Organs** (i.e Located Behind The Peritoneum) Situated On The Posterior Wall Of The Abdomen On Each Side Of The Vertebral Column, At About The Level Of Twelfth Rib.
The Left Kidney Is Slightly Higher In The Abdomen Than The Right, Due To The Presence Of The Liver Pushing The Right Kidney Down.
Each Kidney Measures About 10-12 Cms In Length, 5-7 Cms In Width & 3 Cms In Antero-Posterior ThickNess.

Neuro-Vascular Supply -
Arterial Blood Supply Directly From The Aorta Via The Renal Arteries.
The Indivisual Variations Of Renal Blood Supply & Presence Of More Than One Renal Artery Is Well Documented.
Renal Vein From Either Kidney Drain Into Infereior Vena Cava.
Nervous System & The Renals Communicate Through **The Renal Plexus.**
Sympathetic Nervous System Stimulation Leading To VasoConstriction & Hence Reduce Renal Bood Flow.

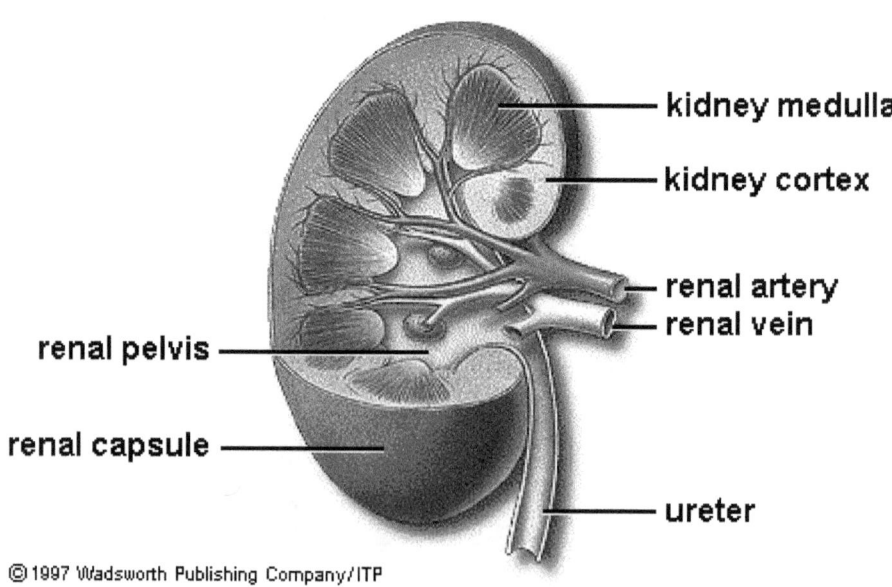

Essentials Of Litho-Tripsy

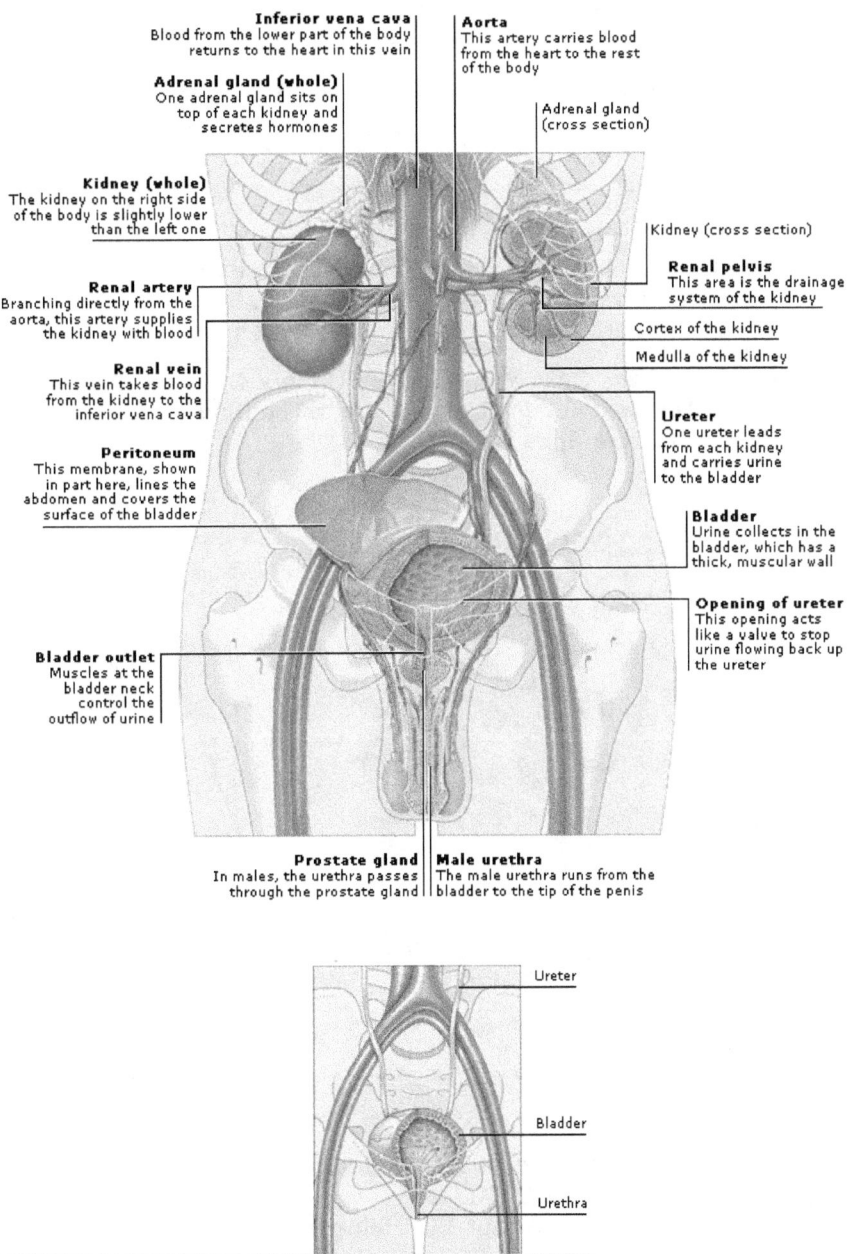

Female Lower Urinary Tract

Source-Medical Encyclopaedia www.aviva.co.uk 600 × 635

Histology-
On Cut Section- Kidney Has A Pale Outer Region- The **Cortex** & A Darker Inner Region- The **Medulla**.

The Medulla Is Costituted Of 8-18 Conical Regions, **The Renal Pyramids**. The Base Of Each Pyramid Starts From The Corticomedullary Border, With The Apex Ending In The **Renal Papilla**, That Merges To Form **The Renal Pelvis** And Then **The Ureter**.

The Renal Pelvis Is Divided Into Two Or Three Spaces -The **Major Calyces**- Which In Turn Further Divided Into **Minor Calyces**, Constituting The **Complete Pelvi-Calyceal System**, Consisting **Superior, Middle & Inferior Calyces**.

The Walls Of The Calyces, Pelvis And Ureters Are Lined With **Smooth Muscles,** Forcing Urine Towards The Bladder With **Peristaltic Contractility**.

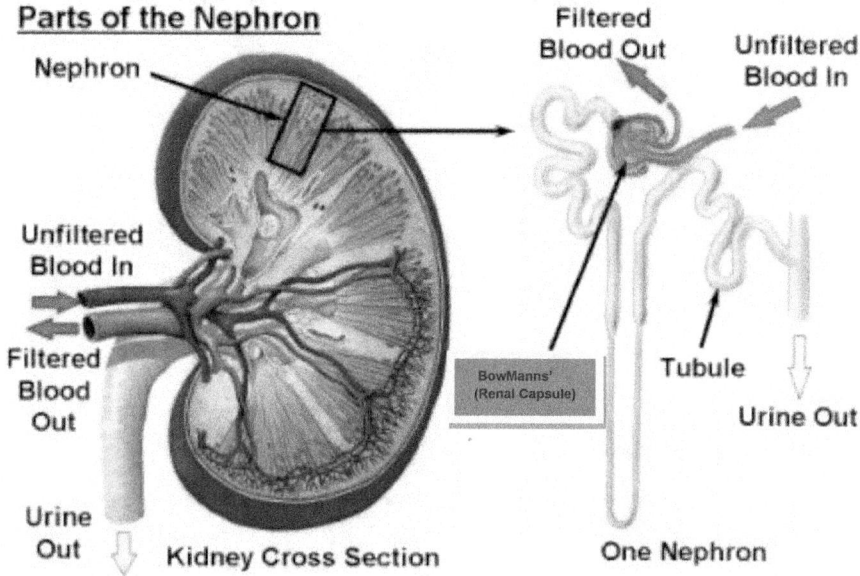

The Cortex And The Medulla Are Made Up Of **'Nephrons'** **(The Functional Units Of Kidney)**.
Each Kidney Contains **About 1.3 Million Nephrons**.

The Nephron Is The Unit Of The Kidney Responsible For **Ultrafiltration Of The Blood And Reabsorption Or Excretion Of Products**, In The Subsequent Filtrate.

Essentials Of Litho-Tripsy

Each Nephron Is Constituted Of:
The Glomerulus (A Filtering Unit) - **125ml/Min Of Filtrate** Is Formed By The Kidneys By **Uncontrolled Filteration** Through These Sieve-Like Structures.
The Proximal Convoluted Tubule - **Controlled Absorption** Of Glucose, Sodium, And Other Solutes Goes On In This Region.
The Loop Of Henle – Is Responsible For **Concentration And Dilution Of Urine** By Utilising A *Counter-Current Multiplying* **Mechanism**. Basically, Being Water-Impermeable, **By Pumping Sodium Out**, Affects The Osmolarity Of The Surrounding Tissues And Thus Affecting The Subsequent Movement Of Water In Or Out Of The **Water-Permeable Collecting Duct.**
The Distal Convoluted Tubule - The Region Along With Joined **Collecting Duct,** Is Responsible,For **Absorbing Water Back Into The Body**. Out Of 125mlUrine Filtered Every Minute, **99% Of The Water Is Normally Reabsorbed**, Leaving Highly Concentrated Urine To Flow Into The Collecting Duct And Then Into The Renal Pelvis.

Urinary System Physiology

Human Body Converts Nutrients From Food InTo Energy.
After The Needed Taken From The Food By The Body ,Waste Products Are Left Behind In The Bowel And In The Blood Stream.
The Blood. Urea Is Produced When Foods Containing Protein, Such As Meat, Poultry, And Certain Vegetables, Are Broken Down In The Body. Urea Is Carried In The Bloodstream To The Kidneys.
The Urinary System By Selective ReAbsorption, Retains Chemicals, Such As Sodium, Potassium And Water In Balance, While Removing Urea, From Bood Stream Into Urine.

Blood Is Returned To The Inferior Vena Cava Via The Renal Veins.
Urine (The Filtered Product Containing Waste Materials And Water) Excreted From The Kidneys Passes Down The
Fibromuscular **Ureters** And Collects In The **Bladder**.
The Bladder Muscle (The **Detrusor Muscle**) Is Capable Of Distending To Accept Urine Without Increasing The Pressure Inside; This Means That Large Volumes Can Be Collected (700-1000ml) Without High-Pressure Damage To The Renal System Occuring.
When Urine Is Passed, The **Urethral Sphincter** At The Base Of The Bladder Relaxes, The Detrusor Contracts, And Urine Is Voided Via The **Urethra**.

Renal functions:
The Kidneys Are **Essentially Regulatory Organs** Which Maintain The Volume And Composition Of Body Fluid By **Filtration Of The Blood And Selective Reabsorption Or Secretion Of Filtered Solutes.**

Thus Regulating Electrolyte Balance Of The Body, Blood Pressure, And Stimulating Red Blood Cell Production, Secretion Of Erythropoietin, Prostaglandins, Vitamin D & Others.

The Various Different Functions Include-
Removal Of Liquid Waste From The Blood In The Form Of Urine.
Excretion Of Waste Products.
Regulation Of Water, Electrolytes & Acid – Base Balance.
Regulate Blood Pressure.
Secretion Of ProstaGlandins.
Erythropoietin Production, Thus Aiding Red Blood Cells Formation.
SynthesisOf VitaMin-D To Active Form.
Renal Clearance.

TWO URETERS
The Two Narrow Tubes On Either Side, Connecting Kidneys To Urinary Bladder, About 22 To 30 Cms Long.
Divided Into Upper, Middle & Lower Ureter, The Upper End Is Known As **Pelvi-Ureteric Junction(PUJ)**, WhileThe Lower Distal End Is Named As Vesico-Ureteric Junction**(VUJ)**/Uretero-Vesical Junction**(UVJ).**

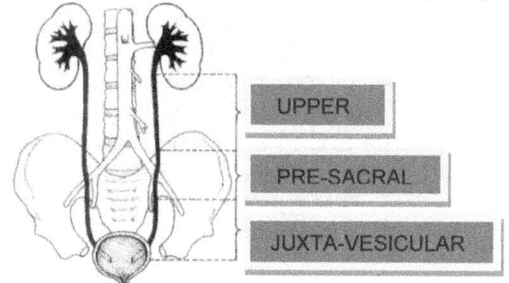

Surgical Anatomy Division Of Ureters
The Schematic Division Became Practically More Reliable, For UreteroScopy & ESWL Management Of UreteroLithiasis, As Compared To Open UreteroLithotomy & Blind Manipulations, In The Past.
Source - JenKins 1990

The **Peristaltic Activity** Produced Due To, Contractility & Relaxation Of Smooth Muscles Of The Ureters, Carry Urine Downwards Into The Urinary Bladder, Away From The Kidneys. About Every 10-15 Seconds, Small Amounts Of Urine Is Emptied Into The Bladder From The Ureters.

The Various Pathologies (Stone,Stricture,Tumour Etc.) Causing,
The **Obstruction In The Urinary OutFlow**, Lead To Stagnation, Infection & Other Obstructive UroPathy Changes.

Essentials Of Litho-Tripsy

URINARY BLADDER

A **Triangle-Shaped, Hollow Organ** Located In Lower Abdomen, Held In Place By **Ligaments**, Attached To Other Organs And Pelvic Bones.
Urinary Bladder Posterior Relations Consists Of Ano-Rectum, In **Males**, While Uterus(With Intervening VesicoUterine-Pouch Of Douglas) & Ano-Rectum In **Females**.
The **Space Of Retzius**, Being In Anterior Relation Of U.B, Peritoneum, In Proximity To Retro-Pubic Space.

In Urinary Bladder, **Urine Collection & Storage** Is By Relaxation & Expansion Of The Bladder's Walls, While Their Contraction & Flattening Lead To **Urine Emptying** Through The Urethra.

The Bladder Is Composed Of Bands Of Interlaced Smooth Muscle **(Detrusor)**.
The **Innervation** Of The Body Of The Bladder Is Different From That Of The Bladder Neck.
The Body Is Rich In Beta Adrenergic Receptors. These Receptors Are Stimulated By The **Sympathetic** Component Of The Autonomic Nervous System (ANS). **Beta** Stimulation, Via Fibers Of The Hypogastric Nerve, Suppress Contraction Of The Detrusor.
Conversely, **Parasympathetic** Stimulation, By Fibers In The Pelvic Nerve, Cause The Detrusor Contraction.
Sympathetic Stimulation Is Predominant During Bladder Filling,
While **Parasympathetic** Causes Emptying.

Urinary Bladder Neck Sphinteric Controls

Two Sphincters Control The Bladder Outlet.
The Internal Sphincter Is Composed Of Smooth Muscle Like
The Detrusor Extending Into The Bladder Neck
Controlled By The ANS Is Normally Closed.
The Primary Receptors In The Bladder Neck Are **Alpha Adrenergic**.
Sympathetic Stimulation Of These **Alpha** Receptors, Via Fibers In
The **Hypogastric Nerve**, Contributes To **Urinary Continence**.

The External Sphincter Is Histologically Different From The Detrusor And Internal Sphincter, Composed Of **Striated Muscle** (Like Skeletal Muscle), Hence Is Under Voluntary Control.
It Receives Innervation From The **Pudendal** Nerve,
Arising From The Ventral Horns Of The Sacral Cord.

During Micturition, Supraspinal Centers Block Stimulation By
The Hypogastric And Pudendal Nerves.
This Relaxes The Internal And External Sphincters And Removes
The **Sympathetic** Inhibition Of The **Parasympathetic** Receptors,
Resulting In Unobstructed Passage Of Urine,
When The Detrusor Contracts.

The Ureters Pass Between The Layers Of The Detrusor And Enter
The Bladder Through The Trigone.
The Propelled Urine By Ureters Into The Bladder, Is Accepted By The
U.B By Passive Expansion.
With The U.B Expansion & Intravesicular Pressure Increase,
The Ureters Are Compressed Between The Layers Of Muscle,
Creating A 'Valve Mechanism',
Responsible For Limiting The Backflow Of Urine.
The Normal Adult Bladder Holding Capacity Is About 500 Cc Of Urine.
After Emptying, About 50 Cc Residual Volume
(Post Void Residue-PVR) May Be Retained.
At About 150 Cc Of U.B Volume, Stretch Receptors In The Detrusor
Begin Signaling The CNS Via Afferent Nerves & At 400 Cc Urinary Urge
Normally Manifests.
The Urinary Bladder Capacity (Volume)For Healthy Indivisuals Has
Variation From 500-750 CC.For Two To Three Hours
Summary: Largely Because The Cerebrum By Suppressing The
Sacral Micturition,The Ability Of Normal Indivisuals Regarding ,
Where & When To Void Is, Maintained.
If The Sacral Reflex Is Unrestrained, Parasympathetic Stimulation Via
The Pelvic Nerve Causes Detrusor Contraction.
Detrusor Contraction Is Suppressed By,
A**lpha** And **Beta Sympathetic** Stimulation Via The Hypogastric Nerve.
In Response To **Afferent** Stimulation,
The Cerebrum Becomes Aware Of The Need To Void. If Appropriate,
It Relaxes & Sympathetic Inhibition To External Sphincter Blocks,
The Bladder Contracts And Urine Is Expelled.

URETHRA
Is A DelcateTubular Organ, Allowing Urine To Pass Outside The Body,
By 'Urethral Orifice'/ External Urinary Meatus.
The Female Urethra Is Shorter Than The Male Urethra,
And Sits Slightly Lower In The Pelvis.
The **Brain Signals** The Bladder Muscles To Tighten, Squeezing
Urine Out Of The Bladder.
Simultaneously Brain Signals To Relax The Sphincter Muscles Allows
Urine Exit From Bladder Through The Urethra.
All The Signals Occuring In The Correct Order,
Normal Urination Occurs.

Essentials Of Litho-Tripsy

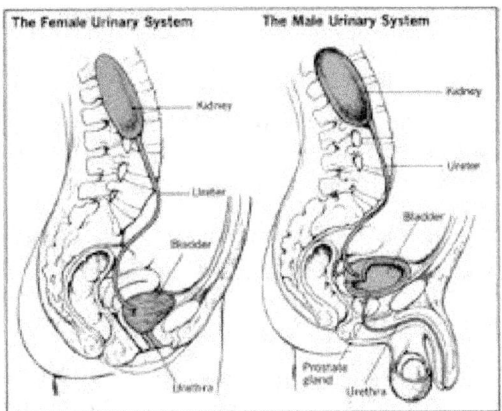

**Male & Female Urinary System
Longitudinal Views**
<u>Source</u> - 2010 revision of the Complete Home Medical Guide © Dorling Kindersley Limited.

Histology

The Urinary System Is Covered In **Transitional Epithelium**, Unlike Other Epithelium, It Does Not Have A Fixed Size & Is Capable Of Flattening And Distending.

Urothelium Covers Most Of The Urinary System, Including The Renal Pelvis, Ureters.
Resting On A Basement Membrane. Urothelial Tissue Is Highly Specific To The Urinary Tract, Characterized By High Elasticity And Trans-Epithelial Electrical Resistance.
Urothelium Consists Of Approximately 3-5 Cell Layers, Accompanied By A Thick Layer Of Protective Glycoprotein Plaques At Its Luminal (Apical) Surface, And Is Classified As Transitional Epithelium.

Urine Formation

Average Urine Production In Adult Humans Is **About 1 – 2 L Per Day**, Depending On State Of Hydration, Activity Level, Environmental Factors, Weight, And The Individual's Health, Too Much Or Too Little Urine Production Needs Medical Attention.

Polyuria- Excessive Production Of Urine (> 2.5 L/Day),
Oliguria - < 400 Ml Production
Anuria - < 100 Ml Per Day Production

Filtration Of Blood In The Kidneys Is The First Step For Urine Formation. In A Healthy Human,The Kidney Receives 12 - 30% Of Cardiac Output, With An Average Of About 20% C.O Or About 1.25 L/Min.

The **Glomerular Filtration Rate (GFR)** Amounts To 180 Litres Per Day. About 99% Of This Filtrate Is Reabsorbed As It Passes Through The Nephron And The Remaining 1% Becomes Urine.

The Urinary System Is Regulated By The Endocrine System Such As Antidiuretic Hormone, Aldosterone, And Parathyroid Hormone. While Urinary Cocentration & Volume Is Influenced By Blood Pressure, Nervous System & Endocrine System.

Antidiuretic Hormone (ADH), Is A **Neurohypophysial Hormone** Found In Most Mammals. Its Two Primary Functions Are **To Retain Water In The Body And To Constrict Blood Vessels**.

Vasopressin Regulates The **Body's Retention Of Water** By Acting To Increase Water Absorption In Collecting Ducts Of Kidney Nephron. Vasopressin Increases Water Permeability Of The Kidney's Collecting Duct And Distal Convoluted Tubule By Inducing Translocation Of **Aquaporin-CD Water Channels**, In The Kidney Nephron Collecting Duct Plasma Membrane.

References

Dugdale, David (16 September 2011). "Female urinary tract". *MedLine Plus Medical Encyclopedia*.

Maton, Anthea; Jean Hopkins; Charles William McLaughlin; Susan Johnson; Maryanna Quon Warner; David LaHart; Jill D. Wright (1993). *Human Biology and Health*. Englewood Cliffs, New Jersey, USA: Prentice Hall. ISBN 0-13-981176-1.

Caldwell HK, Young WS III (2006). "Oxytocin and Vasopressin: Genetics and Behavioral Implications". In Lajtha A, Lim R. *Handbook of Neurochemistry and Molecular Neurobiology: Neuroactive Proteins and Peptides* (3rd ed.). Berlin: Springer. pp. 573–607. ISBN 0-387-30348-0.

Nielsen S, Chou CL, Marples D, Christensen EI, Kishore BK, Knepper MA (February 1995). "Vasopressin increases water permeability of kidney collecting duct by inducing translocation of aquaporin-CD water channels to plasma membrane". *Proc. Natl. Acad. Sci. U.S.A.* **92** (4): 1013–7.doi:10.1073/pnas.92.4.1013. PMC 42627. PMID 7532304.

Baba, T; Murabayashi, S; Tomiyama, T; Takebe, K (1990). "Uncontrolled hypertension is associated with a rapid progression of nephropathy in type 2 diabetic patients with proteinuria and preserved renal function". *The Tohoku journal of experimental medicine* **161** (4): 311–8. doi:10.1620/tjem.161.311.PMID 2256104.

"Peripheral Neuropathy". Patient UK. Retrieved 2014-03-20.

Essentials Of Litho-Tripsy

(2.)(ii)
URINARY STONES:
GENERAL CONSIDERATIONS

Urinary Stones (Urolithiasis):
Anatomical Classification- In The Kidney (Nephrolithiasis), Ureter (Ureterolithiasis), Or Bladder (Cystolithiasis),
  Bio-Chemical Composition Classification- Calcium-Containing, Struvite, Uric Acid Or Other Compounds.

Renal Lithiasis, Kidney Stone Or Renal Calculus (From The Latin *Rēnēs*, "Kidneys," And *Calculus*, "Pebble"), Are Solid Concretions Or Crystal Aggregation Forming Small, Hard Deposits In The Kidneys, Of Variable Composition & Differing Aetio-Pathogenesis, Affecting Any Part Of Urinary Tract From Dietary Minerals In The Urine.

The First Recorded Existence Of Kidney Stones Ranges From Thousands Of Years Ago, With Lithotomy For The Removal Of Stones, As One Of The Earliest Known Surgical Procedures.
In 1901, A Stone Discovered In The Pelvis Of An Ancient Egyptian Mummy , **Dated Back To 4,800 Bc**.
Calculous Disease Has Been Mentioned In All Medical Texts From Ancient Mesopotamia, India, China, Persia, Greece, And Rome.
Part Of The Hippocratic Oath Suggests Of Practicing Surgeons In Ancient Greece To Whom Physicians Were To Defer For Lithotomies.
The Roman Medical Treatise *De Medicina* By Aulus Cornelius Celsus Contained , A Description Of Lithotomy, Serving As The Basis For This Procedure Until 18th Century.[1,2]

Epidemiology
Kidney Stones Affect All Geographical, Cultural, And Racial Groups.
The Lifetime Risk Is About 10 To 15% In The **Developed World**, But Can Be As High As 20 To 25% In The **Middle East**, Due To The Increased Risk Of Dehydration In Hot Climates, Combined With A Diet 50% Lower In Calcium And 250% Higher In Oxalates Compared To Western World, Can Be Accountable Factors For The Overall Higher Risk Of Stone Disease In The Middle East, Uric Acid Stones Being More Common Than Calcium-Containing Stones.

For An Unknown Reason In The **United States,** Over The Past (2) Decades, Urolithiasis Patients Has Been Increasing .
White People Are More Prone Compared To **Coloured Persons.**
Caucasians Have More Incidence Than **African-Americans.**
Age & Sex - Mostly Between The Ages Of 20 And 40.
About 80% Patients Are Men.The Number Of Women Developoing

UroLithiasis, Has Been Increasing Over The Past 10 Years,
Causing The Ratio To Change.

The Number Of Deaths Due To Kidney Stones Is Estimated At 19,000 Per Year Being Fairly Consistent Between 1990 And 2010.
**Once Persons Develop More Than One Stone,
They Are More Likely To Develop Others.**
According To The U.S. National Institutes Of Health (NIH),
Roughly 1 Person In 10 Develops Kidney Stones During Their
Lifetime And Renal Stone Disease Accounts For 7–10 Of
Every 1000 Hospital Admissions.
Kidney Stones Are Most Prevalent In Patients Between The Ages Of 30 And 45, With Men Affected Three Times More Often Than Women. Overall Incidence Declines After Age 50.

AETIO-PATHOGENESIS

Genetic, Environmental And Dietary Factors Contribute In The Pathophysiology Of Nephrolithiasis.
<u>Causes Of Kidney Stones</u>:
The Most Common Type Of Composition Is Calcium Oxalate Crystals, Occurring In About 80% Of Cases, Thus The Factors That Promote The Precipitation Of These Crystals In Urine Are Responsible For The Development Of These Stones.
While, Kidney Stones Associated With Too Many Chemicals,
Easily Dissolvable In The Available Urine.
The Most Common Causes Of This Are:
- A High Level Of Urinary Calcium **(Hypercalciuria),**
- High Urinary Oxalate **(Hyperoxaluria),**
- High Urinary Uric Acid **(Hyperuricosuria),**
- **Insufficient Urinary Citrate,** Or
- **Inadequate Water** Flowing Through The Kidneys.

<u>Risk factors-</u>
(1.) Dietary-Dehydration From Low Fluid Intake Is A Major Factor In Stone Formation. High Dietary Intake Of Animal Protein, Sodium, Refined Sugars, Fructose, And High Fructose Corn Syrup, Oxalate, Grapefruit Juice, And Apple Juice Increase The Risk Of Kidney Stone Formation.

(2.) Metabolic Causes-Underlying Metabolic Predisposing Conditions:
Distal Renal Tubular Acidosis, Dent's Disease, Hyperparathyroidism, Primary Hyperoxaluria, Or Medullary Sponge Kidney(3–20% Of Renal Stones Patients Have Medullary Sponge Kidney).
Kidney Stones Are More Common With **Crohn's Disease**, Due To
Its Association With **Hyperoxaluria And Magnesium Malabsorption.**

Essentials Of Litho-Tripsy

Recurrent Kidney Stones Cases, Need Screening For Such Disorders, Typically Done With A **24-Hour Urine Collection & Analysing Stone Formation Promoting Features.**

CALCIUM

Being One Important Component Of The Most Common Type Of Urolithiasis, Calcium Oxalate Stones.
According To Some Studies Calcium As A Dietary Supplement Increases The Risk Of UroLithiasis, These Findings Were Used As The Basis For Setting The **Reference Daily Intake For Calcium For Adults**, In The United States,
In The Early 1990s, A Study Conducted For Women's Health Initiative,US Found That Postmenopausal Women Consuming 1000 Mg Of Supplemental Calcium And 400 International Units Of Vitamin D Per Day For Seven Years Had A 17% Higher Risk Of Developing Kidney Stones, Than Subjects Taking A Placebo .
The Nurses' Health Study Also Showed An Association Between Supplemental Calcium Intake And Kidney Stone Formation.
Unlike Supplemental Calcium, High Intakes Of Dietary Calcium Do Not Appear To Cause Kidney Stones And **May Actually Protect** Against Their Development., Perhaps Due To Related **Role Of Calcium In Binding Ingested Oxalate In The Gastrointestinal Tract.**
With **Decreased Calcium Intake**, Available Oxalate For Absorption Into The Bloodstream Increases Leading To **Increased Urinary Excretion** By The Kidneys. **The Urinary Oxalate** Is A Very Strong Promoter Of Calcium Oxalate Precipitation—About 15 Times Stronger Than Calcium.
A 2004 Study Found - Low Dietary Calcium Association With A Higher Overall Risk For Kidney Stone Formation.
For Most Individuals, **Other Risk Factors For Kidney Stones, Such As High Intakes Of Dietary Oxalates And Low Fluid Intake, Play A Greater Role Than Calcium Intake.**

OTHER ELECTROLYTES

Calcium Is Not The Only Electrolyte That Influences The Formation Of Kidney Stones. For Example, By Increasing Urinary Calcium Excretion, **High Dietary Sodium** May Increase The Risk Of Stone Formation.**Drinking** Fluoridated Tap Water **May Increase The Risk Of Kidney Stone Formation By A Similar Mechanism,**
Though Further Epidemiologic Studies Are Warranted To Determine Whether Fluoride In Drinking Water Is Associated With An Increased Incidence Of Kidney Stones.
While, High Dietary Intake Of Potassium **Appears To Reduce The Risk Of Stone Formation Because Potassium Promotes The Urinary Excretion Of** Citrate, **An Inhibitor Of Calcium Crystal Formation.**

Kidney Stones Are More Likely To Develop, And To Grow Larger, If A Person Has Low Dietary Magnesium. Magnesium Inhibits Stone Formation.

Animal Protein. Consumption, Creating An Acid Load That Increases,Urinary Excretion Of Calcium ,Uric Acid And Reduced Citrate. **Urinary Excretion Of Excess Sulfurous Amino Acids (Cysteine And Methionine), Uric Acid, And Other Acidic Metabolites** From Animal Protein Acidifies The Urine, **Promoting** The Formation Of Kidney Stones. **The Body Often** Balances This Acidic Urinary Ph By Leaching Calcium From Bones**, Which Further Promotes The Formation Of Kidney Stones.**
Low Urinary Citrate Excretion Is Also Commonly Found In Those With A High Dietary Intake Of Animal Protein, Whereas Vegetarians Tend To Have Higher Levels Of Citrate Excretion. Low Urinary Citrate, Too, Promotes Stone Formation.

VITAMINS
Despite A Widely Held Belief, **The Evidence For A Causal Relationship Between Vitamin C Supplements And An Increased Incidence Of Kidney Stones** Is Inconclusive.
While Excess Dietary Intake Of Vitamin C Might Increase The Risk Of Calcium Oxalate Stone Formation, In Practice This Is Rarely Encountered.
The Link Between Vitamin D Intake And Kidney Stones Is Also Tenuous. Excessive Vitamin D Supplementation May Increase The Risk Of Stone Formation By Increasing The Intestinal Absorption Of Calcium; Correction Of A Deficiency Does Not.

OTHERS
No Conclusive Data Demonstrating A Cause-And-Effect Relationship Between Alcoholic Beverage Consumption And Kidney Stones.
However, Certain Behaviors Associated With Frequent And Binge Drinking Can Lead To Dehydration, That Can In Turn Lead To The Development Of Kidney Stones.[24]

The American Urological Association Has Projected That Global Warming Will Lead To An Increased Incidence Of Kidney Stones In The United States By Expanding The "Kidney Stone Belt" Of The Southern United States. (3-10,19)

Essentials Of Litho-Tripsy

PATHOPHYSIOLOGY

Small Crystals Formed In Kidney, The Most Common Are Made Of Calcium Oxalate, Generally 4-5 mm Size.

(1.) Calcium And Oxalate Come Together To Form The **Crystal Nucleus. Supersaturation Promotes Their Combination (As Does Inhibition.)**

(2.) Continued Deposition At The Renal Papillae Leads To The Kidney Stones Formation.

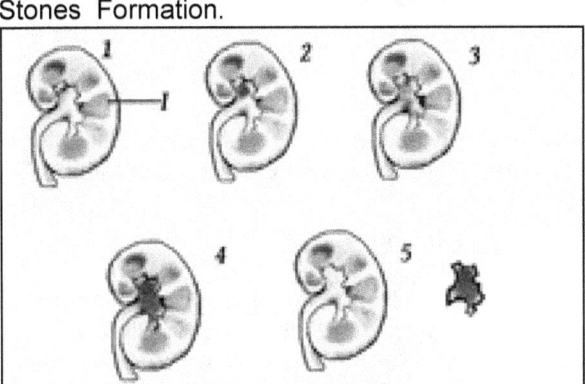

(3.) Kidney Stones Grow And Collect Debris, Blocking All Routes To The Renal Papillae, Can Lead To Severe Discomfort.

(4.) The Complete Staghorn Stone Forms And Retention Occurs. Smaller Solids That Break Off Can Become Trapped In The Urinary Glands Causing Discomfort.

(5.) Displaced Stones Travel Through The Urethra, Either Broken Down, Or Surgically Removed.

Supersaturation Of Urine

Urine Solvent Containing More Solutes Than It Can Hold In Solution, With One Or More Calculogenic (Crystal-Forming) Substances, A Seed Crystal May Form Through The Process Of Nucleation. Heterogeneous Nucleation **(Where There Is A Solid Surface Present On Which A Crystal Can Grow) Proceeds** More Rapidly Than Homogeneous Nucleation **(Where A Crystal Must Grow In Liquid Medium With No Such Surface),** As Less Energy Is Required For Adhering To Cells On The Surface Of A Renal Papilla, **A Seed Crystal Can Grow And Aggregate Into An Organized Mass.**

Depending On The Chemical Composition Of The Crystal,
The Stone-Forming Process May Proceed More Rapidly When The Urine Ph Is Unusually High Or Low.

Supersaturation Of The Urine With Respect To A Calculogenic Compound Is Ph-Dependent, e.g The Solubility Of Uric Acid In Urine At A Ph Of 7.0 Is 158 Mg/100 Ml. While At Ph To 5.0 The Solubility Decreases To Less Than 8 Mg/100 Ml. Hence, The Formation Of Uric Acid Stones Requires A Combination Of Hyperuricosuria (High Urine Uric Acid Levels) And Low Urine Ph(Acidic Medium).

Supersaturation Is Likely The Underlying Cause Of **Uric Acid And Cystine Stones**, But **Calcium-Based Stones** (Especially Calcium Oxalate Stones) May Have A **More Complex Etiology**.

Inhibitors Of Stone Formation

Normal Urine Contains **Chelating Agents**, Such As Citrate, That Inhibit The Nucleation, Growth, And Aggregation Of Calcium-Containing Crystals.

Other **Endogenous Inhibitors** Include Calgranulin (An S-100 Calcium Binding Protein), Tamm-Horsfall Protein, Glycosaminoglycans, Uropontin (A Form Of Osteopontin), Nephrocalcin (An Acidic Glycoprotein), Prothrombin F1 Peptide, And Bikunin (Uronic Acid-Rich Protein). **Biochemical Mechanisms Of Action** Of These Substances, Not Yet Been Thoroughly Elucidated.
However, When These Substances Fall Below Their Normal Proportions, Stones Can Form From An Aggregation Of Crystals.

Sufficient Dietary Intake Of Magnesium And Citrate Inhibits The Formation Of Calcium Oxalate And Calcium Phosphate Stones; In Addition, Magnesium And Citrate Operate Synergistically To Inhibit Kidney Stones. Magnesium's Efficacy In Subduing Stone Formation And Growth Is Dose-Dependent.

The Body Takes Nutrients From Food And Converts Them To Energy. After The Body Has Taken The Food That It Needs, Waste Products Are Left Behind In The Bowel And In The Blood.
The Urinary System Keeps Chemicals, Such As Potassium And Sodium, And Water In Balance, And Removes A Type Of Waste, Called Urea, From The Blood. Urea Is Produced When Foods Containing Protein, Such As Meat, Poultry, And Certain Vegetables, Are Broken Down In The Body. Urea Is Carried In The Bloodstream To The Kidneys. (11-20)

Essentials Of Litho-Tripsy

Renal Stone Classification

Type and main component	%	Other important structural characteristics
Calcium oxalate monohydrate papillary calculi	12.9	core constituted by COM/OM (60.7%) core constituted by HAP/OM (39.2%) size[1]: 2-7 mm
Calcium oxalate monohydrate unattached calculi (formed in renal cavities)	16.4	core constituted by OM (63.3%) core constituted by HAP (29.9%) core constituted by uric acid (6.7%) size[1]: 2-15 mm
Calcium oxalate dihydrate unattached calculi	33.8	containing little amounts of HAP among COD crystals (55.2%) only COD and little amounts of OM (44.8%) can contain variable amounts of COM, even 100%, but it comes from the transformation of COD size[1]: 2-15 mm
Calcium oxalate dihydrate/ hydroxyapatite mixed unattached calculi	11.2	alternative COD/HAP layers (39.6%) disordered COD/HAP deposits (60.4%) size[1]: 3-15 mm
Hydroxyapatite unattached calculi	7.1	containing minute amounts of COD (54.9%) containing only HAP and OM (45.1%) size[1]: 2-15 mm
Struvite infectious calculi	4.1	also contain large amounts of HAP and OM size[1]: 5-50 mm
Brushite unattached calculi	0.6	frequently also contain little amounts of HAP size[1]: 3-15 mm
Uric acid unattached calculi	8.2	mainly anhydrous uric acid (40.7%) mainly dihydrate uric acid (49.0%) uric acid / urates mixed calculi (8.8%) size[1]: 1-20 mm
Calcium oxalate/uric acid mixed calculi	2.6	papillary (12.7%) unattached (non papillary) (87.3%) size[1]: 3-20 mm
Cystine unattached calculi	1.1	also contain minute amounts of OM size[1]: 3-30 mm
Unfrequent calculi	1.9	OM as main component (32.6%) medicamentous (6.1%) post SWEL residues (10.2%) calcium carbonate (14.3%) artefacts (36.7%)

1: Values Of Size Approximately Correspond To The Range Of The Larger Dimension Of Calculi.
Com: Calcium Oxalate Monohydrate.
Cod: Calcium Oxalate Dihydrate.
Om: Organic Matter.
Hap: Hydroxyapatite.
Swel: Shock Waves Extracorporeal Lithotripsy.

Source-Simple Classification Of Renal Calculi Closely Related To Their Micromorphology And Etiology
Felix Grases A,*, Antonia Costa-Bauza´ A, Margarita Ramis A, Vicente Montesinos A, Antonio Conte B Alaboratory Of Renal Lithiasis Research, Faculty Of Sciences, University Of Balearic Islands, Ctra. Valldemossa Km. 7.5,
07071-Palma De Mallorca, Spain
Buniversitary Hospital "Son Dureta", 07071-Palma De Mallorca, Spain
Received 26 November 2001; Received In Revised Form 25 February 2002; Accepted 4 March 2002 Clinica Chimica Acta 322 (2002) 29–36 Www.Elsevier.Com/Locate/Clinchim

Anil K. Sahni

TYPES OF URINARY STONES

Calcium-Containing Stones
CALCIUM STONES- Calcium, A Normal Part Of A Healthy Diet Used In Bones And Muscles, Is Normally Flushed Out With The Rest Of The Urine. However, Excess Calcium Not Used By The Body May Combine With Other Waste Products To Form A Stone,
Most Kidney Stones Are Calcium Stones.

Usually In The Form Of Calcium Oxalate. High Oxalate Levels Can Be Found In Some Fruits And Vegetables, As Well As In Nuts And Chocolate. Liver Also Produces Oxalate.
Dietary Factors, High Doses Of Vitamin D, Intestinal Bypass Surgery And Several Different Metabolic Disorders Can Increase The Concentration Of Calcium Or Oxalate In Urine.
Calcium Stones May Also Occur In The Form Of Calcium Phosphate.

Factors That Promote The Precipitation Of Oxalate Crystals In The Urine, Such As Primary Hyperoxaluria, Are Associated With The Development Of Calcium Oxalate Stones. The Formation Of Calcium Phosphate Stones Is Associated With Conditions Such As Hyperparathyroidism And Renal Tubular Acidosis.

Oxaluria Is Increased In Patients With Certain Gastrointestinal Disorders Including Inflammatory Bowel Disease Such As Crohn Disease Or Patients Who Have Undergone Resection Of The Small Bowel Or Small Bowel Bypass Procedures. Oxaluria Is Also Increased In Patients Who Consume Increased Amounts Of Oxalate (Found In Vegetables And Nuts).
Primary Hyperoxaluria Is A Rare Autosomal Recessive Condition Which Usually Presents In Childhood.

By Far, The Most Common Type Of Kidney Stones Worldwide Contains Calcium. For Example, Calcium-Containing Stones Represent About 80% Of All Cases In The United States; These Typically Contain Calcium Oxalate Either Alone Or In Combination With Calcium Phosphate In The Form Of Apatite Or Brushite.

Calcium Oxalate Stones Appear As 'Envelopes' Microscopically. They May Also Form 'Dumbbells.'

Struvite Stones
About 10–15% Of Urinary Calculi Are Composed Of Struvite (Ammonium Magnesium Phosphate, $NH_4MgPO_4 \cdot 6H_2O$).
Struvite Stones Form In Response To An Infection, Such As A Urinary Tract Infection & Can Grow Quickly And Become Quite Large.

Essentials Of Litho-Tripsy

Struvite Stones (Also Known As "Infection Stones", Urease Or Triple-Phosphate Stones), Form Most Often In The Presence Of Infection By Urea-Splitting Bacteria. Using The Enzyme Urease, These Organisms Metabolize Urea Into Ammonia And Carbon Dioxide. This Alkalinizes The Urine, Resulting In Favorable Conditions For The Formation Of Struvite Stones.
Proteus Mirabilis, Proteus Vulgaris, And Morganella Morganii Are The Most Common Organisms Isolated; Less Common Organisms Include Ureaplasma Urealyticum, And Some Species Of Providencia, Klebsiella, Serratia, And Enterobacter.
These Infection Stones Are Commonly Observed In People Who Have Factors That Predispose Them To Urinary Tract Infections, Such As Those With Spinal Cord Injury And Other Forms Of Neurogenic Bladder, Ileal Conduit Urinary Diversion, Vesicoureteral Reflux,
And Obstructive Uropathies.

They Are Also Commonly Seen In People With Underlying Metabolic Disorders, Such As Idiopathic Hypercalciuria, Hyperparathyroidism, And Gout. Infection Stones Can Grow Rapidly, Forming Large Calyceal Staghorn (Antler-Shaped) Calculi Requiring Invasive Surgery Such As Percutaneous Nephrolithotomy For Definitive Treatment.

Struvite Stones (Triple Phosphate/Magnesium Ammonium Phosphate) Have A 'Coffin Lid' Morphology By Microscopy.

Uric Acid Stones
About 5–10% Of All Stones Are Formed From Uric Acid.
Uric Acid Stones May Occur When Urine Is Too Acidic, As In Certain Conditions, Such As Gout Or Malignancies.
Uric Acid Stones Can Form In People Who Are Dehydrated,
Those Who Eat A High-Protein Diet And Those With Gout. Certain Genetic Factors And Disorders Of The Blood-Producing Tissues Also May Predispose To Uric Acid Stones Formation.

People With Certain Metabolic Abnormalities, Including Obesity,[7] May Produce Uric Acid Stones. They Also May Form In Association With Conditions That Cause Hyperuricosuria (An Excessive Amount Of Uric Acid In The Urine) With Or Without Hyperuricemia (An Excessive Amount Of Uric Acid In The Serum).

They May Also Form In Association With Disorders Of Acid/Base Metabolism Where The Urine Is Excessively Acidic (Low Ph), Resulting In Precipitation Of Uric Acid Crystals.

A Diagnosis Of Uric Acid Urolithiasis Is Supported By The Presence Of A Radiolucent Stone In The Face Of Persistent Urine Acidity, In Conjunction With The Finding Of Uric Acid Crystals In Fresh Urine Samples.[44]

As Noted For Calcium Oxalate Stones, Patients With Inflammatory Bowel Disease (Crohn Disease, Ulcerative Colitis) Tend To Have Hyperoxaluria And Form Oxalate Stones. These Patients Also Have A Tendency To Form Urate Stones.
Urate Stones Are Especially Common After Colon Resection.

Uric Acid Stones Appear As Pleomorphic Crystals, Usually Diamond-Shaped. They May Also Look Like Squares Or Rods Which Are Polarizable.

Patients With Hyperuricosuria Can Be Treated With Allopurinol Which Will Reduce Urate Formation. Urine Alkalinization May Also Be Helpful In These Cases.

Multiple Kidney Stones Are Composed Of Uric Acid And A Small Amount Of Calcium Oxalate

Other Types -

Cystine Stones Consist Of Cystine, One Of The Building Blocks That Make Up Muscles, Nerves, And Other Parts Of The Body.
These Stones Represent Only A Small Percentage Of Kidney Stones.
They Are Formed In A **Hereditary Disorder,** That Causes The Kidneys To Excrete Excessive Amounts Of Certain Amino Acids. **(Cystinuria).**
In Certain Rare Inborn Errors Of Metabolism With Propensity To Accumulate Crystal-Forming Substances In Urine.e.g
Cystinuria, Cystinosis, And Fanconi Syndrome May Form Stones Composed Of Cystine.
Cystine Stone Formation Can Be Treated With Urine Alkalinization And Dietary Protein Restriction.

Xanthine Stones- Affliction With Xanthinuria Often Produce Stones Composed Of Xanthine.
2,8-Dihydroxyadenine Stones, InAdenine Phosphoribosyltransferase Deficiency Affliction.
Alkaptonurics Produce Homogentisic Acid Stones,
Iminoglycinurics Produce Stones Of Glycine, Proline And Hydroxyproline.
Urolithiasis Has Also Been Noted To Occur In The Setting Of Therapeutic Drug Use, With Crystals Of Drug Forming Within The Renal

Essentials Of Litho-Tripsy

Tract In Some People Currently Being Treated With Agents Such As <u>Indinavir</u>, <u>Sulfadiazine</u> And <u>Triamterene</u>.
Other, Rarer Types Of Kidney Stones Can Occur.
Knowledge Of Type Of Kidney Stone Helps To Understand Aetio-Pathogenesis & Prophylaxis To Reduce Risk Of
Getting Additional Kidney Stones. (21-30)

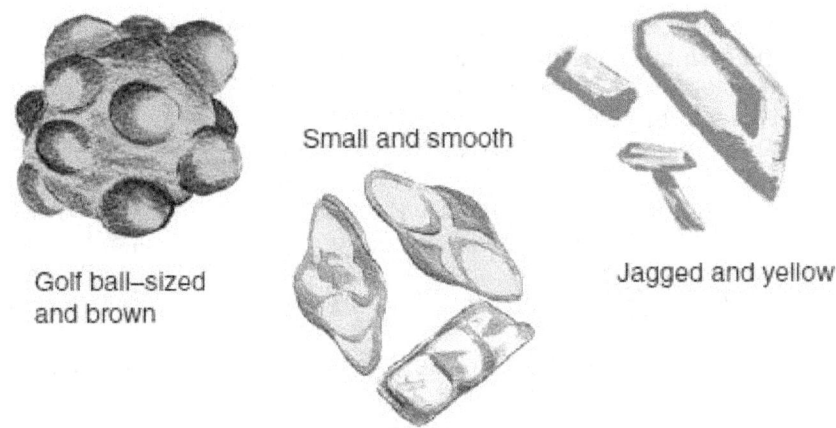

"**Kidney Stones Morphologies**"
Wide Variations Of Shape, Size, Surface, Colour Etc.

CLINICAL MANIFESTATIONS

Urolithiasis, Is One Of The Most Common Disorders Of The Urinary Tract, Clinically Manifesting With Severe, Excruciating Painful Presentations.
According To The Estimations, **About A Million People In The United States, Are Treated For Kidney Stones Each Year**.

Urolithiasis Symptoms
Depend Upon The Anatomical Classification Site-
In The Kidney (**Nephrolithiasis**), Ureter (**Ureterolithiasis**),
Or Bladder (**Cystolithiasis**),

Clinical Presentations-
A Kidney Stone May Not Cause Signs And Symptoms
(**Silent Stones**, Remaining Dormant For Years & Diagnosed By Co-Incidental Investigatory Findings).
Until It Has Moved Into The Ureter — The Tube Connecting The Kidney And Bladder. At That Point, These Signs And Symptoms May Occur:
In Urolitiasis Majority Of Signs And Symptoms, Are Due To- Associated Infection & Or Obstruction Of Urinary Tract.
The Various <u>Signs And Symptoms</u> Include-
- Severe Pain In The Side And Back, Below The Ribs
- Pain That Spreads To The Lower Abdomen And Groin **(Loin To Groin)**.

The Stones That Obstruct The Ureter Or Renal Pelvis Have Excruciating, Intermittent Pain That Radiates From The Flank To The Groin Or To The Genital Area And Inner Thigh. , As **'Referral Pain'** Due To InvolveMent Of Lower Lumbar Nerves.
This Particular Type Of Pain, Known As <u>Renal / Ureteric Colic</u>,
Is Often Described As One Of The Strongest Pain Sensations Known. Renal Colic Caused By Kidney Stones Is Commonly Accompanied By <u>Urinary Urgency</u>, Restlessness, <u>Hematuria</u>, Sweating, Nausea, And Vomiting. It Typically Comes In Waves Lasting 20 To 60 Minutes Caused By <u>Peristaltic</u> Contractions Of The Ureter As It Attempts To Expel The Stone. (3-5)
Renal Colic Is A MisKnowmer, As Kidney Being Solid Organ, While The **'Colic'** Essentially Arises From Hollow Tubular Viscera, Hence More Appropriate Term Being **'Renal Pain'**.
- Pain On Urination
- Pink, Red Or Brown Urine, Mild / Moderate / Severe Haematuria.
- Nausea And Vomiting
- Persistent Urge To Urinate
- Fever And Chills If An Infection Is Present
- Hematuria: Blood In The Urine, Due To Minor Damage To Inside Wall- Kidney, Ureter And/Or Urethra.
- Pyuria: Pus In The Urine.
- Dysuria: Burning On Urination When Passing Stones (Rare).

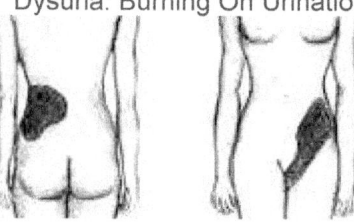

<u>Characterstic 'Ureteric Colic' Radiation Spread (Anterior & Posterior Aspects)</u>

Essentials Of Litho-Tripsy

The Embryological Link Between The Urinary Tract, The Genital System, And The Gastrointestinal Tract Is The Basis Of The Radiation Of Pain To The Gonads, As Well As The Nausea And Vomiting That Are Also Common In Urolithiasis.

The Lower Left Quadrant Pain, Sometimes Needs To Be Differentiated From 'Diverticulitis', As Sigmoid Colon Overlaps The Ureter, Rendering Difficult Identification Of Organ Of Pathology.

Various Grades Of Postrenal Azotemia And Obstructive UroPathy Changes Like U/L & Or B/L Hydronephrosis, Hydro-UreteroNephrosis, Pyelititis, PyeloNephritis, ARF, CRF Can Be Observed Following The Obstruction Of Urine Flow Through One Or Both Ureters. & Or Lower Urinary Tract Syndrome.

Bladder Stones Formation Is Pre-Disposed/ Precipitated By Improper /Incomplete Evacuation Of Bladder Leading To Urine Stasis. Urine Stasis Occurs Commonly In Middle-Aged And Older Men Due To Enlarged Prostate & Can Also Result From Neurogenic Bladder (Loss Of Bladder Control Due To Neurological Causes).
Urinary Tract Infection Being Another Important Precipitating Factor For Bladder Stone Formation.
Bladder Stone Symptoms Include- A Frequent Urge To Urinate (Urgency), Painful Urination, Hematuria, (Blood In The Urine), And Dysuria (Difficulty Urinating). In Some Cases, Bladder Stones Can Cause Potentially Serious Complications.
Urinary Stones:Differential Diagnosis-
Conditions With Similar Symptoms Include Urinary Tract Infection, Kidney Stone, Pyelonephritis, Appendicitis, Sexually Transmitted Diseases & Others.

RELEVANT INVESTIGATIONS
FOR URINARY STONE DISEASE

Appropriate Diagnosis, Assessment , Evaluation Of
'Urinary Stone Disease', For Consideration Of Proper ManageMent Decision, Following Investigations Are Needed-
Laboratory Studies
- Blood Group, Hb,TLC, DLC, ESR
- Anticoagulation Profile (BT,CT,PT/APTT)
- Renal Function Tests- Blood Urea, S.Creatinine, S. Uric Acid
- Urinalysis, With Or Without Urine Culture.
  Pregnancy Test For Childbearing Age Women.
- Other Relevant Investigations For
  Diabetic Profile(Blood Sugar-Fasting,PP, Random),
  Hepatic Dysfunction(LFT), Pancreatic Profile(S.Amylase, S.Lipase)
  & Others

Imaging Studies
- Renal Ultrasonography
- Intravenous Pyelography
- Noncontrast/ Contrast Enhanced CT Scanning
- MRI
- DTPA Renal Scan With/WithOut Diuretics
- DMSA Renal Scan

Other Tests

X-Ray Chest, Abdomen

Routine Electrocardiography - Especially In Patients Older Than 50 Years & Or With A History Of Cardiac Disease

Cardiac Pacemakers Are Also Not Contraindicated, Cardiologist Assistance Should Be Seeked For Needed Help.

Oral Anticoagulants (Eg, Clopidogrel [Plavix] And Warfarin [Coumadin]) Are Discontinued For Normalization Of Clotting Parameters. While For Platelet Function, Discontinuing Aspirin-Containing Products And Nonsteroidal Anti-Inflammatory Drugs (NSAIDS) 7 Days Before Treatment, Is Usually Recommended.

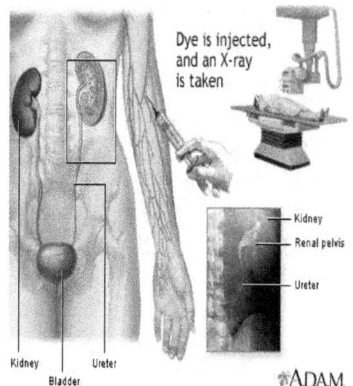

In The Procedure Intravenous Pyelogram (IVP),
The Patient Is Injected With Radiopaque Dye And X-Rays Are Taken As The Dye Travels Through The Urinary Tract.
This Procedure Is Performed To Confirm The Presence Of Kidney Stones, Although Some Stones May Be Too Small To See.
Source-Adams

TREATMENT SELECTION CRITERIA

Stones In The Urinary Tract Are A Common Medical Problem. Fifty Per Cent Of Patients With Previous Urinary Stones Have A **Recurrence** Within 10 Years.

Essentials Of Litho-Tripsy

Treatment For Small Stones With Minimal Symptoms

Most Stones Under 5 Mm (0.20 In) Pass Spontaneously.[18][38]
& Donot Require Invasive Treatment.
Patient May Be Able To Pass A Small Stone By:
Drinking Plenty Of Water, Pain Relievers, Medical Supportive Therapies.
Patient Is Advised To Save The Passed Stone(s),
By Straining(Filtering)The Urine, For **Stone Analysis**,
& Adherence To Dietary Regulations, Accordingly.

Treatment Of Larger Stones

Surgery For Treatement For Large Stones: Is Needed-
Conservative Measures Failure — Either Because They're Too Large To Pass On Their Own Or Because They Cause Bleeding, Kidney Damage Or Ongoing Urinary Tract Infections, Requiring More Invasive Treatment.
Surgical Treatement Remains An Otption To Treat Stones Specially If
1) Causing Urinary OutFlow Obstruction
2) Causing An Ongoing Urinary Tract Infection
3) Damaging Kidney Tissue Or Causing Constant Bleeding

Prompt Surgery May, Nonetheless, Be Required: In Persons With Only One Working Kidney, Bilateral Obstructing Stones, A Urinary Tract Infection And Thus PresumAbly An Infected Kidney, Or Intractable Pain.[70]

Some Of The Treatement Procedures For Larger Stones,
Besides Controversially Successful Various Medical Therapy Regimes, **Extracorporeal Shock Wave Lithotripsy**
And OSS (Classical Open Surgical Stone Extraction),
Other Methods Include:
(1) Percutaneous Nephrolithotomy(PCNL) For Renal Calculi
(2) Retrograde Intra-Renal Surgery (RIRS),
    Retrograde Uretero-Renoscopic Intrarenal Surgery
(3) Ureterorenoscopy (URS) &Lithoclast for Ureteric Calculi,
(4) Laparoscopic Ureterolithotomy
(5) Cystolithopexy/Cystolithoclast For Vesical Calculi,
    Using Lithotrite
(6) Sandwich Technique (ESWL + PNL / Ureterorenoscopic
    Lithotripsy Surgery), Etc.

In The European Association Of Urology (EAU) Guidelines,
For Larger / Large Stones :ESWL And PCNL Are The Recommended Primary Treatment Options For Renal Stones (Stone Size <20mm And 20mm Or More Respectively).

Extracorporeal Shock Wave Lithotripsy (ESWL).

Following Its Introduction In United States In February 1984, ESWL Became, Rapidly And Widely Accepted As, A Treatment Alternative For Renal And Ureteral Stones.

It Is Currently Used In The Treatment Of Uncomplicated Stones Located In The Kidney And Upper Ureter, Provided The Aggregate Stone Burden (Stone Size And Number) Is Less Than 20 Mm (0.79 In) And The Anatomy Of The Involved Kidney Is Normal.
For A Stone Greater Than 10 Mm, ESWL May Not Help Break The Stone In One Treatment; Instead, Two Or Three Treatments May Be Needed. Some 80 To 85% Of Simple Renal Calculi Can Be Effectively Treated With ESWL.

Percutaneous Nephrolithotomy(PCNL): Is EndoScopic Surgical Procedure,To Remove Very Large Kidney Stones,Through A Small Incision(About 1 Cm / Half An Inch) In Back,
Using Nephroscope,LithoClast Under CT Scan Guidance.
PCNL May Be Recommended If ESWL Has Been Unsuccessful Or If Stone Is Very Large.
Anatrophic Nephrolithotomy: Is The Treatment Of Choice For Large Or Complicated Stones (Such As Calyceal Staghorn Calculi) Or Stones That Cannot Be Extracted Using Less Invasive Procedures. [31][38]

Retrograde Intrarenal Surgery (RIRS): The Stone In Ureter Or Kidney Is **Visualized Through The Scope & Using Available IntraCorporeal Devices,** Manipulated Or Crushed By An Ultrasound Probe Or Evaporated By A Laser Probe Or Grabbed, Crushed By Small Forceps Into Small Pieces That Pass With Urine.
Occasionally, A Small Hollow Tube-**Ureteral Stent** Placed In The Ureter For A Short Time For Urinary Drainage & Stone Particles Passage Patency, Is Needed.
Ureteroscopy(URS) Is Often Used For Stones That Migrate From The Kidney To The Ureter.
RIRS Is Performed By A **Specialist EndoUrologist** With Special Expertise In RIRS,Usually Done Under General Or Local(Spinal Anesthesia).
The **Indications Of RIRS** For Renal Stones Are:**1.**Failed Extracorporeal Shockwave Lithotripsy **2.** Radiolucent Stones **3.** Concomitant Ureteric & Renal Stones 4. Anatomical Problems e.g. Infundibular Stenosis **5.** Nephrocalcinosis **6.** Bleeding Disorders
The Main Advantages Of RIRS Over Open Surgery Include,
A Quicker Solution Of The Problem, The Elimination Of Prolonged Pain After Surgery, No Deeper Incision, Less Trauma
And Hence Much Faster Recovery. (30-38)

Essentials Of Litho-Tripsy
References

1. Aulus Cornelius Celsus (1831). "Book VII, Chapter XXVI: Of the operation necessary in a suppression of urine, and lithotomy". In Collier, GF. *A translation of the eight books of Aul. Corn. Celsus on medicine* (2nd ed.). London: Simpkin and Marshall. pp. 306–14.
2. Shah, J; Whitfield, HN (2002). "Urolithiasis through the ages". *British Journal of Urology International* 89 (8): 801–10. doi:10.1046/j.1464-410X.2002.02769.x. PMID 11972501.
3. Wolf Jr. JS (2011). "Background". *Nephrolithiasis*. New York: WebMD. Retrieved 2011-07-27.
4. Preminger, GM (2007). "Chapter 148: Stones in the Urinary Tract". In Cutler, RE. *The Merck Manual of Medical Information Home Edition* (3rd ed.). Whitehouse Station, New Jersey: Merck Sharp and Dohme Corporation.
5. Pearle, MS; Calhoun, EA; Curhan, GC (2007). "Chapter 8: Urolithiasis". In Litwin, MS; Saigal, CS. *Urologic Diseases in America (NIH Publication No. 07–5512)*. Bethesda, Maryland: National Institute of Diabetes and Digestive and Kidney Diseases, National Institutes of Health, United States Public Health Service, United States Department of Health and Human Services. pp. 283–319.
6. [b]Cavendish, M (2008). "Kidney disorders". *Diseases and Disorders* 2 (1st ed.). Tarrytown, New York: Marshall Cavendish Corporation. pp. 490–3. ISBN 978-0-7614-7772-3.
7. Curhan, G. C.; Willett, W. C.; Rimm, E. B.; Spiegelman, D.; Stampfer, M. J. (Feb 1996). "Prospective study of beverage use and the risk of kidney stones". *Am J Epidemiol* 143 (3): 240–7. doi:10.1093/oxfordjournals.aje.a008734. PMID 8561157.
8. Knight J, Assimos DG, Easter L, Holmes RP (2010). "Metabolism of fructose to oxalate and glycolate". *Horm Metab Res* 42 (12): 868–73. doi:10.1055/s-0030-1265145. PMID 20842614.
9. Johri, N; Cooper B, Robertson W, Choong S, Rickards D, Unwin R (2010). "An update and practical guide to renal stone management". *Nephron Clinical Practice* 116 (3): c159–71. doi:10.1159/000317196. PMID 20606476.
10. Moe, OW (2006). "Kidney stones: pathophysiology and medical management". *The Lancet* 367 (9507): 333–44. doi:10.1016/S0140-6736(06)68071-9. PMID 16443041.
11. Thakker, RV (2000). "Pathogenesis of Dent's disease and related syndromes of X-linked nephrolithiasis". *Kidney International* 57 (3): 787–93. doi:10.1046/j.1523-1755.2000.00916.x. PMID 10720930.
12. National Endocrine and Metabolic Diseases Information Service (2006). "Hyperparathyroidism (NIH Publication No. 6–3425)". *Information about Endocrine and Metabolic Diseases: A-Z list of Topics and Titles*. Bethesda, Maryland: National Institute of Diabetes and Digestive and Kidney Diseases, National Institutes of Health, Public Health Service, US Department of Health and Human Services. Retrieved 2011-07-27.
13. ^ Jump up to: [a][b] Hoppe, B; Langman, CB (2003). "A United States survey on diagnosis, treatment, and outcome of primary hyperoxaluria". *Pediatric Nephrology* 18 (10): 986–91. doi:10.1007/s00467-003-1234-x. PMID 12920626.
14. Reilly Jr. RF, *Chapter 13: Nephrolithiasis*, pp. 192–207 in Reilly Jr. and Perazella (2005)
15. Parmar, MS (2004). "Kidney stones". *British Medical Journal* 328 (7453): 1420–4. doi:10.1136/bmj.328.7453.1420. PMC 421787. PMID 15191979.
16. Negri, A. L.; Spivacow, F. R.; Del Valle, EE. (2013). "[Diet in the treatment of renal lithiasis. Pathophysiological basis]". *Medicina (B Aires)* 73 (3): 267–71. PMID 23732207.
17. Goodwin, JS; Mangum, MR (1998). "Battling quackery: attitudes about micronutrient supplements in American academic medicine". *Archives of Internal Medicine* 158 (20): 2187–91. doi:10.1001/archinte.158.20.2187. PMID 9818798.
18. Rodman, JS; Seidman, C (1996). "Chapter 8: Dietary Troublemakers". In Rodman, JS; Seidman, C; Jones, R. *No More Kidney Stones* (1st ed.). New York: John Wiley & Sons, Inc. pp. 46–57. ISBN 978-0-471-12587-7.
19. Brawer, MK; Makarov, DV; Partin, AW; Roehrborn, CG; Nickel, JC; Lu, SH; Yoshimura, N; Chancellor, MB; Assimos, DG (2008). "Best of the 2008 AUA Annual Meeting: Highlights from the 2008 Annual Meeting of the American Urological

Association, May 17–22, 2008, Orlando, FL". *Reviews in Urology* 10 (2): 136–56. PMC 2483319. PMID 18660856.
20. Perazella MA, *Chapter 14: Urinalysis*, pp. 209–26 in Reilly Jr. and Perazella (2005)
21. Knudsen BE, Beiko DT and Denstedt JD, *Chapter 16: Uric Acid Urolithiasis*, pp. 299–308 in Stoller and Meng (2007)
22. Wolf Jr. JS (2011). "Pathophysiology: formation of stones". *Nephrolithiasis*. New York: WebMD. Retrieved 2011-07-27.
23. Coe, FL; Evan, A; Worcester, E (2005). "Kidney stone disease". *The Journal of Clinical Investigation* 115 (10): 2598–608. doi:10.1172/JCI26662. PMC 1236703. PMID 16200192.
24. del Valle, E. E.; Spivacow, F. R.; Negri, A. L. (2013). "[Citrate and renal stones]". *Medicina (B Aires)* 73 (4): 363–8. PMID 23924538.
25. Anoia, EJ; Paik, ML; Resnick, MI (2009). "Chapter 7: Anatrophic Nephrolithomy". In Graham, SD; Keane, TE. *Glenn's Urologic Surgery* (7th ed.). Philadelphia: Lippincott Williams & Wilkins. pp. 45–50. ISBN 978-0-7817-9141-0.
26. Miller, NL; Lingeman, JE (2007). "Management of kidney stones". *BMJ* 334 (7591): 468–72. doi:10.1136/bmj.39113.480185.80. PMC 1808123. PMID 17332586.
27. National Endocrine and Metabolic Diseases Information Service (2008). "Renal Tubular Acidosis (NIH Publication No. 09–4696)". *Kidney & Urologic Diseases: A-Z list of Topics and Titles*. Bethesda, Maryland: National Institute of Diabetes and Digestive and Kidney Diseases, National Institutes of Health, Public Health Service, US Department of Health and Human Services. Retrieved 2011-07-27.
28. De Mais, Daniel. ASCP Quick Compendium of Clinical Pathology, 2nd Ed. ASCP Press, Chicago, 2009.
29. Weiss, M; Liapis, H; Tomaszewski, JE; Arend, LJ (2007). "Chapter 22: Pyelonephritis and other infections, reflux nephropathy, hydronephrosis, and nephrolithiasis". In Jennette, JC; Olson, JL; Schwartz, MM et al. *Heptinstall's Pathology of the Kidney* 2 (6th ed.). Philadelphia: Lippincott Williams & Wilkins. pp. 991–1082. ISBN 978-0-7817-4750-9.
30. Halabe, A; Sperling, O (1994). "Uric acid nephrolithiasis". *Mineral and Electrolyte Metabolism* 20 (6): 424–31. ISSN 0378-0392. PMID 7783706.
31. Kamatani, N (1996). "Adenine phosphoribosyltransferase (APRT) deficiency". *Nippon Rinsho. Japanese Journal of Clinical Medicine* (in Japanese) 54 (12): 3321–7. ISSN 0047-1852. PMID 8976113.
32. Rosenberg, LE; Durant JL, Elsas LJ (1968). "Familial iminoglycinuria. An inborn error of renal tubular transport". *The New England Journal of Medicine* 278 (26): 1407–13. doi:10.1056/NEJM196806272782601. PMID 5652624.
33. Coşkun T, Ozalp I, Tokatli A (1993). "Iminoglycinuria: a benign type of inherited aminoaciduria". *The Turkish Journal of Pediatrics* 35 (2): 121–5. ISSN 0041-4301. PMID 7504361.
34. Schlossberg, D; Samuel, R (2011). "Sulfadiazine". *Antibiotic Manual: A Guide to Commonly Used Antimicrobials* (1st ed.). Shelton, Connecticut: People's Medical Publishing House. pp. 411–12. ISBN 978-1-60795-084-4.
35. Carr, MC; Prien EL Jr, Babayan RK (1990). "Triamterene nephrolithiasis: renewed attention is warranted". *Journal of Urology* 144 (6): 1339–40. PMID 2231920.
36. Shock Wave Lithotripsy Task Force (2009). "Current Perspective on Adverse Effects in Shock Wave Lithotripsy". *Clinical Guidelines*. Linthicum, Maryland: American Urological Association. Retrieved 2011-07-27.
37. Lingeman, J.E., Matlaga, B.R., and Evan, A.P. (2007). Surgical management of urinary lithiasis. In:Campbell-Walsh Urology Edited by AJ Wein, LR Kavoussi, AC Novick, AW Partin, CA Peters. Philadelphia: W. B. Saunders. (pp. 1431–1507)
38. Preminger, GM; Tiselius, HG; Assimos, DG et al. (2007). "2007 Guideline for the management of ureteral calculi". *The Journal of Urology* 178 (6): 2418–34. doi:10.1016/j.eururo.2007.09.039. PMID 17993340

Essentials Of Litho-Tripsy

Further Readings

1. Andreassen KH, Dahl C, Andersen JT, Rasmussen MS, Jacobsen JD, Mogensen P. Extracorporeal shock wave lithotripsy as first line monotherapy of solitary calyceal calculi. Scand J Urol Nephrol 1997;31:245-8.

2. Renner CH, Rassweiler J. Treatment of renal stones by extracorporeal shock wave lithotripsy Nephron 1999;81:71-81.

3. Kane CJ, Bolton DM, Stoller ML. Current indications for open stone surgery in an endourology center. Urology 1994;45:218-21.

5. Gould DL. Holmium: Yag laser and its use in the treatment of urolithiasis: Our first 160 cases. J Endourol 1998;12:23-6.

6. Keeley FX, Gialas I, Pillai M, Chrisofos M, Tolley DA. Laproscopic ureterolithotomy: The edinburgh experience. Br J Urol 1999;84:765-9.

7. Figge M. Percutaneous transperitoneal nephrolithotomy. Eur Urol 1988;14:414-6.

8. Pettersson B, Tiselius HG. Are prophylactic antibiotics necessary during extracorporeal shock wave lithotripsy? J Urol 1990;144:15.

(2.)(ii.)
ESWL:UROLITHIASIS
PROCEDURAL DETAILS

Pre-Procedural Preparations
Properly Established Diagnosis For Stone Disease
Excluding Distal Obstruction,
Ensured Patient Compliance After Comprehensive Awareness Of
Treatment Plan (Needed Ureteral Stenting, Urinary Asepsis Etc.)
With 'Informed Consent', LithoTripsy (ESWL) Is Performed.

Certain Pre-Requisites:

- An Appropriate History And Physical Examination, Including All Aspects Regarding Previous Surgery, Medical Diseases, Drug Allergy Any Medications, Latex, Tape, Or Anesthetic Agents (Local And General).

- A Complete Blood Count (CBC) & Other Relevant Blood Tests, Urine Examination Including Culture, Ensured Within 7 Days Of ESWL.

- Pregnancy Test For Female Under 50.

- A Recent IVP Or CECT Scan & Plain X-Ray Abdomen KUB (After Proper Preparation), On The Procedure Day

- A Recent Electrocardiogram (EKG) & For Over 45 Yrs. Age Or Heart Disease - Day Before Lithotripsy, With Cardiologist Clearance.

- As Intestinal Gas And Bowel Contents Interfere With Localization And Targeting Of Stone, During The 48 Hours Prior To Lithotripsy Procedure, <u>Avoidance Of All Foods That Cause Gas,</u> As Following-
Carbonated Beverages, Milk Products, And Chewing Gum. Fiber Foods Such As Bran, Beans, Peas, Most Fruits, Oatmeal And Whole Grain Breads, Vegetables Such As Cabbage, Broccoli, Cauliflower, Brussels Sprouts, Celery, Cucumbers, Eggplant, Onions And Radishes, Starches Including Potatoes, Corn, Noodles And Wheat.

<u>A Course Of Laxatives(Dulcolax-BisaCodyl, Cremaffin White) Combined With Available AntiFlatulent</u> ; Destronil- Simethicone & Or Charcoal Tabs.H.S For 1-2 Days Before Procedure,
Has Demonstrable Good Results.

Essentials Of Litho-Tripsy

- <u>Avoidance Or Restriction</u> Of Aspirin-Containing Products(As Monitored By BT,CT,INR Etc), Nonsteroidal Anti-Inflammatory Medications & Others.

- The Effects Of Herbal Supplements(Ginkgo Biloba Garlic,Ginseng St. John's Wort,Ephedra Kava,Valerian Echinacea,Vitamin E Fish Oil) On Blood Coagulation Are Not Completely Understood. But They Do Thin The Blood.
  For Safety Interest, The Use Of These Herbal Supplements 7 Days Before ESWL Should Be Discontinued.

- Exclusion And / Or Management Of Pre-Existing Illnesses, Being The Most Important Aspect Of Pre-Procedural Preparations.

- Certain Pre-Existing Urologic And Medical Conditions, Need Cautious Specific Control For The Procedure.

UnderStanding, AwareNess For Limitations Of Treatment:
- Untreated Urinary Tract Infection
- Nonfunctioning Kidney
- Obstruction Of The Ureter Beyond The Stone Being Treated
- Blood Coagulation Disorder, Permanent Anticoagulation Therapy And Certain Drugs
- Cardiac Pacemakers And Implanted Defibrillators In Some Instances
- Anatomies That Prevent Stone Targeting
- Pregnancy

- <u>Pre-Procedural Preparations</u> Including Over-Night Fasting Depending On The Type Of Anesthetic Or Sedation Used. Bowel Preparations, Immediate Bladder Evacuation Etc Are Cautiously Instituted,
  With Provision For Needed Appropriate Transport.

Per-Procedural Details

Lithotripsy May Be Performed As Out-Patient Procedure
& Or SomeTimes In-Door Facilities Are Needed,
Depending Upon Co-Existing Medical Conditions Control,
Need For Ureteral Stenting
& Or Forced Diuresis (Lasix Therapy) Regimes.

Jewellary,Clothes,Especially Radio-Opaque,Conducting Materials
Etc. Are Removed & Patient May Be Asked To Wear A Gown.

Before Treatment, Patient May Be Given Medication,
Either By Mouth(With Restricted Sip Of Water) Or Intravenously,
IV Line & Other Monitoring Devices Are Attached.
Most Treatments Are Done With Sedation.
Anesthesia Is SomeTimes Needed.

PATIENT'S POSITION

Patient Is Placed On Back Or Abdomen On The Treatment Table,
Depending Upon The Location Of The Stone.
(a) Patient Stone Side Toward The Machine
(b) Lies Supine, For Renal And Upper, Mid,Ureteric Calculi
(c) Prone Position, For Lower Ureteric / VUJ Stones.

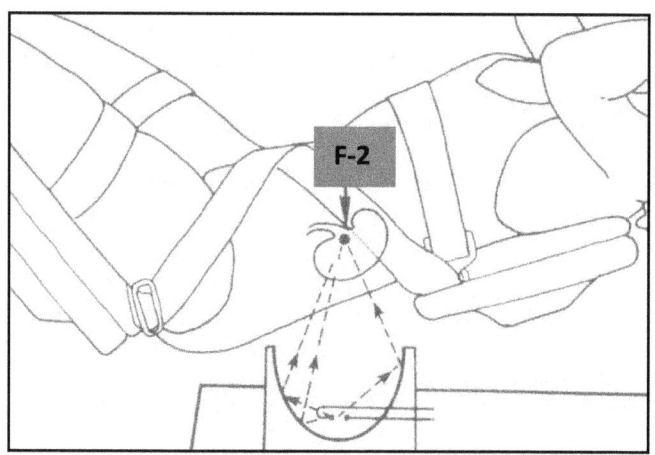

Stone Localization And Focusing HM3 LithoTriptor

Note- The Placements Of Both Arms Above The Patients Head, Pulls
Lungs Above Kidney Regions,Thus Preventing Their Shock Wave Injury.
Lungs, Being Very Susceptible To Multiple Air- Fluid Interfaces Presence.
Source - Chaussy & Fuchs 1987b

The Stone Is Positioned In The Focus Of The Shock Wave,
Using Imaging In Vertical And Oblique Axis Of C-Arm,
Achieved By Anatomical Landmarks(Subcostal Region, Umblicus, Asis,
Pubis And Other Bony Points Pelvis, Vertebrae),
Maneuvering Table Movements,
And May Be Assisted By Patient Movement As A Whole.

Essentials Of Litho-Tripsy

The Shock Tube Is Then Pressed Against Patient Side
And "Coupled" With Some Lubricating Gel-Like Material.

Stand By Anesthesia/Analgesia/Under Sedation

1ml Pentazocine (Fortwin) (+) 2 ml Promethazine(Phenargan),
Diluted To 5 ml By Adding 2 ml Distilled Water,
3 ml Of Preparation Given Slowly Intravenously,
And Remaining 2 ml Given Intramuscularly,
Achieves Almost Complete Sedation And Analgesia
For Conducting Lithotripsy Sitting For About 100 Minutes.

The Total Dose Is Titrated Depending Upon Body Weight,
Patient's Social History (Previous Painkiller Injections, Smoking, Alcohol Etc.) And Associated Medical Problems.
Diazepam Was Supplemented Through Intravenous Or Intramuscular Route, Sometimes, To Facilitate Patient Compliance For Lithotripsy Sitting.

Need & Scope Of GA / SA
Analgesics / Antispasmodics /
Anesthetic Agents (Alfentanil, Midazolam, Propofol, Fentanyl Combinations)
Were Needed Rarely,
Especially In Pediatric Or Apprehensive Patients
With Supportive Use Of Topical Agents, Emla Cream Etc Otherwise.

Special Cares For ESWL In Paediatrics Patients Are Needed.

SHOCK DELIVERY INITIATION

Done After Ensured Patient Compliance,
With An Advice Not To Change Position,
In Cautiously Pre-Prepared Lithotripter,
Treatment Begins, With The Light Tapping Feeling On Patient's Skin.

The Shock Waves Are Delivered At Rates Up To 120/Minute.
Patient Compliance Of Not To Change Posture, Is Extremely Important To Retain The Stone In Focus. Medication Can Be Given For Discomfort During Treatment. The Shocks May Be Interrupted To Move The Table To Keep The Stone In The Target Zone.

REGULAR MONITORING
Continuous Discrete Monitoring For-
(a) Stone Position And Status
(b) Vital Signs, Especially Pulse Respiration Etc
(c) Regulation Shock Mode, Power, And Frequency;

While Maintaining Patient's Compliance Throughout
Are The **Key Components** For The Complete Stone-Free Success Rate.

With Discrete Stone Targetting Achieved By Imaging,
The Stone Can Be Positioned Precisely Into The High-Energy Focus Of The Shock Waves.
The Number Of Shock Waves And Treatments Needed For Breakage Of Stones Depends Upon Their Size And Hardness.
Little Or No Anesthesia Is Usually Needed.
Up To 4,000 Shock Waves Are Used, Until Adequate Pulverization Of Stone Is Demonstrated By Available Imaging.
The Procedure Time Varying From **30–90 Minutes**.

Progress Of The Treatment Depends Upon,
The Size And Hardness Of The Stone.
For Larger Or For Multiple Stones,
Second/Third (Ancillary) Treatment May Be Needed.

INTRAOPERATIVE DETAILS

The Optimal Shockwave Lithotripsy Treatment Is Thought To Be About 80-90 Shocks Per Minute. Faster Rates Have Been Shown To Be Associated With Decreased Stone-Free Rates, Especially For Larger Stones (11-20 Mm).
The Difference In Stone-Free Rates Is Less Significant For Smaller Stones. Conversely, Slower Rates Obviously Increase The
Total Operative Time.

During Shockwave Lithotripsy,Tracking The Stone Burden Becomes An Important Issue, In Part Because Of The Natural Movement Of The Kidney During Respiration, With Subsequent Movement Of The Stone Burden In And Out Of The Focal Zone.
The Smaller Focal Zone Of The Newer Devices Allows For Minimal Anesthesia, But The Patient's Increased Ability And Susceptibility To Cough, Shift, Or Otherwise Move
Requires Vigilance To Ensure The Appropriate Targeting Accuracy In The Application Of Energy To The Stone.
This Means That The Targeting Of The Machine Needs To Be Adjusted More Often.

The Decreased Anesthetic Need During Lithotripsy When Using The Later Generation Devices Provides Obvious Advantages,
Such As Rapid Recovery Time And Rapid Turnover Between Patients.
However, A Balance Must Be Struck Between The Minimal Invasiveness Of The Procedure And The Stone Disintegration Efficacy.
The Optimal Anesthetic Regimen To Facilitate This Remains A Subject Of Debate.

Patient-Controlled Analgesia Has Been Suggested To Enable Urologists To Achieve Better Patient Compliance Through More Accurate Pain Control And, Hence, More Effective TreatMent.
To This End,
Parkin Et Al Studied Preoperative Diclofenac Alone Versus Diclofenac And Alfentanil PCA. Pain Scores Based On A Visual Analog Score (VAS) Were Similar Between The 2 Groups But PCA Patients Showed A Statistically Significant Increased Level Of Satisfaction With The Experience.
Kumar Et Al Compared 3 Forms Of Adjunctive Analgesia For ESWL Patients: Preoperative Diclofenac, Topical Eutectic Mixture Of Lidocaine/Prilocaine (Emla), And The 2 In Combination. Stone Free Rates At 3 Months Were The Highest In The Combination Group At 88.75%, And The Retreatment Rate Was The Lowest, Both Reaching Statistical Significance
Thus, Excellent Stone Free Rates Can Be Achieved With Minimal To No <u>General Anesthesia</u> Using Modern Lithotripters. Analgesic Adjuncts Certainly Have A Role In Facilitating These Outcomes.

<u>Post-Procedure Advice</u>

Minimal Side Effects Occur After ESWL,
After A Necessary Short Observation Period
(For Stable Pulse, Blood Pressure, & Respiration Monitoring And AlertNess From Residual Effect Of Sedation, Analgesia),
Patient May Return Home,
Easily Resuming Normal Activities Within 1–3 Days.

Urinary Antiseptics According To Culture And Senstivity,
Prophylactic Antibiotics, Analgesia And Other Supportive Therapy.[8]

Encouraged Urine Output More Than 2500 Ml In 24 Hrs,
Achieved By Increased Fluid Intake,
Depending Upon Climatic & Working Living Conditions Of Patient
Forced Diuresis, As Indicated.

To Strain(Filter) All Urine And Collect Stone Particles,
For 'Stone Analysis'

Follow Up Of Case, As Advised, For Next Sitting Or Otherwise.
Besides, Noticing Bruising / Petechiae On Flank,Back Or Abdomen & Blood In Urine For Few Days Or Longer, That Is In Normal Process.
Notification To Doctor For Reporting Any Of The Following May Be Needed -
Fever And /Or Chills, Burning With Urination,Urinary Frequency Or Urgency,Extreme Lower Back Pain, Hematuria, And Passage Of Stone Fragments With Associated Renal Colic

For Additional Or Alternate Instructions.
Some Groups Have Initiated Trials Of Pharmacologic Aids Similar To Those Involved In Medical Stone-Passage Protocols To Facilitate Stone Passage. In The Treatment Arm, Pharmacologic Aids (Stone-Free Rate Of 86% With Nifedipine And 82% With Tamsulosin) Were Superior To Placebo (Stone-Free Rate Of 52-57%). Quantification Of Residual Stone Burden And Resolution Of Hydronephrosis Was Defined With Postoperative Radiography Or Ultrasonography. **It Is A Part Of Authenticated Evidence Based Medicine(EBM) Practice**, To Obtain Postoperative Imaging, Typically A KUB Or Ultrasound, Within 6 Weeks Following The Procedure Or Sooner If The Patient Is Symptomatic.

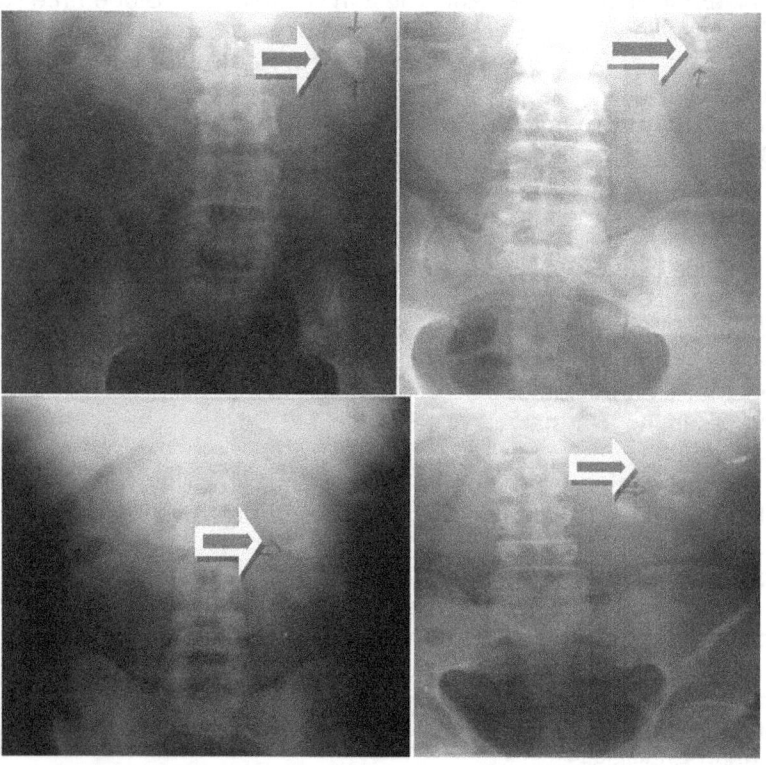

Screening Stages For Subsequent Complete Removal Left Renal Stone About More Than 3 Cms

Essentials Of Litho-Tripsy

TREATMENT ALOGRITHM

Extracorporeal Shockwave Lithotripsy (ESWL) Outcome Is Affected By **Several Stone Related Factors** -

Stone Size
As **Stone Size Approaches 2 Cm**, The Success Rates With ESWL Decrease & The Need For **Retreatment & Adjunctive Therapy** Increase. ESWL Being Most Efficacious In Treating **NonObstructing Renal Calculi. Pre-ESWL Stenting** May Secure Drainage And Prevent Obstructive UroSepsis, In **Large Stone Burden** Cases.

Stone Composition
The **Density And Ability Of A Stone To Resist ESWL**, Partially Depends UpOn The Stone Composition.
Stones Composed Of Calcium Oxalate Dihydrate, Magnesium Ammonium Phosphate, Or Uric Acid Are Comparatively Softer & Fragment More Easily With ESWL.
Stones Composed Of Calcium Oxalate Monohydrate Or Cystine, Are Hand & Hence Less Susceptible To ESWL.

CT Scan Radio-Opacity MeasureMents Of Stones
Can Predict Their Behaviour To ESWL
Recent Retrospective Study Recorded,
That **ESWL Monotherapy** Is More Effective Against Stones With A **Lower Radio-Opacity (551 Hounsfield Units [HU])**
Than With **Higher Radio-Opacity (926 HU)**.

Certain Radiolucent Stones (Uric Acid, Indinavir [Crixivan]) Have Difficult Fluoroscopic Visualization & Hence Either Ultrasonography-Guided Or Retrograde / Intravenous Contrast Localization Is Needed.

Stone Location
Lower-Pole Calculi: Although Fragmented By ESWL, The Resulting Stone-Free Rate Is Decreased Because Of Stone Passage Difficulty From This Location.

Renal Morphologies Associated With **Improved Stone-Free Rates** Studies Include- **Lower Infundibular Length–To–Diameter Ratio** Of < 7, **Lower-Pole Infundibular Diameter** Of >4 Mm, **Single Minor Calyx**.

While,**Decreased Stone-Free Rates Factors** Include-
Infundibulopelvic Angle Of < 70°, **Infundibular Length** Of >3 Cm, **Infundibular Width** Of < 5 Mm.

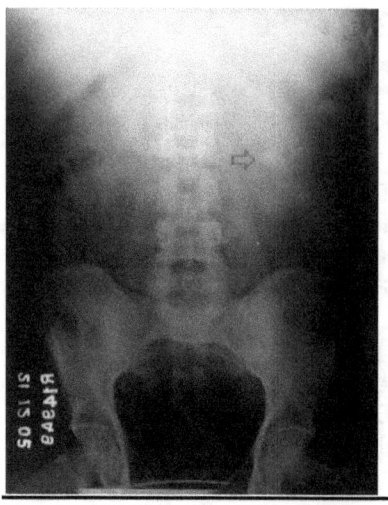
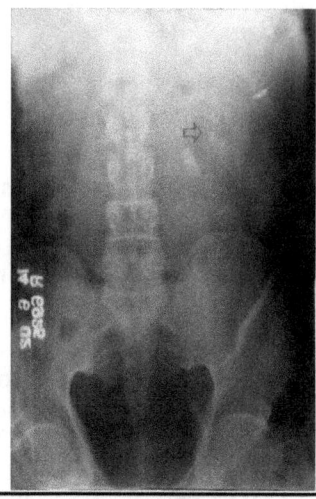
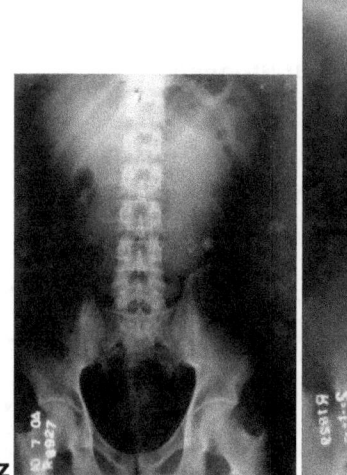
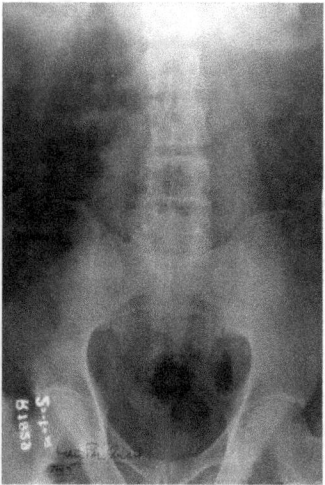

<u>Screening Stages For Subsequent Complete Removal Left Renal Stone About More Than 3 Cms</u>

Regardless Of Anatomy, ESWL Tends To Yield Better Results In Patients With Smaller Stone Burdens.

<u>**Calyceal Diverticula With Infundibular Stenosis**</u>: **Difficult Fragmented Stone Particles Passage Through Obstruction, Caused By Factors Related To Diverticula Or Infundibular Stenosis, Lead To** Resultant Retained Stone Fragments.

Essentials Of Litho-Tripsy

More Invasive Technique Methodology With Available Access For Simultaneous ManageMent Of Obstruction & Stone Disease, Either With **Retrograde** Or **Antegrade Percutaneous** Manner, Are Employed.

Ureteral Calculi: Proximal Stones Fragmentation Is More Effective, Than Mid Or Distal Stones.
When Associated With **Hydronephrosis,**
Ureteroscopy Yields Better Stone-Free Rates
For Stones Larger Than 15 Mm.

Preoperative And Intraoperative Stenting
With Readily Available Access To ESWL And Ureteroscopy,
The **Decreased Indications** For Stenting,
Prior To Definitive Treatment Include-
- Obstructed Pyelonephritis Or Pyelitis &
- Recent Onset Renal Insufficiency Or Renal Failure.
In These Circumstances, The Stent -
1. Assists To Ensure Internal Drainage
2. Allows Passive Dilatation Of The Ureter
Facilitating Future Endoscopic Evaluation.

With The Advent Of Newer And Smaller Ureteroscopic Equipment,
The Rates Of **Endoscopic Complications (ie Strictures)**
Have Subsequently Declined.
For Preoperative Stenting Need, Just Ureteroscopy,
Especially For Ureteral Stones, May Yield Higher Stone-Free Rates
Without Significant Increase In Morbidity, Time, Or Cost.
The Need For Intraoperative Manipulation Of Stones For ESWL
(eg, Stone Pushback) Or Placement Of A Ureteral Catheter,
To Assist With Stone Visualization Has Decreased,
As Newer Machines Are Capable Of Treating Proximal Ureteral Stones
Or Visualizing Radiolucent Stones With Ultrasonography.
Intraoperative Ureteral Stenting, HowEver Should Be Considered In Patients With **Larger Stones,** As The Rate Of **Steinstrasse** (German For "Stone Street") Increases With **Stone Burden**(1-4% In General Vs 10% For Stones >2 Cm).

Thus To Summarize,
Various Factors Influencing ESWL Efficacy, **Include Chemical Composition Of The Stone, Presence Of Anomalous Renal Anatomy And The Specific Location Of The Stone Within The Kidney, Presence Of Hydronephrosis, Body Mass Index, And Distance Of The Stone From The Surface Of The Skin(SSD).**[65]

'Maximal Stone Clearance' With Minimal Co-Morbidities,
(The Basic Fundamental Aim),
The Different Factors Taken Into Consideration Are –
I. Stone Factors: Size Numbers(Total Stone Burden)
             Location Composition Duration.
II. Renal Anatomy Determinants:
  Solitary Kidney
  Aberrant Anatomy & Others.
III. Clinical(Patient) Factors
   Pain
   Infection
   Patient Compliance/ Expectations
IV. Technical Factors

Essentials Of Litho-Tripsy

(2.)(iii.)
INDICATIONS, CONTRAINDICATIONS, ANATOMICAL DETERMINANTS, COMPLICATIONS

INDICATIONS

The Current Options Available For The Treatment Of Renal And Ureteral Calculi Include -
Conservative Management (Watchful Waiting For Spontaneous Passage),
Extracorporeal Shockwave Lithotripsy (ESWL),
Endoscopic Techniques (Rigid Or Flexible Ureteroscopic Lithotripsy),
And Percutaneous Treatments.

The American Urological Association Stone Guidelines Panel Has Classified ESWL As A Potential First-Line Treatment For Ureteral And Renal Stones Smaller Than 2 Cm.
Indications For ESWL Include:

- Individuals Who Work In Professions In Which Unexpected Symptoms Of Stone Passage May Prompt Dangerous Situations (eg, Pilots, Military Personnel, Physicians)
  In Such Individuals, Definitive Management Is Preferred To Prevent Adverse Outcomes).
- Individuals With Solitary Kidneys In Whom Attempted Conservative Management And Spontaneous Passage Of The Stone May Lead To An Anuric State
- Patients With Hypertension, Diabetes, Or Other Medical Conditions That Predispose To Renal Insufficiency

CONTRAINDICATIONS
Absolute Contraindications

- Acute Urinary Tract Infection Or Urosepsis
- Uncorrected Bleeding Disorders Or Coagulopathies
- Pregnancy
- Uncorrected Obstruction Distal To The Stone

Relative Contraindications

- **Body Habitus:** Morbid Obesity And Orthopedic Or Spinal Deformities May Complicate Or Prevent Proper Positioning.
  In These Situations, Attempting To Position The Patient Prior To Anesthetic Induction
  Is Useful To Ensure The Practicality Of The Approach.

- **Renal Ectopy Or Malformations** (eg, HorseShoe Kidneys And Pelvic Kidneys)
- **Complex Intrarenal Drainage** (Eg, Infundibular Stenosis)
- **Poorly Controlled Hypertension** (Due To Increased Bleeding Risk) Relative Renal Hypertension.
    - **Gastrointestinal Disorders:** In Rare Cases, May Be Exacerbated After ESWL Treatment.
    - **Renal Insufficiency:** Stone-Free Rates In Patients With Renal Insufficiency Were Significantly Lower Than In Patients With Better Renal Function
    - **Aortic Or Renal Artery Aneurysm**
    - **Preexisting Pulmonary And Cardiac Problems** Are Not Contraindications, Provided They Are Appropriately Addressed Both Preoperatively And Intraoperatively.

In Patients With A **History Of Cardiac Arrhythmias**,
The Shockwave Can Be Linked To Electrocardiography (ECG),
Thus Firing Only On The R Wave In The Cardiac Cycle, Coinciding With The Refractory Period Of The Cardiac Cycle Known As-'Gated Lithotripsy'.

Ganem And Carson Retrospectively Reviewed Patients Treated With **Gated And Ungated Lithotripsy**.
The Study Population Included Those With Preexisting Hypertension And Cardiac Disease And Those Taking Cardiac Medications.*

Eaton And Erturk- Patients With **Preexisting Cardiac Arrhythmias. Premature Ventricular Contractions (PVC)** Intraoperatively Had **Troponin** Measured 24 Hours Postoperatively.

Investigators Concluded That ESWL-Induced Ventricular Ectopy Was Probably Reflective Of Mechanical Stimulation Of The Myocardium Rather Than Myocardial Injury.*

However, The Authors Caution That As Rare Reports Exist Of **Myocardial Injury After ESWL**, One Should Exercise Caution When Treating Patients With Renal Stones Who May Be At Increased Risk For Cardiac Damage.*

Based On These Studies, Patients With Preexisting Cardiac Disease, Not Including Documented Preoperative Arrhythmia, Can Probably Undergo **UnGated Lithotripsy** Safely.
Close Monitoring Is Imperative As Those Who Develop Arrhythmias Can Be Safely Converted To **Gated Lithotripsy**.

Essentials Of Litho-Tripsy

- *Ganem JP, Carson CC. Cardiac arrhythmias with external fixed-rate signal generators in shock wave lithotripsy with the Medstone lithotripter. *Urology*. Apr 1998;51(4):548-52. [Medline].

- *Eaton MP, Erturk EN. Serum troponin levels are not increased in patients with ventricular arrhythmias during shock wave lithotripsy. *J Urol*. Dec 2003;170(6 Pt 1):2195-7. [Medline].

REFERENCES

1. [PDF] shock wave lithotripsy monotherapy for renal calculi - International ...www.brazjurol.com.br/.../Paterson PDF/Adobe Acrobat
RF PATERSON – 2002 JAMES E. LINGEMAN. Methodist Hospital Institute for **Kidney Stone** Disease, Indianapolis, Indiana, USA and ... endourology, as well as the **limitations** of **ESWL**, have fueled a ... number, composition and location), renal **anatomical** factors, and ...

2. **Limitations** of extracorporeal shockwave **lithotripsy** for lower caliceal ...
www.ncbi.nlm.nih.gov/.../7981732 FJ Sampaio - 1994
Limitations of extracorporeal shockwave **lithotripsy** for lower caliceal **stones:anatomic** insight. ... Department of **Anatomy**, State University of Rio de Janeiro, Brazil.... degrees formed between the lower infundibulum and the **renal** pelvis, and in ...

3. [Efficacy and **limitations** of piezoelectric extracorporeal **lithotripsy** in ...
www.ncbi.nlm.nih.gov/.../2383048   FJ Burgos - 1990
[Efficacy and **limitations** of piezoelectric extracorporeal **lithotripsy** in **kidneys** with ... in 40 **renal** units with the following **anatomic** anomalies: solitary **kidney** (10), ... **stone**fragmentation was achieved in 80% of the patients with solitary **kidney**; ...

4. Less-invasive ways to remove **stones** from the **kidneys** and ureters
www.ccjm.org/content/76/.../592.fu   MK SAMPLASKI - 2009
Each has advantages and **disadvantages**, depending on the location, size, and composition of the stone and on the patient's renal **anatomy**, body habitus, ...**Lithotripsy** is generally indicated for **renal stones** smaller than 2 cm,20 especially ...

5. **Lithotripsy** - The National **Kidney** Foundation: A to Z Health Guide
www.kidney.org/.../lithotripsy.cfm Extracorporeal shock wave **lithotripsy** is a technique for treating **stones** in the **kidney**and ... What are the advantages and **disadvantages** of this treatment? ... If **anatomical**abnormalities prevent this, other methods of **stone** removal may have to ...

6. Shock Wave **Lithotripsy** (SWL) - **Kidney Stone** Clinic
www.kidneystoneclinic.com.au/sho..
Shock wave **lithotripsy** is a technique for shattering stones such as **kidney stones** or... Check more info on SWL advantages and **disadvantages**. ... stone types, and unfavourable kidney **anatomy**; Recent concerns regarding increased long ...

7. [PDF]
Current Perspective on Adverse Effects in Shock Wave **Lithotripsy**
www.auanet.org/resources.cfm?ID..

RENAL ANATOMY
"PREDICTIVE FACTORS"/ "DETERMINANTS"
Various Parameters:
Anatomical Features (Landmarks) [32-34]

- Lower Pole Infundibulopelvic Angle (LIP): Lower Border Of Pelvis With The Medial Border Of Lower Pole Infundibulum Is Equal To Or More Than 70–90°.[30,35]

- Ureteropelvic Axis: Central Point Of Renal Pelvis And Central Point Of The Proximal Ureter.

- Diameter Of Infundibulum (IW): More Than 4–5 Mm.

- Infundibulopelvic Length (IL): < 3 Cm.

- Spatial Distribution Of Calyces, Distorted Calyces System

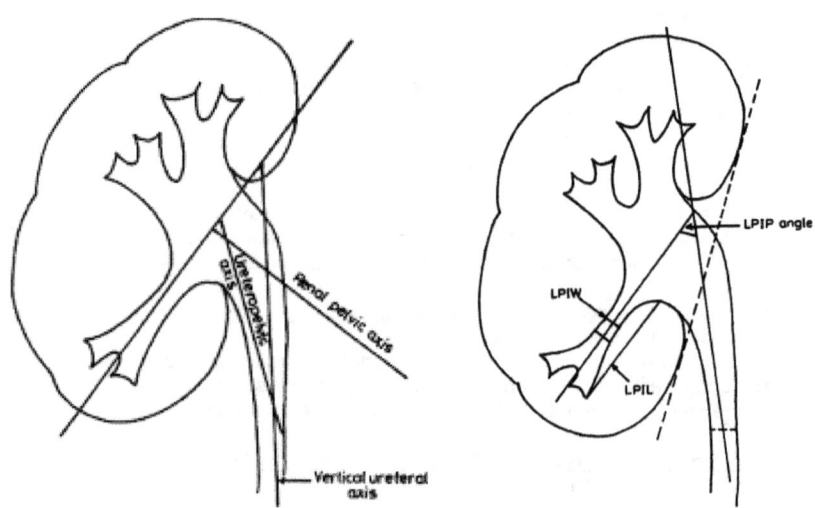

"Diagrammatic Illustrations"
(Anatomical Determinants)
Source- Medical EncyloPaedia:Wikipedia

Essentials Of Litho-Tripsy

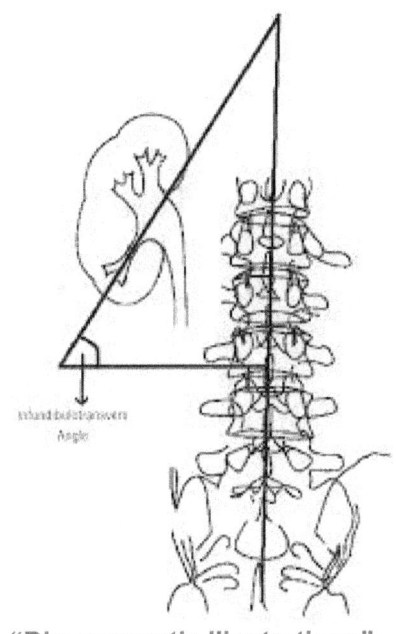

"Diagrammatic Illustrations"
(Anatomical Determinants)
Source- Medical EncyloPaedia:Wikipedia

Studies Have Delineated,
Renal Morphology Associated With Improved Stone-Free Rates,
For Example-
Lower Infundibular Length–To–Diameter Ratio Of < 7,
Lower-Pole Infundibular Diameter Of >4 Mm, Single Minor Calyx

While,Factors Associated With Decreased Stone-Free Rates
Infundibulopelvic Angle Of < 70°, An Infundibular Length Of >3 Cm,
An Infundibular Width Of < 5 Mm

The Lower Infundibulopelvic Angle (IPA) Was Measured By Two Different Methods Based Either On Measuring The Angle Between Vertical Pelvis Axis And Vertical Axis Of Lower Infundibulum Or Finding The Angle Between The Ureteropelvic Axis And Vertical Axis Of Lower Infundibulum.
40° For The IPA-Ureteropelvic Axis Method And 90° For Sampaio's Method Was Most Useful To Determine The Clearance Of Lower Pole Fragments.
The Impact of Radiological Anatomy in Clearance of Lower Calyceal Stones after Shock Wave Lithotripsy in Paediatric Patients
Corresponding author. Present address: Elçi Sokak 19/18, Y. Ayrancı, 06550, Ankara, Turkey. Fax: +90-312-2230528.
Copyright © 2002 Elsevier Science B.V. All rights reserved.

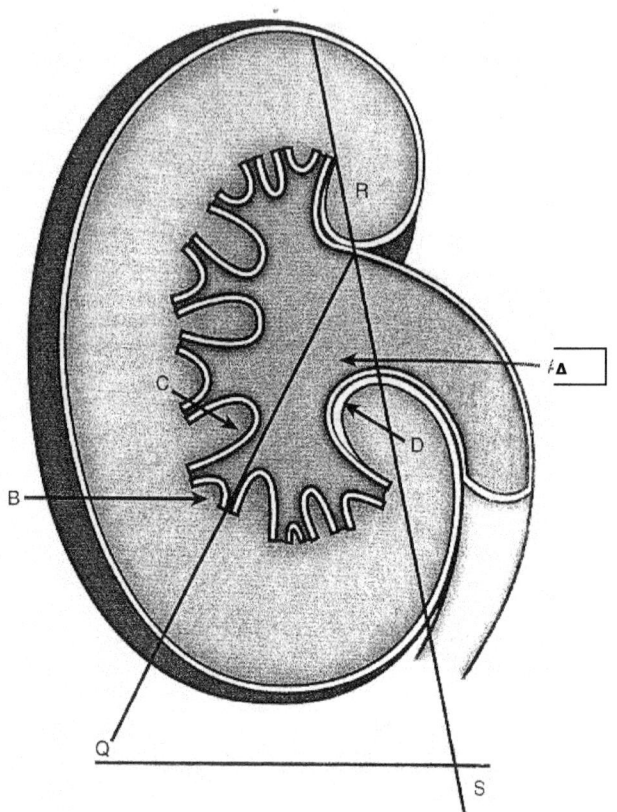

Lower Pole Anatomy MeasureMent Scheme
LPIL (Lower Pole Infundibular Length)-Measurement From A To B
LPIW (Lower Pole Infundibular Widthth)-Measurement From C To D
LPIP (Lower Pole InfundibuloPelvic) Angle-Measure QRS Angle

Source – AlBala DM, Assimos DG, ClayMan RV, et al.
Lower Pole I:A Prospective Radomized Trial Of ExtraCorporeal Shock Wave LithoTripsy & PerCutaneous NephrostoLithotomy For Lower Pole NephroLithiasis-Initial Results.
J Urol 2001;166:2072-80.

AGE RELATED CHANGES IN ESWL 'RESISTIVE-INDEX'.[31]

1. Presence Of Distal Obstructions: Obstructive Uropathy, Urolithiasis, Hydronephrosis; Poor Results Of ESWL, And Other Important Reasons For Residual Fragments,
2. Febrile Urinary Tract Obstruction,
3. Distal Calculi In Females,
4. Morbid Obesity (More Than 100 Pounds): However, The Patient Body Weight Limit For Dorniers H3 Lithotripter Is About 280 Pounds.
5. Other Associated Anatomico Functional Problems: Spinal Deformity, Limb Contractures, Etc.

REFERENCES

Limitations of extracorporeal shockwave lithotripsy for lower caliceal ...
www.ncbi.nlm.nih.gov/.../7981732
FJ Sampaio - 1994 - 94
Limitations of extracorporeal shockwave lithotripsy for lower
caliceal stones:anatomic insight. ... Department of Anatomy, State University of Rio de Janeiro, Brazil.... degrees formed between the lower infundibulum and the renal pelvis, and in ...

Current Perspective on Adverse Effects in Shock Wave Lithotripsy
www.auanet.org/resources.cfm?ID...
PDF/Adobe Acrobat
upper urinary tract calculi; that is, an aggregate stone burden of <2 cm in kidneys with normal renal anatomy. Shock wave lithotripsy is also considered an ...

Extracorporeal Shockwave Lithotripsy Treatment & Management
emedicine.medscape.com/.../44455...
22-08-2012 – The density and ability of a stone to resist ESWL is based in part on the composition of the stone. ..... not show any difference in stone-free rates based onrenal anatomy, ... Limitations of extracorporeal shock wave lithotripsy.

Bay Area Lithotripsy-Kidney Stone Treatment - Pacific Urology
www.pacificurology.com/lithotripsy
A non-invasive way to remove kidney stones Extracorporeal shock wave lithotripsy(ESWL) is a technique for treating stones in the kidney and ureter that ... What are the advantages and disadvantages of this treatment? ... If anatomical abnormalities prevent this, other methods of stone removal may have to be considered.

Sabnis RB, Naik K, Patel SH, Desai MR, Bapat SD. Extracorporeal shock wave lithotripsy for lower caliceal stones: Can clearance be predicted? Br J Urol 1997;80:853-7.

Sampaio FI, Aragao AH. Inferior pole collecting system anatomy:Its probable role in extracorporeal shock wave lithotripsy. J Urol 1992:147:322-4.

Sampaio FI, Aragao AH. Limitations of extracorporeal shockwaves lithotripsy for lower calyceal stones: Anatomic insight. J Endourol 1994;8:241-7.

Keeley FX Jr, Moussa SA, Smith G, Tolley DA. Clearance of lower-pole stones following shock wave lithotripsy: Effect of the infundibulopelvic angle. Eur Urol 1999;36:371-5.

Knapp R, Frauscher F, Helweg G, zur Nedden D, Strasser H, Janetschek G, et al. Age-related changes in resistive index following extracorporeal shock wave lithotripsy. J Urol 1995;154:955-8.

Sampaio FJ, d'anunciacao AL, Silva EC. Comparative follow-up of patients with acute and obtuse infundibulum-pelvic angle subjected to extracorporeal shock wave lithotripsy for lower calyceal stones: Preliminary report and proposed study design. J Endourol 1997;11:157- 61.

ESWL: COMPLICATIONS
A. RENAL COMPLICATIONS

There Are (4) Potential Renal &UrinaryTract Complications Of ESWL:

(i.) Incomplete Stone Fragmentation, Formation And Passage Of Lithiasic Fragments, May Lead To Urinary Tract Obstruction
(ii.) Renal Parenchymal Injury, The Effects On Kidney Function, A Decline In Glomerular Filtration Rate
(iii.) Infective Complications
(iv.) An Elevation In Blood Pressure

(i.)INCOMPLETE STONE FRAGMENTATION

Complications Related to the Formation and Passage of Lithiasic Fragments — The Main Aim Of SWL Is The **Pulverisation Of Stones And Asymptomatic Elimination Of Fragments.**.
This Procedure **May Not Always Be Completely Successful Due To Incomplete Fragmentation**, With Residual Fragments Of A Significant Size, And **Ureteral Blockage By Fragments (Steinstrasse)** Which Ends Up With An Obstruction To The Urinary Flow.

The Ureteral Obstruction Rates, When ESWL Was Used To Treat Single Stones ≤2 Cm In Diameter Was 2.1 Percent For Kidney And Upper Ureteral Stones And 2.1 Percent For Middle And Lower Ureteral Stones At Three Months [3]. The Incidence Of Ureteral Obstruction Varies With The Type Of Machine And The Number Of Shocks.

Clinically Insignificant Residual Fragments(CISF): Are Diagnosed By USG, Radiology, Nephrotomography, Nephroscopy,CT Scan, Etc. They Are Important Contributory Factors For Recurrence By Providing 'Nidus' For Future Stone Formation And Should Be Avoided By Proper Procedural & Supportive Techniques.
Necessary Management Is Achieved By Available Medical Therapy Regimes, With Ingredient-Specific Medications (Role Of Specific Alkalizers), Diet Regulations Etc.[41-43] Routine Urine Test For Crystalluria, Sediments, And Casts Provides Useful Index Besides Various Metabolic Evaluators.

Factors Responsible For The Level Of Fragmentation After A Lithotripsy, And Therefore Real Risk Factors For SWL Failure Are –

1.Stone Composition - The Stones Made By **Struvite, Uric Acid & Dehydrated Calcium Oxalate** Tend To **Fragment Into Tiny Parts** That May Be Easily Passed.

Essentials Of Litho-Tripsy

While, **Dehydrated Calcium Phosphate Stones (Brushite) And Monohydrate Calcium Oxalate Stones** Tend To **Produce Larger Fragments** Which Are Hence Much Harder To Pass.
Cystine Stones Are Particularly Difficult To Treat,
As Like Other Organic Compound, Has Acoustic Features Similar To Those In The Surrounding Tissues.

2. Volume - SWL Treatment Success Is Related To **'Stones Volume'**.
Better "Stone Free Rate" For Stones <2 Cm, Decrease With Increase Of Stone Size & Further Again For Staghorn Stones
Besides 'Stone Burden', **Stone Composing Ingredients** Is Important Determinant Factor.

3. Number And Site - All Other Characteristics Being Same,
For **Lower Pole Kidney Stones**, The Success Rates Are Less,
Often Requiring Multiple Treatments For Clearance.
Multiple Stones Management,
Recorded Larger Number Of Relapses After SWL
For **Ureteral Stones**, Overall Success Rates Are Not As High In Absolute Terms And Depends Primarily, On The Segment Of Stone Location:
Proximal Ureter 82%, Medial Ureter 73%, And Distal Ureter 74%

4. Frequency and Strength of Shock Wave - Although The Effects Of Shock Wave Frequency On The Efficacy Of The Treatment Were Not Clinically Widely Evaluated
In Vitro Studies Demostrated, **A Reduction In Frequency Improves The Possibility Of Fragmentation** &
Increased Voltage Supplied, Results InTo A **Reduction In Lesser Volume Fragments**.

Comparative Results For Different Energy Font Used:
ElectrohydraulicLithotripsy Supplied Fragments <2 Mm In 91% Cases,
While **An Electromagnetic** In Only 65% Of The Cases.
For **Different Models Of Same Energy Font**, Success Rates Range Of 63% - 83% Were Recorded, (1-15)

'Steinstrasse'(Street Of Stone), Is Directly Related Complication To Incomplete Fragmentation, With Variable Incidence Rate Due To MutiFactorial Causes
The Incidence Of Accumulation Of Stone Fragments Obstructing Ureter After ESWL Being 2–10%,
Large Stone Burden Staghorn Calculii, Bilateral ESWL, Pre-Existing Ureteral Obstruction Are Known Risk Factors.

Diagnosed By Radiology, Nephrotomography, USG, CT scan Etc .
A Radiological Or Ultrasound Examination Should Be Carried Out Routinely 4–6 Weeks After The SWL Treatment.

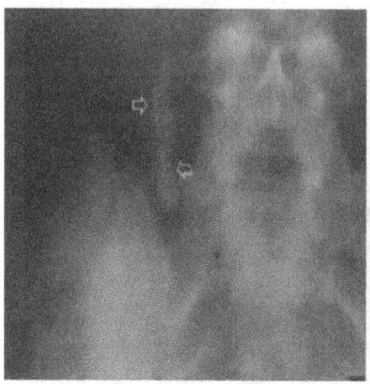 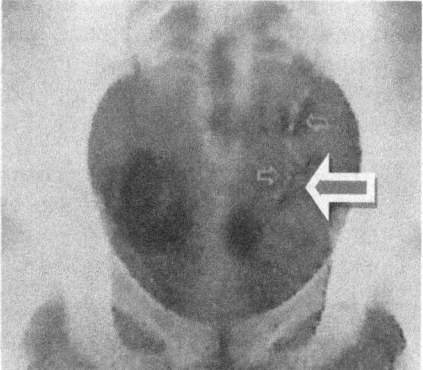

<u>Stone particles passage Rt. Mid ureter
Depicting Stone Particles Passage In Lower Ureter
Phenomenon Known As "Stone/ Steine Strasse"</u>

Role Of Ureteral Stenting

<u>Pre-ESWL Ureteral Stenting Significantly Decreases But
Do Not Eliminate Steinstrasse (Controversial Reports)</u>.
Amongst Differently Available Ureteral Stenting Devices,
"DJS"Is Commonly In Use.

With AvailAble **Modern Efficient LithoTriptors**,
Adequately Powered And Frequency (Time Spaced),
Shock Delivery With Discrete Coherence Upon Stone
Throughout The Procedure Being Key To Success.
As Minutely Shattered Stone Particles Passing With Urine
Spontaneously,Thus, Avoiding Obstructive Complications
And Hence Minimizing The Need Of **'Ureteral Stenting'**
(Various Availables)Including **Double J Stent** Insertion,
Besides Exclusion And/Or Management Need For Pre-Existing Illnesses.

However, In Large, Hyperdensity Stones, Double J Stenting
May Be Of Great Importance Preventing Obstructive Processes Like
"Stone/Steine Strasse."

Indications Include:
(1) Obstructive Uropathy Of Cosiderable Duration
(2) Associated Infection
(3) DTPA Renal Scan, With/Without Diuresis Or Other Indices,
    Revealing Decreased Renal Function.

Essentials Of Litho-Tripsy

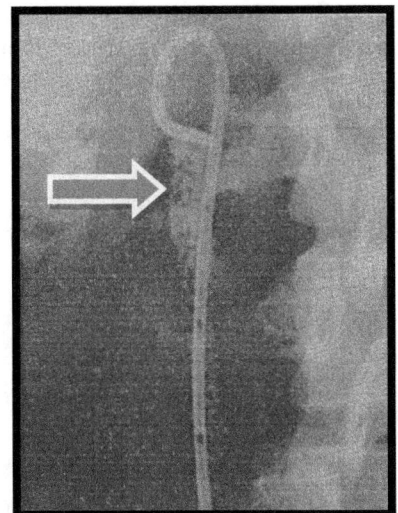

Complex Proximal Stein-A-Strasse

Other SideEffects/Complications Of 'Ureteral Stenting':

1.Stent Symptoms; LUTS, UTI, Pain,Urgency,Dysuria,Haematuria, Back Pain Etc.
>80% Patients Experience- Stent Related Pain Affecting Daily Activities, 32% Patients Report Sexual Dysfunction, 58% Patients Complains Reduce Work Capacity(Joshi et al.2003).
Pathophysiolgy Of StentSymptoms Has Not Been Clearly Elucidated, But According To The Common Belief, The Adverse Stent Symptoms Are Induced By Urinary Bladder Mucosal Irritation By The Distal End Of Stent, Smooth Muscle Spasm & Urinary Reflux Leading To Flank Pain (Haleblian et al.2008).
The Anatomic Postion Of The Stent Curl, If Located In A Calyx or If Crosses The MidLine Of UriNary Bladder, Is Reported To Lead To Increased Stent Symptoms(EJ Nahas et al.2006)
Incomplete Distal Curl Also Increase Stent Symptoms(Rane & Colleagues,2001).
Stent Composition DoesNot Effect Stent Symptoms, With Presently Available Stent Materials(Pryot Et Al 1991).
Pharmacological Approaches-Oral AntiCholinergics, Phenazopyridine,& Standard Analgesic Medications Are Use(Nottis et al.2008).
IntraVesical Instillation Of Ketorlac Or OxyButynin For Pain Decrease After Stent Insertion(Beiko et al.2004)
The Use Of **Alpha$_1$ AdrenoReceptor Blockers**(Tamsulosin & Afuzosin), Are Beneficial For Stent Symptoms & Pain
(Deliveliotis et al.2006,Damiano et al. 2008).

2. Other Complications-Incorrect Placement, Migration, Stent Blockage, Encrustations, Forgotten Stent Etc, Are Not Very Uncommon & Are **Managed By** Radio-Diagnostic Assessment Guidance, Utilizing Different Endo-UrologyTechniques e.g.
SWL & PNL For Proximal Stone Burden & Encrustations, While For Distal Stent Ecrustations, Cysto-Lithoclast & Urteo-Renoscopy Are Emplyed. Eno-Urology Treatment In Single or Multiple Stages, Is SuccessFul In Removing Up To 85%-97% Of The Stents(Bultitude Et Al.2003:Gonzalez RamiRez et al.2009).
Chemolysis(Sulby Solution Or HemiAcridin),As An AlterNative To Invasive TreatMent For Stent Encrustations, Should Be Reserved As Last Resort Doe To Its Irritating Effects On Urinary Tract & Potential Electrolyte Imbalance On Systemic Absorption(Vanderbrink & Colleagues,2008).

SteinStrasse Management

Spontaneous Stone Clearance Occurs In 60–80% Cases.
Necessary Management Is Achieved By-

- Available Medical Therapy Regimes With Ingredient-Specific Medications (Role Of Specific Alkalizers).
- Increased Fluids InTake With Forced Diuresis(Lasix Therapy).
- Suitable Pain Control Therapy(An Round The Clock Coverage By An Approriate Combination Of Analgesia & Spasmolytics)
- Diet Regulations Etc.
- Routine Urine Test For Crystalluria, Sediments, And Casts Provides Useful Index Besides Various Metabolic Evaluators.
- Specific Medical Treatment Comprising-
  Alpha-Blockers, Bladder Out Flow Obstruction Releivers (Tamsulosin 0.4 Mgm OD & Finasteride(10)Mgm Or DutaSteride(2)Mgm OD Alone Or In Combination, Preferably With BreakFast)
  Corticosteroids(DeflazaCort), Nifedipine Etc.
  May Accelerate The Clearance Of Fragments. With Symptoms & Steinstrasse No Longer Than 2.5 Cm.

- **ESWL Aimed For Fragmentation Of Steinstrasse** Has A High Success Rate With Minimal Complications.
  Especially Where Larger Distal Fragments Are Present, Steinstrasse Has Effectively Been Treated With Repeated Sessions Of SWL Showing Positive Results In 90% Of Cases.
  With **Ureteral Meatotomy** Results Have Also Been Satisfactory.

Failure To Resolve Within 3–4 Weeks Time & Recurrent Colics, **With Special Indications** Like Bilateral Obstruction, Solitary Kidney, Severe Refractory Pain Or Infected Hydronephrosis,

Necessitates Intervention Aiming **Prompt Urinary Track Decompression**, By Ureteral Stenting, URS (Retrograde Or Anterograde Percutaneous Ureterorenoscopy) Management Including Basket Extraction Of Stone Particles Etc.
Renal Function Maintainence ThroughOut The Course Is Ensured.
Ultimately With Severe Infections And Complete Obstructions **Nephrostomy Tube Drainage**, Becomes The Tt Of Choice.

(ii.) <u>INFECTIVE COMPLICATIONS</u>

During Extracorporeal Lithotripsy, One Of The Forces Applied To The Stone Comes From **Cavitation Bubble Collapse**. This Force, However, May Cause Damage To The Small Renal Vessels That Would Result In **Microhaemorrhage**, The Release Of **Cell Mediator Of Phlogosis** & The **Infiltration By Inflammatory Response Cells**.
These Tiny Lesions May Also Allow The Passage Of Bacteria, Present In The Urine Or Inside The Stones Themselves, Into The Blood Stream Leading To Other Related Problems.

"**Infection**" Is Harmful Colonization Of A Species Unknown To The Host Organism That Responds To The Infection With Inflammation.
"**Sepsis**" Refers To A Serious Medical Condition, Characterised By Generalised State Of Inflammation, Called **SIRS (Systematic Inflammatory Response Syndrome)**, And By The Definite Or Suspected Presence Of An Infection.

Bacteriuria Evidence Is Present In Up To 23.5% Of Patients.
While A Real Clinical Urinary Infection Is More Frequently Observed In Patients With Either Multiple Or Complex Struvite Stones.

Bacteremia Is Less Common, Developing In Up To 14% Of Patients, With Fewer Than 1% Developing Clinical Sepsis (Although This Number Increases To 2.7% In Patients With Staghorn Calculi).

Sepsis Development After Bacteremia Is Relatively Low In Absolute Terms, <1% Of Cases, Although It Is Considerably Higher In The Presence Of Staghorn Stones
The Risk Of Infection Is Naturally Greater, Where Urinoculture Is Positive Or Where Urinary Obstruction Exists.

There Are No Truly Trustworthy Signs Attesting To The Early Onset Of Bacteremia Or Bacteriuria: White Cells Blood Count, Speed Of Erythrosedimentation, And A Positive Culture Are All Useful Signs, **Unfortunately They Generally Tend To Show Up Positive When The Patient Is Already Symptomatic.**

For Infective Complications Reduction & OverAll Cost EffectiveNess Of Involved Treatment,
Antibiotic Prophylaxis Use Is Proposed, But Has Not Been Confirmed In Other Randomised Controlled Studies For Patients Without Preexisting UTI Or Infected Stones. To Sum Up,
Antibiotics Should Only Be Administered To Patients With Positive Urine Culture, With Staghorn Or Low Density Struvite Stones, With A History Of Struvite Stones Or Recurring Urinary Infections, To Patients Who Will Undergo A Contemporary Instrumental Procedure, And Finally To Those With A Nephrostomy Or A Stent In Place.

The Present Discussed Study Concludes That,
Proper Management With Broad-Spectrum/Specific Antibiotics (C And S), Along With Spasmolytics, Analgesics Etc, Is Recommended,
Especially In Obstructive Uropathy, Infected Stone Nidus Cases,
In Consideration With OverAll Infection Rate, Bacterial Flora Status
Of The Involved InfraStructure, Appliances & ManPower.

Incomplete Stone Fragmentation Being The Most Important
Factor For The Failure Rate & Consequent Infection,
Can Be Prevented By Appropriate Discrete Shock Delivery In Patient Compliance, With Proper AntiBiotic Coverage,
In Appropriate Doseage & Duration.

(iii.) <u>EFFECTS ON KIDNEY</u> The Most Evident Expression Of Kidney Trauma Is **Haematuria** That Generally Passes In A Few Days.
Collections Of Symptomatic Fluids Or Perirenal, Subcapsular,
Or Intrarenal Haematomas Are Rare And Occur In >1% Of Patients.
If, However, Patients Have Systematically Undergone A CT Scan Or MRI
Then Evidence Of Haematoma Rises To 25%
Other Lesions Show In X-Rays In Most Patients: **An Increase In Kidney Volume**, A **Loss In Corticomedullary Demarcations** [30], And A **Reduction In The Signal In The PeriRenal Fat**.
These Signs Express Lesions Such As **Haemorrhages, Generally Focalised, And Oedema Within And Around The Kidney** [31].

Perirenal Collections Typically Disappear After A Few Days,
While A Period Of Between 6 Weeks And 6 Months Is Required For **Subcapsular Lesions**. It Is Rare To See Lesions For Any Longer Than That.

<u>**Characteristic Evidences On Microscopic Examination:**</u>
Haemorrhagic Lesions Are Preferentially Localised In The
Corticomedullary Joint, Probably Due To Differences In The Density Of The Tissue At That Level [33];

Moreover, Signs Of Damage Are Immediately Visible From The Thin **Vascular Walls And The Glomeruli** [34].
Haemorrhage Leads To Tissue Hypoxia, Which Can Play A Role In The Development Of **Apoptosis**, But It Has Been Experimentally Shown That Shock Waves Administration Does Not Affect The **Apoptosis Index** In Normal Rats After 2000 And 4000 Shock Waves [35] And After 1-2 Weeks Signs Of Reorganisation May Be Noticed, While After 1 Month Signs Of **Glomerular Atrophy And Sclerosis** Are Noticeable In Tiny Areas Of **Fibrosis**. However, Most Of The Parenchyma Appears Normal [32], **Leading To The Conclusion That Damage Due To SWL** Is A Focal Process That Leaves Most Of The Parenchyma Intact.
A Short Pretreatment With 10–20 Shockwaves Could Further On Reduce The Renal Tissue Damage, Probably Due To
Reflex Local Vasoconstriction.
Renal Atrophy, Although Uncommon, Can Result From Renal Vascular Or Severe Atherosclerotic Disease. Patients With Underlying Renal Parenchymal Disease Are At A Higher Risk Of Renal Atrophy. However, Studies Of ESWL In Patients With A Solitary Kidney Have Shown No **Statistical Evidence Of Renal Function Deterioration Secondary To Shockwave Lithotripsy**.

Renal Complications, Thus Can Be Summarized As Below-
1.Haemorrhage:
Post-Lithotripsy Hematuria: Varying Severity And Duration, Usually Controlled By Medical Therapy, Including Hemostats, e.g., Tranexamic Acid Up To 2 – 4 Gm/Day Doses,
Have Shown Very Good Result Besides Other Supportive Measures Including Cause Evaluation And Management.
2.Hemorrhage And Edema: Peri-Renal, subcapsular, and Intra-Parenchymal Of Varying Severity.
Need Increased Caution In Bleeding—Diasthesis, Hemophilia, Polycystic (Autosomal Dominant) Kidney Disease, Hydronephrosis Etc.
3.Histological Damage: Acute/Chronic Renal Injury: Structural/ Functional Changes, AC. & Chr. Histologic Changes,Extent Of Renal Trauma & Other Associated Factors.Various Studies,
Variable Results Are Available.
ESWL Is Recognized As A Form Of Trauma Similar To Renal Contusions With Occasional Resultant Adverse Sequelae.
In The Absence Of Human Error,The Latest Sophisticated Versions Of Lithotripters, Especially Dornier's Lithotripter, Renal Injury And Other Adverse Bio-Effects Are Negligibly Minimal In Normal Individuals.
HowEver, Longterm Adversre Effect Study,
Is Not Available For Justification. (16-25)

(iv.) CARDIOVASCULAR APPARATUS EFFECTS
The **Incidence Of Arrhythmia** During An SWL Varies From Between 11% And 59%, And Is, In General, Related To Minor Premature Ventricular Beats. Evidence Of **Ischemic Lesions** Is Very Rare, And This **Incidence May Be Further Reduced By Synchronising The Supply Of Shock Waves With Pulsations**.

There Is **No Documented Relationship Between The Onset Of Arrhythmia** And Age, Sex, Cardiopathy, Site, Volume Of The Stone, Onsite Stent Or Nephrostomy, With Or Without Anaesthesia, The Number Of Shock Waves, And The Type Of Lithotripter.

Even Those **Patients With Pace Makers** May Undergo An SWL With Necessary Precautions And Cardiological Supervision.

Although Clinical And Experimental Data Indicates That Patients With **Aortic Or Renal Aneurisms** May Be Treated Successfully, Literature Has Reported Some Cases Of Breakage After An SWL.

It Is Clear, As In Other Similar Cases, That A Careful Examination Of The Cost/Benefit Relationship Is Necessary And That Where The Procedure Is Embarked Upon Each And Every Possible Development Must Be Considered Beforehand.
Cases Of **Serious Venous Thrombosis** After SWL Have Also Been Recorded, The Exact Pathogenesis Of Which Is Still Badly Defined; However, It Is Probably Caused By Haematological Disorders, Even If This May Just Be To A Small Extent.

The Association Between SWL And Arterial Hypertension Has Always Been A Controversial Argument And Debated.
The Diagnosis Of Hypertension After SWL Has Been Reported In 8% Of Cases, That Does Not Differ Greatly However From The Incidence Of About 6% Of New Diagnosis In The Overall Population.
An Increase In Diastolic Pressure After An SWL Was Also Noted, And A Relationship Between This And The Number Of Shock Waves Was Therefore Hypothesised Upon,
A Large Retrospective Study Has Analysed Patients Who Underwent An SWL, Controlled Against Patients Who Underwent An Ureterorenoscopy Or A Percutaneous Lithotripsy Without Being Able To Show, Within One Year Of The Treatment, Any Significant Differences In The Incidence Of Hypertension (2.4% Versus 4%), And Even After 4 Years, The Differences Were Not Particularly Significant (2.1% Versus 1.6%); However, A Statistically Significant Increase In Diastolic Pressure Showed Up After SWL.
The Real Causes Of Hypertension After SWL Are More Likely To Have Many Different Factors, And There Is No Clear Evidence Whether There Is

Essentials Of Litho-Tripsy

Any **Direct Relationship Between Hypertension And The Procedure**. Even If One Considers More Recent Studies That Have Demonstrated, With A Followup Of 24 Months, How It Is The **Presence Of Stones Rather Than The Modality Of Treatment That Determines The Increase In Pressure**.
Many Of The Studies That Have Been Documented Are Retrospective. Limiting Oneself To Randomly Controlled Studies There Is No Evidence That SWL Treatment Determines Changes In Arterial Pressure
In Fact, It Is Possible That The **Extracorporeal Lithotripsy Is Responsible For Hypotension**, And Likewise For Alterations In Renal Metabolism Determined By The Treatment And Function Of The Number And Strength Of Shock Waves Administered.

There Is Variable Evidence That ESWL Results In Hypertension. However, Studies Reveal That With Successful Management Of Stone Disease, The **Pre-Existing Hypertension (? Cause) Management** Needs Comparatively Less Or To The Extent Of No Medication.

Studies For **Resistive Index, Renovascular Status** (Altered Plasma Flow Intra Renal Blood Flow Changes), Blockage By Aminophylline, Nifedipine, And Allopurinol Have Been Reported.
Regarding **Plasma Renin Activity Phenomenon** And Other Factors, Various Study Reports Are Available.

(v.) GASTROINTESTINAL APPARATUS EFFECTS
Several Gastrointestinal Lesions Of Various Types Have Repeatedly Been Recorded Following An SWL With A Global Incidence Of 1.8%.

A Specific Study Has Shown **Gastroduodenal Erosions** In 80% Of Patients Who Underwent A Pre- And Post-SWL Endoscopic Study.
The Exact Mechanism Of The Lesions Is, As Of Yet, Unknown, However, The Majority Were Observed In Patients Subjected To Treatment In **Prone Position** And In Patients Who Had Undergone A Number Of Shock Waves That Exceeds What Is Recommended.

(vi.) FERTILITY AND PREGNANCY
A Sufficiently High Amount Of Clinical And Experimental Evidence Exists To **Exclude Any Permanent Effects On Testicular Or Ovarian Function** To Thus Confirm That There Are No Existing **Correlations Between SWL And Fertility**
Pregnancy, However, Constitutes An Absolute Contraindication To The Procedure Itself Because Of Any Potentially Harmful Effects To The Foetus From Shock Waves, As Has Repeatedly Been Shown In The Results Of Many Experimental Studies.

(vii) MEDICAL COMPLICATIONS

Hypertension Is An Unusual Complication Of ESWL But May Occur As A Sequelae Of A Large Perinephric Hematoma (Ie, Page Kidney).
Older Patients Who Undergo ESWL May Have A Slightly Higher Likelihood Of Eventually **Developing Hypertension And Diabetes** Than Patients Who Undergo Other Therapies For Stone Removal,

Krambeck Et Al. 2006 Study, Retrospectively Identified 630 Patients Who Were Treated With ESWL 19 Years Prior, And Queried Them Regarding Development Of Hypertension And Diabetes Mellitus. Compared With A Control Group Treated Conservatively For Nephrolithiasis At The Same Time,
Diabetes And Hypertension Were More Common, A Finding That Persisted In Multivariate Analysis When BMI Was Controlled For. Authors Suggested **Pancreatic Islet Cells Injury By The Shock Waves** As An Explanation For This Observation.

Wendt-Nordahl Et Al Measured **Pancreatic Enzymes Post-ESWL** In Patients Treated For Proximal Ureteral And Renal Stones To Evaluate For **Acute Pancreatic Injury**.
The Control Group Consisted Of Patients Treated With ESWL For Lower Ureteral Stones And No Difference Was Demonstrated Between The 2 Groups.
Thus Concluding That The Hypothesis That ESWL Causes Acute Trauma To Pancreatic Islet Cells, Leading To An Endocrine Insufficiency Resulting In DM, Therefore Seems Unlikely.

Makhlouf Et Al Examined A Cohort Of Almost 2000 Patients Who Underwent ESWL Between 1999 And 2002.
The Control Group Consisted Of Matched Individuals From A National Database. At 6 Years Of Follow-Up,
The Number Of Patients In The Study Group And The Control Group Who Had **Developed DM** Were The Same.

Based On These Studies, The Relationship Between ESWL And The Development Of Diabetes, Remains Unclear. One Of The Criticisms Of Krambeck Et Al Is That The Study Patients Were Treated With **First Generation Lithotripters**, With Significantly Wider Focal Areas Than Current Lithotripters.
On The Other Hand, This Study Was Based On 19 Years Of Follow-Up While Antoine Et Al Only Reported On 6 Years Of Follow-Up. Further Studies Are Necessary To Elaborate This Relationship.

(26-38)

(vii) OTHER POSSIBLE COMPLICATIONS
Less-Common Complications May Include-
(1) **Pulmonary Contusion**
(2) **Pancreatitis**
(3) **Splenic Hematoma**
(4) **Elevated Liver Functions (Transient)**
(5) **Biliary Colic With Inadvertent Fragmentation Of Adjacent Biliary Stones.**

Extrarenal Tissue Injuries:
Liver, Skeletal Muscles Trauma, Evident By Serum Bilirubin, Lactic Dehydrogenase, Glutamic Transaminase & Creatinine Phosphokinase.
Upper GIT; Gastric, Duodenal Erosion,
Most Common Extra-Renal Complication
Pancreatitis Single Case In 6800 Cases, **AcuteFatal Pancreatitis**, Lithotripsy For Renal Calculi, BJU International (2001) Reported.
People Who Had Undergone ESWL, Compared With Age And Gender-Matched People Who Had Undergone Nonsurgical Treatment.
Whether Or Not Acute Trauma Progresses To Long-Term Effects Probably Depends On Multiple Factors That Include The Shock Wave Dose (i.e., The Number Of Shock Waves Delivered, Rate Of Delivery, Power Setting, Acoustic Characteristics Of The Particular Lithotriptor, And Frequency Of Retreatment),
As Well As Certain Intrinsic Predisposing Pathophysiologic Risk

Factors. **To Address These Concerns**, The American Urological Association Established The **Shock Wave Lithotripsy Task Force** To Provide An **Expert Opinion** On The Safety And Risk-Benefit Ratio Of ESWL. The Task Force Published A White Paper Outlining Their Conclusions In **2009**. They **Concluded The Risk-Benefit Ratio Remains Favorable For Many People**.
The Advantages Of ESWL Include Its Noninvasive Nature,
The Fact That It Is Technically Easy To Treat Most Upper Urinary Tract Calculi, And That, At Least Acutely, It Is A Well-Tolerated, Low-Morbidity Treatment For The Vast Majority Of People.
However, They **Recommended Slowing The Shock Wave Firing Rate From 120 Pulses Per Minute To 60 Pulses Per Minute** To Reduce The Risk Of Renal Injury And Increase The Degree Of Stone Fragmentation.

Shock Wave Lithotripsy Task Force (2009). "Current Perspective on Adverse Effects in Shock Wave Lithotripsy". *Clinical Guidelines*. Linthicum, Maryland: American Urological Association. Retrieved 2011-07-27.

References

1. C. Chaussy, E. Schmiedt, and J. Schuller, "Extracorporeal shock-wave lithotripsy (ESWL) for treatment of urolithiasis," Urology, vol. 23, no. 5, pp. 59–66, 1984.
2. C. Türk, T. Knoll, A. Petrik, et al., "Guidelines on Urolithiasis," European Association of Urology, pp. 6–106, 2010.
3. S. B. Streem, A. Yost, and E. Mascha, "Clinical implications of clinically insignificant stone fragments after extracorporeal shock wave lithotripsy," The Journal of Urology, vol. 155, no. 4, pp. 1186–1190, 1996. View at Publisher · View at Google Scholar · View at Scopus
4. T. Egilmez, M. I. Tekin, M. Gonen, F. Kilinc, R. Goren, and H. Ozkardes, "Efficacy and safety of a new-generation shockwave lithotripsy machine in the treatment of single renal or ureteral stones: experience with 2670 patients," Journal of Endourology, vol. 21, no. 1, pp. 23–27, 2007. View at Publisher · View at Google Scholar · View at PubMed · View at Scopus
5. J. E. Lingeman, T. A. Coury, D. M. Newman et al., "Comparison of results and morbidity of percutaneous nephrolithotomy and extracorporeal shock wave lithotripsy," The Journal of Urology, vol. 138, no. 3, pp. 485–490, 1987. View at Scopus
6. J. Graff, W. Diederichs, and H. Schulze, "Long-term followup in 1,003 extracorporeal shock wave lithotripsy patients," The Journal of Urology, vol. 140, no. 3, pp. 479–483, 1988. View at Scopus
7. J. E. Lingeman, "Prospective randomized trial of extracorporeal shock wave lithotripsy and percutaneous nephrostolithotomy for lower pole nephrolithiasis: initial long-term follow up," Journal of Endourology, vol. 11, article 95, 1997.
8. A. P. Evan and J. A. McAteer, "Q-effects of shock-wave lithotripsy," in Kidney Stones: Medical and Surgical Management, F. L. Coe, M. J. Favus, C. Y. C. Pak, J. H. Parks, and G. M. Preminger, Eds., pp. 549–570, Lippincott-Raven, Philadelphia, Pa, USA, 1996.
9. K. Madbouly, A. M. El-Tiraifi, M. Seida, S. R. El-Faqih, R. Atassi, and R. F. Talic, "Slow versus fast shock wave lithotripsy rate for urolithiasis: a prospective randomized study," The Journal of Urology, vol. 173, no. 1, pp. 127–130, 2005. View at Publisher · View at Google Scholar · View at PubMed · View at Scopus
10. A. Greenstein and H. Matzkin, "Does the rate of extracorporeal shock wave delivery affect stone fragmentation?" Urology, vol. 54, no. 3, pp. 430–432, 1999. View at Publisher · View at Google Scholar · View at Scopus
11. Y. Zhou, F. H. Cocks, G. M. Preminger, and P. Zhong, "The effect of treatment strategy on stone comminution efficiency in shock wave lithotripsy," The Journal of Urology, vol. 172, no. 1, pp. 349–354, 2004. View at Scopus
12. S. F. Graber, H. Danuser, W. W. Hochreiter, and U. E. Studer, "A prospective randomized trial comparing 2 lithotriptors for stone disintegration and induced renal trauma," The Journal of Urology, vol. 169, no. 1, pp. 54–57, 2003. View at Scopus
13. A. J. Portis, Y. Yan, J. G. Pattaras, C. Andreoni, R. Moore, and R. V. Clayman, "Matched pair analysis of shock wave lithotripsy effectiveness for comparison of lithotriptors," The Journal of Urology, vol. 169, no. 1, pp. 58–62, 2003. View at Scopus
14. C. F. Ng, L. McLornan, T. J. Thompson, and D. A. Tolley, "Comparison of 2 generations of piezoelectric lithotriptors using matched pair analysis," The Journal of Urology, vol. 172, no. 5, pp. 1887–1891, 2004.View at Publisher · View at Google Scholar · View at Scopus
15. A. F. Bierkens, A. J. M. Hendrikx, W. A. J. G. Lemmens, and F. M. J. Debruyne, "Extracorporeal shock wave lithotripsy for large renal calculi: the role of ureteral stents. A randomized trial," The Journal of Urology, vol. 145, no. 4, pp. 699–702, 1991. View at Scopus
16. M. P. Wirth, M. Theiss, and H. G. W. Frohmuller, "Primary extracorporeal shock wave lithotripsy of staghorn renal calculi," Urologia Internationalis, vol. 48, no. 1, pp. 71–75, 1992. View at Scopus
17. J. L. Weinerth, J. A. Flatt, and C. C. Carson, "Lessons learned in patients with large steinstrasse," The Journal of Urology, vol. 142, no. 6, pp. 1425–1427, 1989. View at Scopus
18. V. Naja, M. M. Agarwal, A. K. Mandal et al., "Tamsulosin facilitates earlier clearance of stone fragments and reduces pain after shockwave lithotripsy for renal calculi; results from an open-label randomized study," Urology, vol. 72, no. 5, pp. 1006–1011, 2008. View at Publisher · View at Google Scholar · View at PubMed · View at Scopus
19. 19.S. K. Bhagat, N. K. Chacko, N. S. Kekre, G. Gopalakrishnan, B. Antonisamy, and A. Devasia, "Is there a role for tamsulosin in shock wave lithotripsy for renal and ureteral

calculi?" The Journal of Urology, vol. 177, no. 6, pp. 2185–2188, 2007. View at Publisher · View at Google Scholar · View at PubMed · View at Scopus

20. M. Sigman, V. Laudone, and A. D. Jenkins, "Ureteral meatotomy as a treatment of Steinstrasse following extracorporeal shock wave lithotripsy," Journal of Endourology, vol. 2, article 41, 1988.

21. M. M. Levy, M. P. Fink, J. C. Marshall et al., "2001 SCCM/ESICM/ACCP/ATS/SIS international sepsis definitions conference," Critical Care Medicine, vol. 31, no. 4, pp. 1250–1256, 2003. View at Publisher ·View at Google Scholar · View at PubMed · View at Scopus

22. V. G. O. Müller-Mattheis, D. Schmale, M. Seewald, H. Rosin, and R. Ackermann, "Bacteremia during extracorporeal shock wave lithotripsy of renal calculi," The Journal of Urology, vol. 146, no. 3, pp. 733–736, 1991. View at Scopus

23. C. Dincel, E. Ozdiler, H. Ozenci, N. Tazici, and A. Kosar, "Incidence of urinary tract infection in patients without bacteriuria undergoing SWL: comparison of stone types," Journal of Endourology, vol. 12, pp. 1–3, 1988.

24. A. F. Bierkens, A. J. M. Hendrikx, K. Ezz El Din et al., "The value of antibiotic prophylaxis during extracorporeal shock wave lithotripsy in the prevention of urinary tract infections in patients with urine proven sterile prior to treatment," European Urology, vol. 31, no. 1, pp. 30–35, 1997. View at Scopus

25. N. B. Dhar, J. Thornton, M. T. Karafa, and S. B. Streem, "A multivariate analysis of risk factors associated with subcapsular hematoma formation following electromagnetic shock wave lithotripsy,"The Journal of Urology, vol. 172, no. 6, pp. 2271–2274, 2004. View at Publisher · View at Google Scholar ·View at Scopus

26. R. B. Dyer, N. Karstaedt, and D. L. McCullough, "Magnetic Resonance imaging evaluation of immediate and intermediate changes in kidney treated with extracorporeal shock wave lithotripsy," in Shock Wave Lithotripsy II: Urinary and Biliary Lithotripsy, J. E. Lingeman and D. M. Newman, Eds., pp. 203–205, Plenum Press, New York, NY, USA, 1989.

27. J. E. Lingeman, J. A. McAteer, S. A. Kempson, and A. P. Evan, "Bioeffects of extracorporeal shock-wave lithotripsy," Urologic Clinics of North America, vol. 1, article 89, 1987.

28. G. Seitz, K. Pletzer, D. Neisius, W. Dippel, and T. Gebhardt, "Pathologic-anatomic alterations in human kidneys after extracorporeal piezoelectric shock wave lithotripsy," Journal of Endourology, vol. 5, no. 1, pp. 17–20, 1991.

29. F. Recker, W. Hofmann, A. Bex, and R. Tscholl, "Quantitative determination of urinary marker proteins: a model to detect intrarenal bioeffects after extracorporeal lithotripsy," The Journal of Urology, vol. 148, no. 3, pp. 1000–1006, 1992. View at Scopus

30. G. Zanetti, F. Ostini, E. Montanari et al., "Cardiac dysrhythmias induced by extracorporeal shockwave lithotripsy," Journal of Endourology, vol. 13, no. 6, pp. 409–412, 1999. View at Scopus

31. D. D. Albers, F. E. Lybrand, J. C. Axton, and J. R. Wendelken, "Shockwave lithotripsy and pacemakers: experience with 20 cases," Journal of Endourology, vol. 9, no. 4, pp. 301–303, 1995. View at Scopus

32. E. Neri, G. Capannini, F. Diciolla et al., "Localized dissection and delayed rupture of the abdominal aorta after extracorporeal shock wave lithotripsy," Journal of Vascular Surgery, vol. 31, no. 5, pp. 1052–1055, 2000. View at Scopus

33. M. Brodmann, H. Ramschak, F. Schreiber, G. Stark, E. Pabst, and E. Pilger, "Venous thrombosis after extracorporeal shock-wave lithotripsy in a patient with heterozygous APC-resistance," Thrombosis and Haemostasis, vol. 80, no. 5, p. 861, 1998. View at Scopus

34. M. A. S. Jewett, C. Bombardier, A. G. Logan et al., "A randomized controlled trial to assess the incidence of new onset hypertension in patients after shock wave lithotripsy for asymptomatic renal calculi," The Journal of Urology, vol. 160, no. 4, pp. 1241–1243, 1998. View at Publisher · View at Google Scholar ·View at Scopus

35. Maker and J. Layke, "Gastrointestinal injury secondary to extracorporeal shock wave lithotripsy: a review of the literature since its inception," Journal of the American College of Surgeons, vol. 198, no. 1, pp. 128–135, 2004. View at Publisher · View at Google Scholar · View at PubMed · View at Scopus

36. M. A. Al Karawi, A. R. El-Sheikh Mohamed, K. E. El-Etaibi, M. S. Abomelha, and R. F. Seed, "Extracorporeal shock-wave lithotripsy (ESWL)-induced erosions in upper gastrointestinal tract. Prospective study in 40 patients," Urology, vol. 30, no. 3, pp. 224–227, 1987. View at Google Scholar ·View at Scopus

37. M. Murad Basar, M. Murat Samli, M. Erbil, O. Ozergin, R. Basar, and A. Atan, "Early effects of extracorporeal shock-wave lithotripsy exposure on testicular sperm morphology," Scandinavian Journal of Urology and Nephrology, vol. 38, no. 1, pp. 38–41, 2004. View at Publisher · View at Google Scholar ·View at PubMed · View at Scopus
38. J. Vieweg, H. M. Weber, K. Miller, and R. Hautmann, "Female fertility following extracorporeal shock wave lithotripsy of distal ureteral calculi," The Journal of Urology, vol. 148, no. 3, pp. 1007–1010, 1992.View at Google Scholar · View at Scopus

Further Readings-

Al-Awadi KA, Abdul Halim H, Kehinde EO, Al-Tawheed A. Steinstrasse: Comparison of incidence with and without J Stenting and the effect of J Stenting on subsequent management. Br J Urol Int 1998;84:618-21.

Fedullo LM, Pollack HM, Banner MP, Amendola MA, Van Arsdalen KN. The development of steinstrasse after ESWL: Frequency, natural history and radiologic management. AJR Am J Roentgenol 1988;151:1145-7.

Claro JA, Lima ML, Ferreira U. Blood pressure changes after extracorporeal shock wave lithotripsy in normotensive patients. J Urol 1992;147:553-8.

Lingeman JE, Woods JR, Nelson DR. Commentary on ESWL and blood pressure. J Urol 1995;154:2-4.

Strohmaier L, Koch J, Balk N. Limita

tion of shock-wave-induced renal tubular dysfunction by nifedipine. Eur Urol 1994;25:99-104.
45. Lechevallier E, Siles S, Ortega JC, Coulange C. Comparison by spect of renal scars after extracorporeal shock wave lithotripsy and percutaneous nephrolithotmy. J Endourol 1993;7:465-7.

Shigeta M, Kasaoka Y, Yasumoto H, Inoue K, Usui T, Hayashi M, *et al.*Fate of residual fragment after successful extracorporeal shock wave lithotripsy. Int J Urol 1999;6:169-72.

Streem SB, Yost A, Mascha E. Clinical implications of clinically insignificant stone fragments after extracorporeal shock wave lithotripsy. J Urol 1996;155:1186-90.

Back EM, Riehle RA. The fate of residual fragments after extracorporeal shock wave lithotripsy monotherapy of infection stones. J Urol 1991;145:6-9.

Cicerello E, Merlo F, Gambaro G, Maccatrozzo L, Fandella A, Baggio B, *et al.* Effect of alkaline citrate therapy on clearance of residual stone fragments after extracorporeal shock wave lithotripsy in sterile calcium and infection nephrolithiasis patients. J Urol 1994;151:5-9.

Newman LH, Seltzman B. Identification of risk factors in the development of clinically significant subcapsular hematomas following shock wave lithotripsy. In: Lingeman JE, Newman DM, editors. Shock wave lithotripsy 2: Urinary and biliary lithotripsy. New York: Plenum Press; 1989. p. 207-10.

Preminger GM, Kettelhut MC, Elkins SL, Seger J, Fetner CD. Ureteral stenting during extracorporeal shock wave lithotripsy: Help or hindrance? J Urol 1989;142:32-6.

Pryor JL, Jenkins AD. Use of double-pigtail stents in extracorporeal shock wave lithotripsy. J Urol 1990;143:475-8.

Nicely ER, Maggio MI, Kuhn EJ. The use of a
cystoscopically placed cobra catheter for direct irrigation of a lower pole calyceal stones during extracorporeal shock wave lithotripsy. J Urol 1992;148:1036-9

Essentials Of Litho-Tripsy

PRECAUTIONS TO AVOID COMPLICATIONS-

Proper Case Selection Is Very Important. Only Those Patients Would Be Ideal For Treatment If **Complete Stone Clearance** Can Be Achieved In Less Than Three Sessions Of ESWL.
Proper Case Selection Should Also Help In Avoiding **Steinstrasse**.
The Need For **Frequent Endourological Treatment Of Steinstrasse** Is A Definite Sign Of Wrong Case Selection For ESWL.
Thorough Pre-ESWL Evaluation Including **Complete Urological Investigations** Like Sonography, Intravenous Urography And Other Radiological Tests When Indicated; Complete Coagulation Profile, Urine Culture And Sensitivity Tests.

Best Results Of ESWL Are Obtained When ESWL Is Conducted, By An Experienced Urologist Who **Uses Adequate Number Of Shockwaves And Utilizes Enough Fluoroscopy Time** For Accurate Tareting Of The Calculi.
Altered Cardiac Rhythm, Both Brady & TachyArrhythmias, During ESWL, **Cardiac Arrest** Are Known After ESWL, (Available Ample Reports In Literature),
In View Of These Findings,
All Patients Must Have A **Continuous ECG And Blood Pressure Monitoring** During The **First ESWL Session**.
In Subsequent Sessions Monitoring Is Done In Elderly Patients, Patients With Previous Cardiac Ailments,
Or Patients Showing ECG Changes In First Session.
Adequate Analgesia Whenever Needed Should Be Provided.
Need For Analgesia Is Higher In Women, Younger Patients Or Patients Where A Higher Voltage Is Applied.

Patients Need Some **Evaluation Before Every Subsequent Session** Of ESWL. This Is The Time When Evaluation Is Commonly Missed.
It Is Necessary To Look For **Control Of Diabetes And Urinary Infection**. Complications Like Renal Hematoma And Infections Are Also Common In **Second Session** Of ESWL.

Appropriate Space Between ESWL Sessions, Is Necessary.
Minimal Safe Spacing Between ESWL Session Is At Least 48 Hours.
Longer Space Of 1-3 Weeks Or More Are Given,
Depending Upon Clinician Patient Compliance, InfraStructural & S Other Availabilities.
Antibiotic Cover Is Necessary For Each Session Of ESWL.

Further Evaluation Is Necessary If Patient Presents With **Unexplained Symptoms** Like Pain, Backache Or Fever.

References

Gallagher HJ, Tolley DA. 2000 AD: Still a role for the intravenous urogram in stone management ? Curr Opin Urol 10(6): 551-555, Nov 2000.

Al-Awadi KA, Abdul Halim H. ehinde EO, Al-Tawheed. A Steinstrasse : a comparison of incidence with and without J-stenting and the effect of J-stenting on subsequent management. BJU Int 84(6): 618-21, Oct 1999.

Logarakis NF, Jewett MA, Luymes J, Honey RJ. Variation in clinical outcome following shock wave lithotripsy. J Urol 163(3): 7215. March 2000.

Fujita K, Mizuno T, Ushiyama T, Suzuki K. Hadano S, Satoh S. Kambayashi T. Mugiya S, Nakano M. Complicating risk factors for pyelonephritis after extracorporeal shock wave lithotripsy. Int J Urol 7(6): 224-30. Jun 2000.

Candau C. Saussine C, Lang H. Roy C. Faure F. Jacgmin D. Natural history of residual renal stone fragments after ESWL. Eur Urol 37(1): 18-22. Jan 2000

Collado Serra A, Huguet Perez J, Monreal Garcia de Vicuna F. Rousaud Baron A. Izquierdo de la Tone F. Vicente Rodriguez J. Renal hematoma as a complication of extracorporeal shock wave lithotripsy. Scand J Urol Nephrol 33(3): 171-5. Jun 1999.

Further Readings

1. **Shock Wave Lithotripsy and Renal Hemorrhage**
   www.ncbi.nlm.nih.gov/.../PMC255...
   J Silberstein - 2008 - 8
   Abstract. Although **shock wave lithotripsy** is a safe and efficacious treatment for nephrolithiasis, the most common acute **complication** is renal hemorrhage. Shock ...
2. Renal **complications** of extracorporeal **shock wave lithotripsy**
   www.uptodate.com/.../renal-**compli**... -
3. **Complications** From Extracorporeal **Shock Wave Lithotripsy** ...
   www.livestrong.com/.../68669-**com**...
   28-03-2011 – **Complications** From Extracorporeal **Shock Wave Lithotripsy**. Kidney stones are very painful and can cause blockage of the urinary tract, leading ...
4. Acute **complications** during and after extracorporeal **shock wave** ...
   www.indianjurol.com/article.asp?...
   ME Schmidt - 2001
   Acute **complications** during and after extracorporeal **shock wave lithotripsy**. Indian J Urol [serial online] 2001 [cited 2013 Feb 25];17:118-20. Available from: ...
5. Extracorporeal **Shockwave Lithotripsy**
   emedicine.medscape.com/.../44455...
   22-08-2012 – Prior to the introduction of extracorporeal **shockwave lithotripsy** ...Extracorporeal **shock wave lithotripsy** 25 years later: **complications** and their ...
6. [PDF]
   Extracorporeal **Shock Wave Lithotripsy** 25 Years Later - American ...
   www.auanet.org/.../...
   PDF/Adobe Acrobat
   A Skolarikos - 2006 - 95
   Extracorporeal **Shock Wave Lithotripsy** 25 Years Later: **Complications** and Their Prevention. Andreas Skolarikos a, Gerasimos Alivizatos a, Jean de la Rosette b, ...

2.(v.) EMPHASIS MANAGEMENT STONES

URETERAL STONES

In 1984, With The Approval By U.S FDA For General Clinical Use Of Dornier HM3 LithoTriptor ,Only Renal & **Upper Ureteric Stones Above The Iliac Crest Were Being Treated.**

Initial Studies,For Ureteral Stones Insitu Treatment,
Reported 50% Success Rate(Chaussy et al.1981),
Most Of The Stones Were DisIntegrated But Pieces Were Held Together By Oedematous Ureteral Mucosa,
Especially In Patients With Complete Ureteral Obstruction For More Than 6 Weeks,Needing open Surgical Removal Of Fragments.

The Observation Led To Comparatively Short History Based,
Case Selection Criteria For UreteroLithiasis ESWL Management.
Subsequent Studies Documented Passage Of A Ureteral Catheter
In All Cases & Pushing The Stone Up Into Collecting System,
To Be Managed By ESWL.
If Ureteral Catheter Can Not Be Negotiated, Attempted Passage Of
(4) French Stent Around The Stone Was Recommended,
With A View That Additional Space Will Facilitate
More SuccessFul Stone DisIntegration.

Assessment Of Fragmentation

**UretroLithiasis ManageMent With ESWL,
Needs Specific Care Due To Its Surgical Anatomy.**

In Recent Clinical Practice, With Available LithoTriptors,
For Majority Of Ureteral Stones Disintegration,
Usually1500-3000 Shocks Are Needed.

Cautious Discrete Supervision,
For Stone Shattering Into Minute Particles,
Rendered More **Efficient By Available CT Monitoring**
& Sophisticated LithoTriptors,
Is Capable Of Providing Safety Profile For Single Sitting & Or Ancillary Procedure Regimes, In Accordance To Stone Density, Volume, Impaction Status And Other Determinants.

Ureteral Stone DisIntegration Bio-Physics
Expansion Space Theory

The Presumed Theory Regarding Action Of Shock Waves On A Stone Is The Creation Of InterActing Compressive &Tensile Forces At Fluid- Stone InterFaces, With Stone Material Being Torn Off In Layers.

The Fact That, Clinically, Impacted Ureteral Stones
Behave More Resistantly, As Compared To Capacious Renal Pelvis Forms
The Basis For FundaMental Bio-Physics Regarding
'Expansion Space Theory', As Depicted By Following Illustrations-

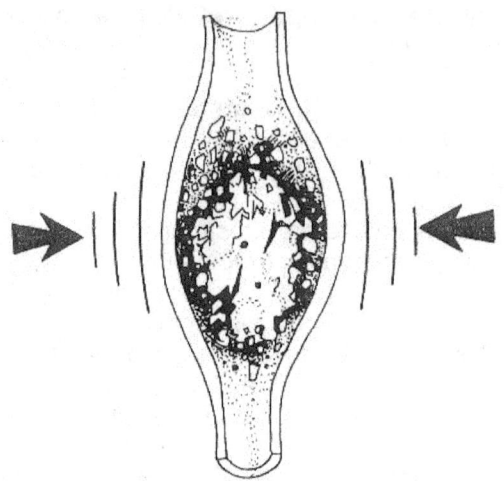

Partially Fragmented Impacted Ureteral Stone.
Multiple Fluid-Stone Interfaces Creation, In Fragments' Outer Layer,
Absorb Subsequent Shock Wave Energy, ThereBy Preventing
Fragmentation Of Solid Core.
Source- Mueller et al. 1986
And Williams & WilKins Publishers.

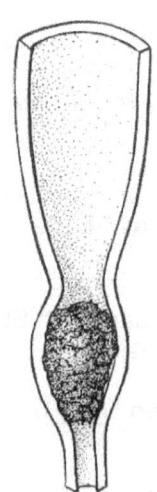

Impacted UreteralStone With No Expansion Space
Theoretically, Such Stone Respond Poorly To InSitu ESWL.
Source-Jenkins 1988.

Essentials Of Litho-Tripsy

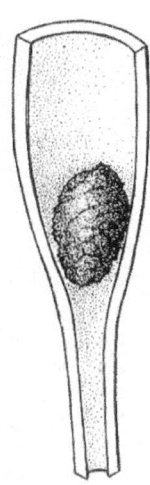

UreteralStone With Natural Expansion Space
Theoretically, Such Stone Respond Well To InSitu ESWL.
Source-Jenkins 1988.

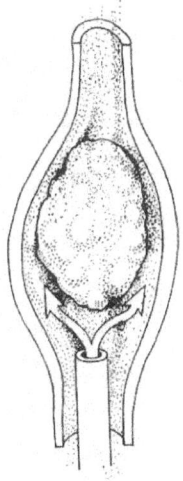

**Fluid Injected Through A Ureteral Catheter,
Placed Just Distal To Stone.**
Results In Artificial Expansion Space Creation, Along With Newly Fragmented Stone Particles Flushing Away From The Solid Stone Core.
Source- Griffith1987.

Surgical Management of Upper Urinary Tract Calculi
Brian R. Matlaga, James E. Lingeman . Jan 2012: 1357-1410

Illustrations Depicting 'Patient Positionings' Specialized Manovures For Ureteric Stones

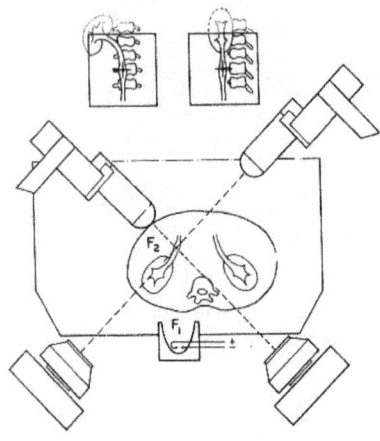

SuperImposition Of A Ureteral Stone Over Vertebral Body & Transverse Process.
Source – Fuchs et al. 1987

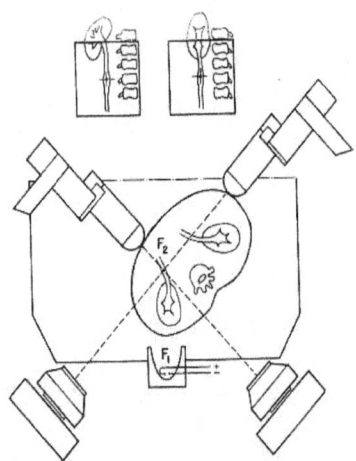

Correction Of SuperImposition Of A Ureteral Stone Over The Spine By Rotating The Patient
The Manovure Is Not Uniformly SuccessFul.
Source – Fuchs et al. 1987

Essentials Of Litho-Tripsy

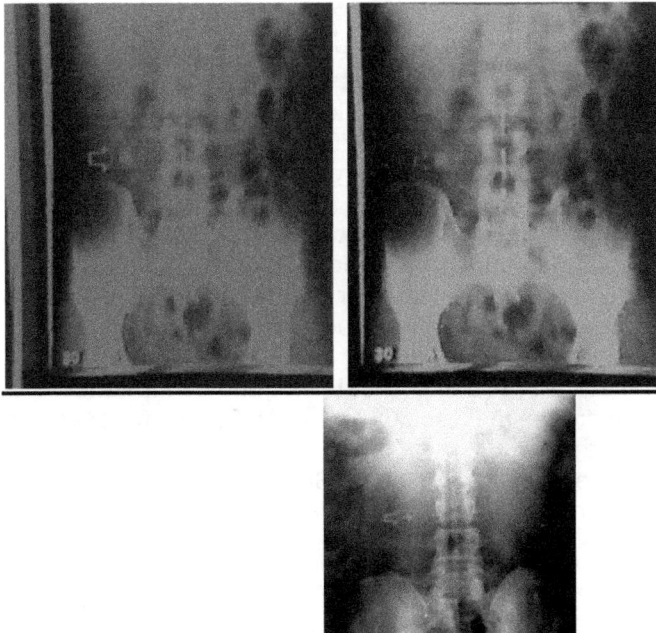

**Ureteric Stones Completely Removed By ESWL
(1-2 Sittings Average)**

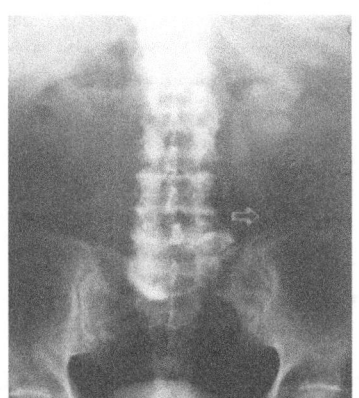

**IVP Film –
Left Mid Ureteric Stones With Hydroureteronephrosis
Subsequent IVPs After About > 6 Months:WNL,
Single Sitting Clearance.**

LOWER URETERIC STONES

Being Technically Difficult Eitherwise, Have Comparatively Low Success Rate Usually, And Are Less Attempted By Lithotripsy. However, ESWL Gives Good Result Yield, And Not Uncommonly Performed In Patients Demanding Specific Treatment Modality, Reluctance, Or Contraindication For Surgery.

Patient's Position Being Prone, Cautious Shock Power Delivery In View Of Adjacent Anatomical Structures, Especially In Females, With Advice For Empty Urinary Bladder Etc Are Useful Precaution Guidelines For Success.

Properly Administered Forced Diuresis Regime Compliance, Have Shown Manifold Increase In Result Outcome As Supportive Measure, Minimizing The Use Of 'DJS',
Avoiding Obstructive Phenomenon, e.g., Stein-A-Strasse,
By Expelling Out Minutely Shattered Stone Particles.[12,13]

12. Bierkens AF, Hendrikx AJ, De La Rosette JJ. Treatment of mid-and lower ureteric calculi: Extracorporeal shock-wave lithotripsy vs. laser ureteroscopy. A comparison of costs, morbidity and effectiveness. Br J Urol 1998;81:31-5.
13. Clayman RV. Outpatient treatment of middle and lower ureteroscopic laser lithotripsy. J Urol 1999;162:1876-7.

Illustrations Depicting 'Specialized Patient Positionings' For Lower Ureteric Stones

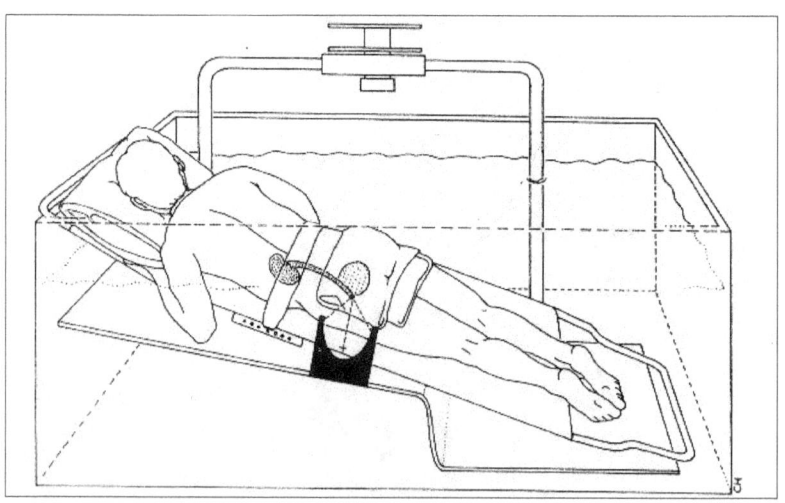

Prone ESWL Positioning For Pre-Sacral Calculus
HM3 Lithotriptor Non-Motorized Patient Chair Modified With Stryker Frame
Source- Lesson From Jenkins & GillenWater 1988
And The Publishers Williams & WilKins, BaltiMore

Essentials Of Litho-Tripsy

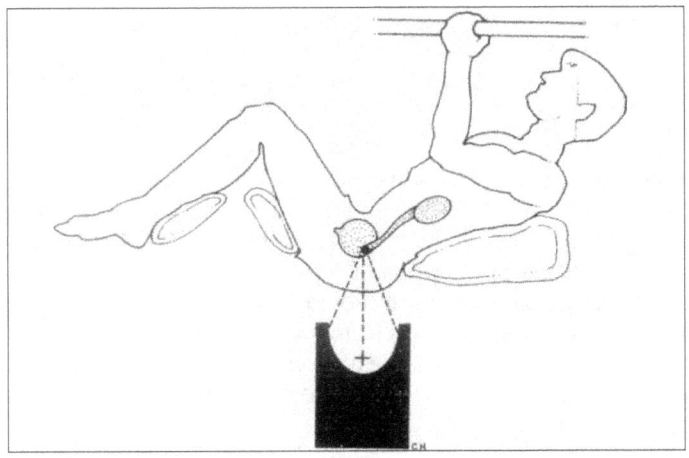

HM3 Lithotriptor: Patient's Sitting Position For Juxta-Vesicular Stone

Source-Jenkins 1990

INFERIOR CALYCEAL STONES, LOWER POLE KIDNEY STONES

Can Be Managed EitherWise Or
By ESWL, As Discussed With The Special Emphasis Supportive Measures & MethodologyTechniques.
SWL Is The Preferred Tratment Methodology ,For Most Of Patients With Symptomatic Upper Urinary Tract Calculii,Yet There is Cosiderable Controversy Regarding Management Of LPS With SWL (Trolley & Downey,1994), As Stone Free Rate Achieved With PNL Were Superior To ESWL.
According To Documented Meta-Analytic Study By
LingeMan & Associates (1994) Low Treatment Reult OutComes,
For LPS & Inf. Calyceal Stones Of <1, 1-2 & >2 Cms Size,
By Differing SWL, URS & PCNL Techniques.

The Regression Analysis Demostrated, Increasing Stone Burden Association With Progressively Less SuccessFul Stone Free Rate Rates With SWL, While PNL Treated Patients Stone Free Rate Rates Remained Costant ThroughOut Different Categories.

The Impact Of Lower Calyceal Anatomy Studies, Revealed Changes In Stone Distribution Explained By The Tendency Of Small, Radio-Graphically UnDetectable Fragments, To Gravitate To More Dependendent Calyx After SWL Therapy
& Act As A Nidus For New Stone Growth(Carr et al.1996).

The Reasons For Poor Clearance Of Fragments From LPS After SWL Are Unclear & Include-
i. Gravty Dependent Position Of Lower Pole Calyx May Impede The Passage Of Various Stone Fragments(Elbahnasy et al.1998b).
ii. Important Role Of Anatomic Features In The Evacuation Of Stone Fragments From Lower Positions-

Sampaio & Aragao(1992,1994) Studied The Lower Anatomy Using Polyester EndoClasts Of The IntraRenal Collecting System Obtained From Adult Cadavers & Hypothesized That-
1. A Lower Pole With Multiple Infundibula Might Have Poor Drainage & Consequently Low Possibility Of Eliminating The Stone Fragments, tHan A single Infundibulum Receiving Receiving Fused Calyces.
2. Small Diametre Of Lower Pole Infundibulum Might Hinder Stone Fragments Passasge.
3. The Angle Formed Between Lower Infundibulum & The Renal Pelvis & Hypothesized That An Angle Greater Than 90^0 (Obtuse) Should Facilitate Drainage Of Segments From The Lower Pole.

Other Studies Have Reported Anatomical Factors Alone, In Combination May Pomote Stone Clearance,
The Other Study Group Recorded No Effect Of Anatomical Factors In Predicting Result Out Comes, May Be Due To Disparity In The ParaMetre MeasureMent Techniques.

Pace & Colleagues(2000) Studied Wide Variation In Lower Calyceal Infundibuar Width(LCIW) MeasureMents,During Different Phases Of IntraVenous Pyelography & Reported Greatest LCIW During Compression Film & Smallest On The Post Void Film, Prompting The Suggestion Of Standarized Time For Infundibular Width MeasureMent During IntraVenous UroGraphy.

The Other Sources Of Result OtCome Variability Inclded- Type Of LithoTriptor Appliances, Stone Composition, Stone Volume, Burden Etc.

Regarding The Discrete Study Of Other Lower Pole Anatomic Features, As Predictive Factors Of Stone Clearanc,e May Be Some Computronics Modelling Assistance Is Of Immense Help In Near Future.
Polakis & Associates(2003) Developed An Artificail Neural NetWork, Incorporating Both Anatomic Features & Dyanamic Movements, For Accurately Predicting SuccessFul OutComes By SWL.

McCullough(1989) AnecDotally Reported Postural Drainage Support,, While Brownie& Associates(1990), Subsequently Treated LPS Fragments By- Controlled Inversion Therapy,SuppleMenting IV Hydration, Inversion &Percussion.

Essentials Of Litho-Tripsy

The Role Of Percussion, Inversion & Furosemide Forced Diuresis For Lower Pole & Or Inferior Calyceal Stones ManageMent Comparative Analytical Studies Are Available, In Several 20th Century Studies.

RetroSpective Studies Have Confirmed The Previous Observations That Results Of SWL For LPS Are Inferior To PNL, With Specially Poor Results Of Stone Clearance, As Stone Size Increased Above 10mm Size.

UreteroReoscopy, One Of Latest UseFul Advent In Endo-Urology, Has Been Recognized For Its UseFul Applications, Including UroLithiasis, Especially In Lower, Middle Ureter Stone Disease Cases & Also For Displacement Of Ureteric & Renal Stones To Appropriate Positionings For Fragmentations & Subsequent Clearance.

In Consideration Of Different Available Comparative Statistical Data Involving- LPS, Inf. Calyceal Stones Management (Of Varying Anatomical MeasureMents, Stone Composition, Size, Volume, Burde & Other Factors), TreatMent Methodologies, Namely-SWL, PNL, URS & Others-

Choice Of Patients, Anatomical And/Or Other Determinants,Consideration With **Postprocedural Period Advice; For Foot End Elevation (To Gain Gravitational Support), Aided By Proper Forced Diuresis Regime For About 1–3 Days**, The Discussed Study,Have Shown Considerably Good Results To Flush Out Minute Stone Particles, Leaving Stone-Free Patients [Figure 5].[15,19,20]
During/After Procedure 'Inverse Positioning','Shake-Up' Methodology Techniques Had Synergistic Result Outcome Effects.

References

Lingeman JE, Siegel YI, Steele B, Nyhuis AW, Woods JR. Management of lower pole nephrolithiasis: A critical analysis. J Urol 1994:151:663

Karlin GS, Smith AD. Approaches to the superior calyx: Renal displacement technique and review of options. J Urol 1989;142:774-7.

Küpeli B, Biri H, Sinik Z, Karaca K, Tuncayengin A, Karaoğlan U, et al.Extracorporeal shock wave lithotripsy for lower calyceal calculi. Eur Urol 1998;34:203-6.

Rodrigues Netto N Jr, Claro JF, Cortado PL, Lemos GC. Adjunct controlled inversion therapy following extracorporeal shock wave lithotripsy for lower pole calyceal stones. J Urol 1991;146:953-4.

Karlin GS, Smith AD. Approaches to the superior calyx: Renal displacement technique and review of options.
 J Urol 1989;142:774-7.

Küpeli B, Biri H, Sinik Z, Karaca K, Tuncayengin A, Karaoğlan U, et al.Extracorporeal shock wave lithotripsy for lower calyceal calculi. Eur Urol 1998;34:203-6.

May DJ, Chandhoke PS. Efficacy and cost-effectiveness of extracorporeal shock wave lithotripsy for solitary lower pole renal calculi. J Urol 1998;159:24-7.Talic RF, El Faqih SR. Extracorporeal shock wave lithotripsy for lower pole nephrolithiasis: Efficacy and variable that influence treatmentoutcome. Urology 1998;51:544-7.

Pace KT, Tariq N, Dyer SJ, Weir MJ, D'A Honey RJ. Mechanical percussion, inversion and diuresis of or residual lower pole fragments following shock wave lithotripsy. A prospective, single blinded randomized controlled trial.
 J Urol 2001;166:2065-71.

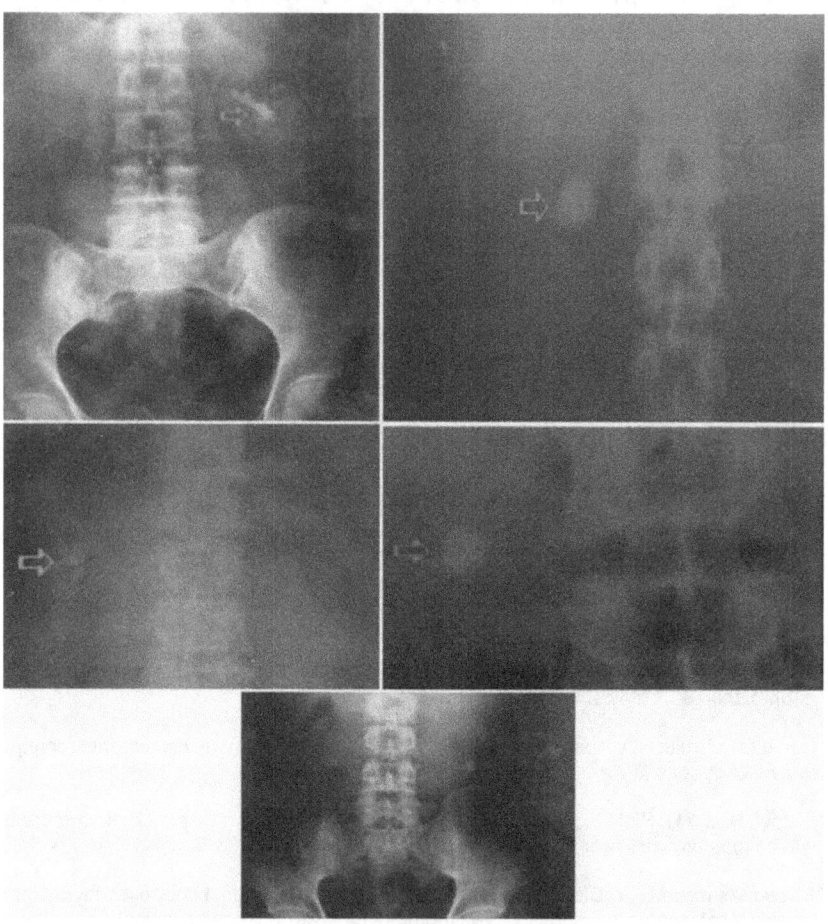

Kidney And Ureteric Stones Of Different Sizes, Locations(LPS Etc.) Removed Completely

Essentials Of Litho-Tripsy

THE MANAGEMENT OF CALULI IN ASSOCIATION WITH PELVIURETERIC JUNCTION OBSTRUCTION

In Patients, With Calculus Or Calculi, In Association With 'Pelvi-Ureteric Junction Obstruction', Both Elements Of The Problem Must Be Treated.
Open Surgery Has Been Used For The Management Of This Situation With Excellent Results. The Wide Exposure Obtained After Renal Pelvis Exposure For PyeloPlaty, Provides Excellent Access To The Inside Of The Renal Pelvis And The Calyces, Rendering Good Visualization And Removal Of All Of The Fragments Of Stones Situated In The Kidney, Subsequently Standard Pyeloplasty Performed,
With Excellent Long-Term Results.

ESWL, Has No Role In The Management Of Stones In Association With Pelvi-Ureteric Junction Obstruction, For The Obvious Reason That After Pulverization Of The Stone, The Fragment Would Be Unable To Pass Into The Ureter, Hence Increased Obstruction With Subsequent Pyonephrosis May Occur. In The Longer Term, An Almost Certain Recurrence Of The Stone Is Reported.

The Surge In Endourological Procedures, Due To The Significant Technological Advances Leading To Advent Of SuccessFul Less Invasive Technique Methodolologies, Comparable To
Open Surgical Procedures.
Renal Calculi In Association With Pelviureteric Junction Obstruction Management, Is An Important Example.
Endoscopic Division & Repair Of The Pelviureteric Junction
Has Been Given A Veriety Of Names: Percutaneous Pyelolysis, Percutaneous Intubated Ureterotomy, Percutaneous Intubated Ureterotomy, Percutaneous Endopyelotomy, Endouretero-Pyelotomy, And Endoureteroplasty Etc.
The Technique Itself Has Been Refined And Is Now Well Established (Wickham & Kellett 1983, Badlani Et Al 1986).

The Comparabilities Of Renal Scans(DTPA With /WithOut Forced Diuresis Etc.), Before & After Definite Duration Of Open / EndoScopic Procedures, Determines Success Extent Of OverAll Result OutComes.

In Cases Of Ureteropelvic Junction Obstruction, In Addition To Anatomic Obstruction, Coexistent Metabolic Abnormalities Are Contributing To Stone Formation.[4]
Suggestive Treatments For PUJ Obstruction With Stone;
Classical Open Surgical Stone Extraction And Pyeloplasty,
PNL With Concomitant Endopyelotomy,
And Recently Laparoscopically(An Antegrade Approach Preferred With Existing Stone, Although Retrograde Can Be Performed) [Figure 6].

<u>CONG. ANOMALIES</u>: Include Ureteropelvic Junction Obstruction, Horse Shoe Kidneys, Other Ectopic Or Fusion Anomalies, Hydronephrosis, And Calyceal Diverticulae[9,10]

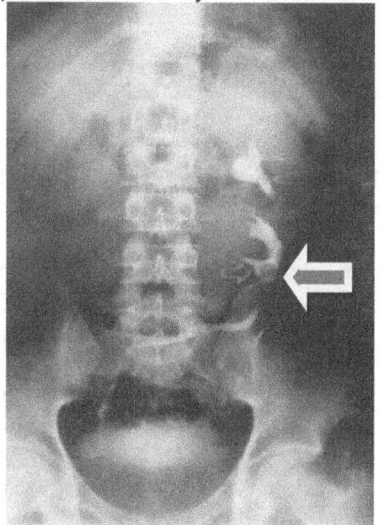

IVP Film –
Horse Shoe Shaped Kidney, Renal Ectopia Pelvic Kidney,
(Renalpelvis Stone About 1.5 Cms
With Non Obstructive Collecting System Drainage)
Subsequent IVPs After About > 6 Months:WNL,
Single Sitting Clearance.

The Anatomic Abnormalities Of **Horseshoe Kidneys** Cause Some Difficulties In The Use Of SWL ,
Although Adequate Fragmentation Can Be Achieved In Stone-Bearing Horseshoe Kidneys, The Anatomic Abnormalities Prevent Fragment Passage In A Substantial Number Of Patients.

Essentials Of Litho-Tripsy

CALCULI IN HORSESHOE KIDNEY

The Horseshoe Kidney Is One Of The Commonest Congential Renal Anomalies And Is The Commonest Anomaly Of Fusion Of The Kidney.
With An Incidence Of I In 400 To I In 1800,
Has An Association With Other Systems Anomalies,
& Is Often Complicated By Hydronephrosis,Infection,Or Renal Calculi.
Reported Renal Calculi Occurrence In Horseshoe Kidneys Being 20% ,With Unknown Exact Aetiology.
The Increased Incidence May Be Associated With The Unusual Drainage Of Urine From The Horseshoe Kidney Caused By eg.
The High Insertion Of The Ureter Over The Renal Substance.
The Possibility Of An Associated Metabolic Abnormality In Patients With Horseshoe Kidney Has Also Been Noted (Evans & Resnik 1981).

The Management Of Stones In Horsehoe Kidneys,
Especially With The Less Invasive Methods Of
Percutaneous Nephrolithotomy, Or The Non-Invasive Method Of ESWL
Encountered Difficulties Include-
More Anterior Position Of The Horseshoe Kidney Than The Normal Kidney And If The Patient Is Obese,
The Position Of The Kidney May Be Too Far Anteriorly To Allow Access To The Nephroscopist.
This Problem Is Further Compounded, With The Stone Is Lying In The Middle Calyx Or At The Lower Pole.
Therefore, Discrete CT Scanning Of The Renal Areas, For Accurate Localization Of Stones, Within The Kidney Is StronglyRecommended.

ESWL Failure Are Due To Same Reasons,
Middle Calyx Stones Positioning, Overlying The Spine,
Prevents Shock Waves Delivery Access, Is Another Problem.
Again The Stone May Be Too Far Forward For The Focal Point Of The Machine To Coincide With It.

CALCULI IN CALYCEAL DIVERTICULA

Calyceal Diverticulitis:
This Occurs When Congenital Eventrations Of The Renal Collecting System Is Lined ByTransitional Cell Epithelium.
Calcyceal Diverticula Occur Uncommonly And Are Present In Less Than 0.5%
Treatments Include Traditional Open Surgical Nephrostomy
With Infundibulum Closure And Diverticular Cavity Fulguration,
Invasive Surgical PNL Ureteroscopy, ESWL, And Laparoscopy.

Reported Stone Free Rate For Calyceal Diverticular Stone Treatment
With ESWL Averages Only 21%.

In Intravenous Urography, Stones Are Thought To Occur,
In About 10% Of Calcyeal Diverticula.
In Many Cases They Are Asymptomatic,
But Sometimes Associated With Chronic Loin Pain,
Necessitating Surgical Removal.
Calculi In Calyceal Diverticula May Be Present In Association With
Other Calculi In The Same Kidney, Needind Simultaneous Removal.

These Stones Have Been Managed By **Traditional Open Removal**,
Involving Kidney Exposure & A **Nephrotomy Over The Diverticulum**
With Removal Of The Calculi Followed By Obliteration Of The Cavity,
Achieved By **Marsupialization Of The Diverticulum** And Closure Of
Its Neck With Sutures, Or By **Fulguration**.
Extracorporeal Shock Wave Litho-Tripsy, Is Of Limited Help In The
Management Of Stones In Calyceal Diverticula,
As In Most Cases The **Neck Of The Diverticulum** Is Extremely Narrow,
Not Permitting The Passage Of The Stone Fragments Into The Main
Collecting System.
In Some Cases, With Wide Neck Of The Diverticulum,
ESWL Is Of Value, Particularly Where The Diverticulum Is High
And Relativery In Accessible.

Percutaneous Approach As The Method Of Choice For
Calyceal Diverticular Calulii Removal, 10 Patients Case Series,
Review Study By Hulbert &Colleagues1986, Reported, That With
Direct Diverticular Puncture Approach,
Guidewire Could Not Be Negotiated Through The Narrow Calyceal
Neck Into The Main Collecting System & Coiled Up Within The
Diverticulum During The Dilatation Of The Track.
After Removal Of The Calculi From The Diverticulum,
The Guidewire Passed Under Direct Vision Into The Collecting System
And The Neck Of The Diverticulum Dilated In Order To Allow A
Nephrostomy Tube To Be Passed Through It.
The Lining Of The Diverticula Subsequently Became Obliterated By
Granulation Tissue Growing Around The Tube.
While In,**Indirect Diverticulum Approach Technique**, Renal Pelvis
Access Is Achieved Via An Initial Puncture Was Made Through A Different
Calyx. Using Flexible Nephroscope The Diverticular Opening Located And
Then Either Dilated Or Cut In Order To Remove The Contained Stone.
In Both Methods, C-Arm Fluoroscopy Unit Use Is Extremely Helpful.
The Study Concluded, Direct Puncture Of The Diverticulum To Be The
Preferable Method Of Access, With The Advantage Of Satisfactoy
Obliteration Of Diverticulum.

Essentials Of Litho-Tripsy

In Most Upper Pole, Direct Puncture Was Possible Between The 11th And 12th Ribs.
Small Calyceal Stones In The Vast Majority, Are Asymptomatic & Require NoTreatment Unless Associated With Haematuria, Urinary Tract Infection, Or Are Found To Be Enlarging Or Causing Pain.
The Last Indication Is Controversial,
Loin Pain And A Small Calyceal Stone Fragment ManageMent, Especially By Open Surgery Is CumberSome & Was Avoided,
Due To Difficulty Of Stone Localization Within The Kidney At The Time Of Operation &The Resultant Large Painful Surgical Scar To Remove Such A Small Stone.

The Changing Attitudes For Relieving Loin Pain By Removing Calyceal Stones, Has Been Observed,Following Introduction Of Less Invasive Techniques (Percutaneous & Others) For Treating Urinary Calculi. Small Non Obstructing Calyceal Stones Percutaneous Or ESWL Removal Render Pain Relief, To A Considerable No. Of Patients.

The Small Non-Obstructing Calyceal Stones Seen In Clinical Practice Are Responsible For Sometimes Associated Lion Pain,Is Virtually Impossible To Prove,Needing Lot Of Time Performing Complicated Diagnostic Tests At Regular Intervals During Medical Therapy Regimes,Supports ESWL Acceptablity For ManageMent Of Small Non-Obstructing Calyceal Stones.

MoreOver,Percutaneous Removal Of Multiple Calyceal Stones Is Further Complicated By Often Required Multiple Puctures, In Addition To Requiring A Flexible Nephroscope And Other Instruments To Dilate Or Incise Narrow Calyceal Infundibula (Lange Et Al 1984).
In These Instances, When ESWL Is Not Available, It Preferable To Manage These Stones Conservatively.

References

Effectiveness Of Extracorporeal Shockwave Lithotripsy In The Management Of Stone-Bearing Horseshoe Kidneys
ZIYA KIRKALI, A. ADIL ESEN, And M. UĞUR MUNGAN. Journal Of Endourology. February 1996, 10(1): 13-15. DOI:10.1089/End.1996.10.13.
Published In Volume: 10 Issue 1: March 30, 2009

Shockwave Lithotripsy In Patients With Horseshoe Kidney: Determinants Of Success
A. Andrew Ray, Daniela Ghiculete, R. John D'A. Honey, Kenneth T. Pace
Journal Of Endourology. Mar 2011, Vol. 25, No. 3: 487-493

Factors Affecting Outcomes Of Percutaneous Nephrolithotomy In Horseshoe Kidneys
Abdulkadir Tepeler, Priyanka D. Sehgal, Tolga Akman, Ali Unsal, Ekrem Ozyuvali, Abdullah Armagan, Stephen Y. Nakada
Urology. Oct 2014

Outcomes Of Retrograde Flexible Ureteroscopy And Laser Lithotripsy For Stone Disease In Patients With Anomalous Kidneysİbrahim Mesut Ugurlu, Tolga Akman, Murat Binbay, Erdem Tekinarslan, Özgür Yazıcı, Mehmet Fatih Akbulut, Faruk Özgör, Ahmet Yaser Müslümanoğlu Urolithiasis. Aug 2014

Management Of Stones In Abnormal Situations Yung K. Tan, Doh Yoon Cha, Mantu Gupta Urologic Clinics Of North America. Feb 2013, Vol. 40: 79-97

Retrograde Intrarenal Surgery In Patients With Horseshoe KidneysGokhan Atis, Berkan Resorlu, Cenk Gurbuz, Ozgur Arikan, Ekrem Ozyuvali, Ali Unsal, Turhan Caskurlu Urolithiasis. Feb 2013, Vol. 41: 79-83

Urolithiasis in the horseshoe kidney: a single-centre experience Stephanie J. Symons, Anil Ramachandran, Abraham Kurien, Ramen Baiysha, Mahesh R. Desai
BJU International. Dec 2008, Vol. 102, No. 10.1111/bju.2008.102.issue-11: 1676-1680

Extracorporeal Shockwave Lithotripsy in Anomalous KidneysBORA KÜPELİ, KENAN İSEN, HASAN BİRİ, ZAFER SINIK, TURGUT ALKİBAY, ÜSTÜNOL KARAOĞLAN, İBRAHİM BOZKIRLIJournal of Endourology. Jun 1999, Vol. 13, No. 5: 349-352

Urolithiasis In Kidneys With Abnormal Lie, Rotation Or FormArvind P Ganpule, Mahesh R DesaiCurrent Opinion In Urology. Mar 2011, Vol. 21: 145-153

Stones In Patients With Renal AnomaliesAlana Desai, Ramakrishna Venkatesh
. Sep 2009: 212-228

Percutaneous Nephrolithotomy In Renal Anomalies Of Fusion, Ectopia, Rotation, Hypoplasia, And Pelvicalyceal Aberration: Uniformity In HeterogeneityAbdul Majid Rana, Jai Parkash Bhojwani Journal Of Endourology. Apr 2009, Vol. 23, No. 4: 609-614
European Urology. Jan 2008, Vol. 53: 201-202

Management Of Urolithiasis In The Congenitally Abnormal Kidney (Horseshoe And Ectopic) Robert J Stein, Mihir M Desai Current Opinion In Urology. Mar 2007, Vol. 17: 125-131

Treatment Of Stones Associated With Complex Or Anomalous Renal Anatomy
M GUPTA, M LEE Urologic Clinics Of North America. Aug 2007, Vol. 34: 431-441

Management Of Stones In Patients With Anomalously Sited Kidneys
Andreas J. Gross, Megan Fisher Current Opinion In Urology. Mar 2006, Vol. 16: 100-105

Shock Wave Lithotripsy For Urinary Stones And Non-Calculus Applications
Kenneth Ogan, Margaret Pearle . Jan 2005: 395-424

Stones In Anomalous Kidneys: Results Of Treatment By Shock Wave Lithotripsy In 150 PatientsLUTFI TUNC, HUSNU TOKGOZ, MUSTAFA OZGUR TAN, BORA. KUPELI, USTUNOL KARAOGLAN, IBRAHIM BOZKIRLIInternational Journal Of Urology. Oct 2004, Vol. 11, No. 10.1111/Iju.2004.11.Issue-10: 831-836

Rutchik SD, Resnick MI. Ureteropelvic junction obstruction and renal calculi. Pathophysiology and implications for management. Urol Clin North Am 1998;25:317-21.

Küpeli B, Isen K, Biri H, Sinik Z, Alkibay T, Karaoğlan U,
et al. Extracorporeal shock wave lithotripsy in anomalous kidney. J Endourol 1999;13:349-52.

Kirkali Z, Esen AA, Mungan MU. Effectiveness of extracorporeal shockwave lithotripsy in the management of stone-bearing horseshoe kidneys. J Endourol 1996;10:13-5.

PEDIATRIC STONE DISEASE

Although Kidney Stones Do Not Often Occur In Children, The Incidence Is Increasing Prior To 1990, Nephrolothiasis Was Responsible For 1 In 1000 To 1 In 7600 Hospital Admission Annually Throughout The United States (Nimkin Et Al. 1992.) **In Recent Years, However, A Dramatic Increase In Pediatric Urolithiasis Has Been Observed** (Srivastavs And Alon, 2005),Especially Among Adolescents Without Known Metabolic Disturbance. The Speculations Are That Sodium And Carbohydrates Rich Diets May Contribute To The Etiology Of Urolithiases.

Paediatric Urolithiasis Is, Often Related To A **Pre-Existing Inherited Metabolic Defect, Or Congenital Anatomical Anomaly, Vesicoureteric Reflux** Etc.

These Stones Are In The Kidney In Two Thirds Of Reported Cases, And In The Ureter In The Remaining Cases. Older Children Are At Greater Risk Independent Of Age And Sex.
As With Adults, Most Pediatric Kidney Stones Are Predominantly Composed Of Calcium Oxalate; Struvite And Calcium Phosphate Stones Are Less Common. Calcium Oxalate Stones In Children Are Associated With High Amounts Of Calcium, Oxalate, And Magnesium In Acidic Urine.

"Diet and Definition of Kidney Stones, Renal Calculi". Retrieved 2013-10-11.

Kirejczyk, JK.; Porowski, T.; Filonowicz, R.; Kazberuk, A.; Stefanowicz, M.; Wasilewska, A.; Debek, W. (Aug 2013). "An association between kidney stone composition and urinary metabolic disturbances in children". *J Pediatr Urol.* doi:10.1016/j.jpurol.2013.07.010. PMID 23953243.

NeoNatal NephroCalciNosis Is Frequently Caused By Loop Diuretics. Cessation Of The Medicine Is Essential & May Be Reversed By The Use Of Thiazides.

Special Considerations In The Endourologic Management Of Stone Disease In Children Include-
Preservation Of Renal Development And Function,
Prevention Of Radiation Exposure,
& Minimizing The Need For Re-Treatment.

Despite Advances In Endourology Equipment And Technique, **Controversy Remains** Regarding The Contribution Of SWL To Future Development Of Diabetes Or Hypertension,
And Whether Ureteric Otifice Dilation During Ureteroscopy (URS) Leads To Ureteral Stricture Formation Or Development Of Vesicoureteral Reflux.

International Consensus Is Lacking As To The Most Effective Surgical Management Of Pediatric Stone Disease Due To Lake Of Prospective Randomized Comparative Trials.
The Presence Of Residual Stone Fragments Is Associated With Adverse Outcomes (Afshar Et Al, 2004). And Every Attempt Should Be Made To Achive A Stone-Free Status.
The Surgeon's Experience & Decision Regarding The Most Efficacious Primary Treatment Modality Must Be Individualized Per Child Based On Age, Anatomy, Location, And Composition Of The Stone Burden.

The Ideal Management Of Stones In Children Should Include A Technique Which Combines The Efficient And Complete Removal Of All Of The Stone In Addition To Ensuring Minimal Morbidity And Minimal Renal Damage. **The Impact Of ESWL** On The Management Of Calculi In Children Has Been Considerable. A Number Of Series Have Shown That This Can Be Carried Out Safely And Effectively Using Either The Dornier HM3 Lithotriptor, The Wolf Piezolith And The Siemen's Lithostar (Newman Et Al 1986, Kramolowsky Et Al 1987, Marberger Et Al 1989, Neisius Et Al 1989 Thornhill Et Al 1990).

Antibiotic Use
In Accordance With The 2008 American Urologic Association's Best Practice Statement On **Antibiotic Prophylaxis**, Less Than Or Equal To 24 Hours Of Perioperative Antibiotics Are Indicated In All Patients Undergoing Upper Tract Instrumentation (Wolf Et Al, 2008).

In Children, Appropriate AntiMicrobial Include Trimethoprim-Sulfamethazole, First- And Second-Generation Cephalosporins, & Amplicillin In Combination With An Aminoglycoside.
A Urine Culture Is Mandatory Before All Upper Tract Procedures To Determine If The Urine Is Sterile, And Culrute Result Are Used To Guide Preoperative Antibiotic Therapy, Particularly For Percutaneous Procedures, Patients With High-Grade Obstruction, Or Patients With An Indwelling Stent (Wu And Docimo, 2004).
According To A Study,For Children With A Negative Urine Culture Undergoing Uncomplicated URS Procedures Receive Perioperative Cefazolin, And All Children Undergoing A Percutaneous Procedure Or Who Have A Preexisting Ureteral Stent/Nephrostomy Tube Receive A Fluroquinolone Or Ampicillin/Gentamicin.
Postoperative Antibiotics Use Is Controversial And Is Determind On An Individual Basis, Especially With Recent Data Demonstrating An Increased Risk Of Developing Resistant Bacterial Strains With Prolonged Use Of Antibiotics Prophylactic Therapy (Conway Et Al, 2007).

SHOCK WAVE LITHOTRIPSY

The Emergence Of Shock Wave Lithotripsy (SWL) Revolutionzed The Minimally Invasive Treatment Of Adult Urolithiasis During The Early 1980's. Since The Initial Report On Successful SWL Use In Children In 1986 (Newman Et Al, 1986), Large Series Have Reported Complication, Safety And Stone-Free Rates Comparable To Adult Cohorts (Myers Et Al, 1995; Elsobky Et Al, 2000; Ather And Noor, 2003; Muslumanoglu Et Al, 2003; Rizvi Et Al, 2003; Aksoy Et Ala, 2004; Raza Et Al, 2005; Demirkesen Et Al, 2006).

As A Primary Treatment Option For Upper Tract Calculi, SWL Efficacy Ranges From 68% To 84% (Rizvi Et Al, 2003;Myers Et Al, 1995; Defoor Et Al, 2005b).

SWL Has Been A Preferred Treatment Modality For Uncomplicated Renal And Proximal Calculi Less Than Or Equal To 15 Mm In The Pediatric Population.

In A Contemporary Series Of 216 Children (Mean Age 6.6 Years) With A Mean Stone Stone Size Of 14.9 Mm And Who Were Undergoing SWL With The Dornier HM3 Lithotripter, Landau And Colleagues (2009) Reported A 3-Month Stone Free Rate Of 80%, Demonstrating That Efficacious Stone-Free Rates Can Be Achieved In Appropriate Candidates.

Complications Rate Are Minimal And Range In Severity From Hematuria And Ecchymisis To Obstruction With Sepsis (Farhat And Kropp, 2007).

Although Well Tolerated In Children, Current Stone-Free Rates With SWL Are Difficult To Interpret From The Existing Body Of Data Due To Discrepancies Between Studies Regarding Type Of Lithotripter, Numbe Of Shock Administered, And Re-Treatment Rates.

Recent Data Suggest That Stone Free Rates In Children With A History Of Urologic Condition Or Urinary Tract Reconstruction Are Quite Low (12.5%), And, With Alternative Surgical Techniques Available, Children May Be Better Served With URS Or PCNL (Nelson Et Al, 2008).

Despite Encouraging Results, SWL Has Not Been Approved By The Food And Drug Administration For Use In Children, Although It Is A Widely Accepted Treatment Modality.

SWL Procedural Technique In Children

General Anesthesia Is Administrered In A Majority Of Smaller Children To Avoid Both Patient And Stone Motion And The Need For Repeated Repositioning. With Modern Lithotripters, **Intravenous Sedation** Has Been Successfully Employed In Select Older Children (Aldridge Et Al, 2006).

Bowel Preparation Is Seldom Used In Order To Avoid Dehydration And Electrolyte Imbalance Postoperatively.

The Number Of Shocks Delivered And The Kilovoltage Used Vary Per Lithotripter, But The Current Consensus Is That Low-Power Settings (17 To 22 Kv) Should Be Used To Prevent Stone Migration During The Procedure, With 3000 Shock Waves Per Session (<2000 In Very Young Children) (Farhat And Kropp, 2007).

In A Recent Report AssessMent & Comparison, The Number And Intensity Of Shock Wave Reuired For Stone Fragmentation In 44 Children (Mean Age 5.9 Years) And 562 Adults (Mean Age 40.9 Years). With An Equivalent Number Of Session (1.1 Vs. 1.1), The Mean Number Of Shock Waves (950 Vs. 1262, P <.001) And The KV Required (11.8 Vs. 12.4, P<.001) Were Significantly Reduced In The Pediatric Cohort (Kurien Et Al, 2009).

Whether Or Not To Place A Ureteral Stent Prior To ESWL In Children Remains Controversial And Is A Matter Of Personal Preference.
It Is Currently Unclear If Placement Of A Ureteral Stent Prior To SWL Facilities Fragment Passage And Improves Stone-Free Outcomes. Although Pre-Stenting Rates Are Not Consistent Across Series.

Current Relative Indications Include Cases Of Solitary Kidneys, Staghorn Calculi, Obstruction, Or Abnormal Anatomy And Are Not Based On Total Stone Burdern.
Ureteral Catheters With Retrograde Opacification Are Occasionally Employed By Some To Aid In The **Localization Of Radiolucent Calculi**.

Stone Size, Location, Composition, And Patient Age

Although **Early Series** Focused Primarily On The Feasibility, Safety, And Efficacy Of SWL In Children,
Recent Effort Are For Identifying Demographic, Anatomic, And Stone-Related Prognostic Factors For Treatment For Upper Tract Calculi Less Than Or Equal To 15 Mm In Children (Farhat And Kropp, 2007),
But Evidence Supporting This Stone Size CutOff Is Lacking. Ather And Noor (2003).

Recently, Shouman And Colleagues (2009) Reported On A Series Of Stone-Free And Complication Rates As 83.3% And 25%, Respectively. **Although It Is Possible To Treat Very Large Stone Burdens With SWL,** Concerns Include The Necessity Of More Shock Treatments, More Frequent Re-Treatment Session, And Increased Risk Of Postoperative Obstruction.
Further Study Delineating **A Clear Size Cutoff** For Uncompleted Upper

Tract Stone Burden The Most Effective First-Line Therapy For Renal Calculi Between 1 And 1.5 Cm.

Renal Anatomy And Stone Location

The Most Effective Management Of **Lower Pole Calculi In Children** Has Yet To Be Determined. Stone-Free Rates From Initial Small Retrospective SWL Series Range From 56 % To 61% (Ozgur Tan Et, Al, 2003; Onal Et Al, 2004).

SWL Failure And Re-Treatment Rates Were Associated With **Increased Mean Stone Burden** (Ozgur Tan Et Al, 2003), **And An Infundibulopelvic Angle Greater Than 45 Degree** (Ozgur Tan Et Al, 2003)

Staghorn Calculi Are Uncommon In Children And Represent A Management Challenge. Although Monotherapy Success Rates Are Low In Adults, Acceptable Stone-Free Rates In Children Have Been Achieved With SWL.
Al-Busaidy And Colleagues (2003) Reported An Overall Stone-Free Rate Of 79%. Although Stent Placement Did Not Affect Stone-Free Rates, They Found That Stent Placement Significantly Reduced The Major Complication Rate.
The Superior Success Rates With SWL Monotherapy Inchildren Compared With Adults Have Been Attributed To Softer Stone Composition, Smaller Relative Stone Volume, Increased Ureteral Compliance To Accommodate Stone Fragments, And Smaller Body Volume To Facilitate Stock Transmission.

SWL Safety And Efficacy Have Been Demonstrated Even In Very Young Children. Mclorie And Colleagues (2003) & In Most Pediatric Series, Although Ureteral Stenting Is More Commonly Employed To Aid In Stone Localization And Clearance (Myers Et Al, 1995) .

Treatment Of Mid To Distal Ureteral Calculi Had Historically Been Avoided In Children Due To Difficulties With Localization Over The **Sacroiliac Joint** And Concern Regarding Possible Injury To **Developing Reproductive Systems.**
The Greater And Lesser Sciatic Foramen Has Been Explored As A Potential Blast Path To Treat Distal Stones In Children.

SWL Success By Stone Composition Is Similar Between The Adult And Pediatric Populations, **Cystine Stones** Are Uniquely Challenging Due To Their Durability And High Recurrence Rates.
Although SWL Monotherapy Has Demonstrated Variable Results In

Adults, There Are Few Reports In The Pediatric Population.
Slavkovic And Colleagues (2002) Reported A 50% Stone-Free Rate In 6 Children With A Cystine Stone Burden Ranging From 0.2 To 2.5 Cm. Although Stone-Free Rates Were Low, Fragmentation Was Achieved In 100% Of Patients, And The Stone Dissolution Was Achieved With Medical Therapy In The Remaining Children Following SWL.
Farhat And Kropp, 2007 Have Proposed That Cystine Stones Formed Within 2 Years Of Therapy May Be More Easily Fragmented With SWL And That Stone Number, And Not Diameter,
May Be More Predictive Of Success

Limitation And Concerns

In Children, There Is **Currently No Consensus** Regarding The **Maximum Size Of Residual Stone Fragments (RF)** That Are Considered Clinically Significant, And As A Result, There Is No Clear Definition As To What Constitutes " **Stone-Free" Status**
(Wu And Docimo, 2004; Farhat And Kropp, 2007).

Although Children Have Been Shown To Have A **Greater Capacity To Clear Fragment That Adults** (Gofrit Et Al, 2001),
The **Presence Of RFs** Have Been Correlated With Adverse Clinical Outcomes (Afshar Et Al, 2004).
Afshar And Colleagues (2004) Followed Series -Asymptomatic With No Fragment Growth, Adverse Clinical Outcomes, Including RF Growth Or Clinical Symptoms. Patients &The Presence Of Metabolic Disorders Was Associated With RF Growth (Afshar Et Al, 2004).
For These Reasons, **Metabolic Evaluations** Are Now Routinely Being Performed In Children With A History Of Calculi, And Every Attempt Should Be Made To Achieve Stone-Free Status.

Although **SWL Is Well Tolerated In Children** With Few Complications, Stone-Free Rates Following Single-Session Monotherapy Can Remain As Low As 44% (Muslumanoglu Et Al, 2003).
As A Result, Children Are Subjected To Multiple Treatments Requiring General Anesthesia (Aldridge Et Al, 2006).
The Need For Multiple Treatment Sessions Is Concerning, Because The Effects Of Shock Waves On Renal Tissue Are Unclear. A Growing Body Of Evidence In Adults Indicates That Shock Waves Result In Renal Vessel Vasoconstriction And That Renal Tubular Injury And Subcapsular Hematoma From Cavitation And Shear Forces Are Dependent On The Kilovoltage Applied (Lingeman Et Al, 2003).
In A Large Series Of Adult Patients With A Mean Follow-Up Of 19 Years Post –SWL, (Krambeck And Colleagues Mellitus Related To Bilateral Treatment, Number Of Administered Shocks, And Treatment Intensity.

Although These Results Are Concerning, **Difference Between Pediatric And Adult Populations And Limitations** Inherent To A Questionnaire-Based Retrospective Study Make Application Of These Data In Children Difficult.

Retrospective Studies With Limited Follow-Up In Children Have Reported That SWL And PCNL Do Not Cause **Renal Morphologic Or Functional Alteration As Measured By Glomerular Flow Rate (GFR) And Serial Dimercaptosuccinic Acid (DMSA) Functional Studies** (Wadhwa Et Al, 2007),
But Long-Term Data Are Unavailable To Date. To Eliminate Confounding Variables And Fully Address The Risks Of Chronic Renal Damage From SWL, Long-Term Prospective Data In Children Are Clearly Required.

Research Directions-The Questions Which Have Not Been Answered Are Those Which Will Have To Be Studies Over A Long Time Period. **Pre- And Postithotripsy Functional Studies Will Have Be Examined In Detail, As Will Any Potential Effect On Renal Growth And Possible Damage To Surrounding Tissues.** The Vexed Question Of Hypertension Also Remains Unsolved. It Would Appear That, In The Short Term, Studies Will Need To Be Performed Before The Anxieties Are Put To Rest.

STONE DISEASE DURING PREGNANCY

Incidence Of Symtomatic Urinary Calculii Has Been Calculated To Be The Same For Pregnant Women As For Non Pregnant Women Of Child Bearing Age (Coe et al, 1978Hendricks et al.1991).

The Acute Evaluation Of A Pregnant Women With Suspected Renal Colic NeedsThrough **Clinical History And Physical Examination**.
Presenting Symptoms Include- Vague Abdominal Pain, Unexplained Fevers, Recurrent Urinary Tract Infections, Persistent Bacteriuria, Or Microscopic Hematuria.

A CareFul **Previous History Of Nephrolithiasis** Is Important,
As The Increased Dilation Of The Ureters During Pregnancy May Increase The Risk, For A Preformed Stone Attempt To Pass During Pregnancy.

Upper Tract Dilatation Is Seen InUpto 90% Of Pregnant Women By The Third Trimester And May Persist For As Long As 12 Weeks Post-Partum(Boridy et al, 1996).

The Right Ureter Tends To Be More Dilated Than The Left & The Dilatation Rarely Is Observed Distal To Pelvic Brim(ShulMan & Herlinger.1975).

Humoral As Well As Mechanical Factors Have Been Implicated For The Etiology Of HydroNephrosis In Pregnant Women. The Circulating Progesterone, A Humoral Factor, Increased During Pregnancy, Causes Relaxation Of Ureteric Smooth Muscles & Reduce Peristalsis.

The Normal Range Of Serum Creatinine And Blood Urea Nitrogen Are Approximately 25% For The Pregnant Patient.

Renal Plasma Flow & GFR Increases.The Filtered Load Of Sodium, Calcium & Uric Acid, Causing A State Of HyperCalciuria & HyperUricosuria (Boyle et al,1966;Howarth et al,1977;Gertner et al,1986).
HyperCalciuria Further Exacerbation Due To Suppression Of Para-Thyroid Hormone & Increase In Circulating 1,25-DiHydroxy CholeCalciferol Produced By Placenta, Increases Intestinal Absorption of Calcium.

24 Hour Urine Chemistries Performed Amongst Pregnant Women, Elevated Urinary ph Is Demostrable, More Dramatically During Second TriMester(Resim et al, 2006).
Urine-Analysis- Signs Of Active Urinary Tract Infection May Be Present.

These **Potentially Lithogenic PhysioLogic Changes** Are OffSet By An Increase In The Excretion Of Urinary IInhibitors Such As Citrates & Magnesium, As WellAs Increase In Urine OutPut(Biyani & Joyce, 2002).

It Has Been Postulated That Metabolic Alterations In The Urine May Contribute To The **Accelarated Encustation Of Ureteral Stents** During Pregnancy(Denstedt &Razvi, 1992;LoughLin.1994).

Ross & Asociates(2000) Reported That, Stones During Pregnancy Are **Calcium Phosphate** In Composition, Explained By Relatively Elevated Urinary Ph & HyperCalciuria Occuring During Pregnancy.

During First Trimester, The Period Of Early OrganoGenesis & Rapid Cell Division, The Embryo Is Sensitive To The Effects Of Radiation(Swartz & ReichLing. 1978).

AlThough The Foetus Has Diminished Sensitivity To The TeraTogenic Effects Of Radiation In The II & III Trimester, Such Exposures May Increase The Risk For DevelopMent Of ChildHood Malignant NeoPlasia(Harvey et al. 1985).

Essentials Of Litho-Tripsy

USG Ultrasonography Is The Standard Initial Imaging Study In Evaluation Of A Pregnant Patient Thought To Be Experiencing Renal Colic.
Horrigan & Associates,1996 Reported That **Renal Resistive Index** Remains Unchanged From The NonPregnant State ThroughOut The Course Of Pregnancy & Also Is UnAffected By The PhysioLogic HydroNephrosis Of PregNancy, Suggesting The UseFullNess Of USG Modality For Detection Of Acute Obstructive Lesions In This Population.
Trans Vaginal USG Can Provide Imaging Of The Distal Ureter.

Intra-Venous PyeloGraphy If Needed, Limited Study Is Recommended.
Conventional CT Should Be Avoided During Pregnancy,
As The Radiation Dose Is Particularly High.

Radiation Exposure To The Fetus Should Be Avidly Avoided. Therefore, Ultrasongraphy Has Become The First Line Imaging Study To Search For Calculi During Pregnancy. Although This Modality Provides Adequate Images Of The Kidney, It Can Be Difficult To Fully Discern The Ureters And Their Contents. In Addition, Hydronephosis From And Obstructing Calculus. **Limited Intravenous Pyelography May Be Performed That Consists Of One Scout Image Followed By One Plate Taken Approximaterly 30 Minutes After The Injection Of Contrast Material. Each Plain Film Exproses The Fetus To 0.1 To 0.2 Rad, Well Below The Threshold Of 1.2 Rad, When The Risk Begins To Increase.** Radiation Exposure Should Be Particularly Avoided In The First Trimester During The Time Of Organogenesis And The Greatest Fetal Risk.
Treatment Urinary Calculi During Pregnancy:

- Ultrasonography Is The Standard Initial Imaging Study In Evaluation Of A Pregnant Patient.
- Improvements In Ureteroscopy Technology Now Permit Ureterscopic Access To And Treatment Of Stones At Any Location In The Collecting System Of The Pregnant Patient.
- It Is Important To Minimize Ionizing Radiation Exposure To The Pregnant Patient During Ureteroscopy By Use A Below Table X-Ray Source And To Shield The Fetus With A Lead Apron Placed Below The Patient.

Approximaterly 66% To 85% Of Pregnant Women With Ureteric Colic Spontaneously Pass The Calculi When They Are Treated Conservatively With Hydration, Analgesics, And, If Infected, Antibiotics (Jones Et Al, 1979; Stothers And Lee, 1992) Some Studies Have Demonstrated Increased Encrustation Of Stents, Requiring Frequent Changes. In Some Instances The Stents Migrated Down The Ureter Because Of The Physiologic Dilation (Stothers And Lee, 1992) . Stents Are

Often Exchanged Every 4 To 6 Weeks To Avoid Excessive Encrustation And The Risk Of Obstruction.

Since Many Expectant Mothers Take Calcium Supplementation, A More Stone-Friendly Form Of This Mineral Has Been Developed (Citra Cal Prenatal Rx). In This Formulation, Calcium Is Bound To Citrate, Which Delivers Extra Stone Inhibitor Into The Urine, Thereby Offsetting The Effects Of Worsening Absorptive Hyper Calciuria. Iron And Foliate Are Also Added To Complete The Elements Commonly Found In Prenatal Multivitamin Supplements. Although There Are No Randomized Data To Support To Use Of This Supplement, Its Use Does Make Intuitive Sense For Patients At Risk For Recurrent Calculi During Pregnancy.
A Full Decussion Of The Surgical Management Of Calculi During Pregnancy Is Beyond The Scope Of This Chapter. **There Is Growing Evidence, Though, That Ureteroscopy, With Holmium Laser Lithotripsy Performed Laterduring Pregnancy, Is Safe And Free Of Increased Risk** (Lifshitz And Lingeman, 2002; Watterson Et Al, 2002). Indeed, The Dedinitive Nature Of One Uncomplicated Urereroscopy Probably Represents Less Risk Than The Anesthesia Associated With Multiple Stent Changes Plus The Infectious Risk Of An Indwelling Foreign Body.

CYSTINE CALCULI

The Management Of Cystine Calculi Presented A Therapeutic Challenge To The Urologist Over The Years. Cystine Stones Are A Feature Of Cystinuria, Which Is An **Inherited Disorder Characterized By Abnormalities In Renal Handling Of Cystine, Ornithine, Arginine And Lysine**. Only The High Concentration Of Cystine In The Urine Gives Rise To Trouble, As It Is The Only One Of These Four Which Precipitates In The Urine, Thus Giving Rise To Urinary Calculi.
Much Important Work Has Been Performed Into The Urinary Excretion Of Cystine And Its Solubility Characteristics; These Have Resulted In The Knowledge That A High Fluid Intake Associated With A Maximally Alkalinized Urine Can Increase The Solubility Of Cystine.

The X-Ray Appearance Of Such Stones On The Straight Addominal X-Ray Is Described As **Ground Glass**. In Addition, Bony Structures Such As The Ribs Can Be Seen Through The Stone, And These Characteristic Enable A Reasonably Confident Diagnosis Of Cystine Calculi To Be Made On The Straight Abdominal X-Ray,
It Is This Very **Semiopaque Nature Of The Stones** That Makes Them **Difficult To Localize** Within The Kidney, Needing Contrast Radiology For Proper Assessment.

Essentials Of Litho-Tripsy

With The Introduction Of **Various Types Of Energy To Fragment Calculi**, The Difficulties Have Become Compounded By The **Crystal Structure Of Cystine Calculi** Render Them Resistant To Fragmentation By The Various Types Of Energy.

The Basic Management Of Cystine Calculi Rests On The Use Of Hydration And Alkalinization. The Urine Ph Should Be Kept At Eight Or Less Because Of The Risk Of Precipitation Of Calcium With Higher Levels Of Alkalinization.
D-Penicillamine (Crawhall Et Al 1963) And Alpha- Mercptopropionylglycine (Hautmann Et Al 1977, Pak Et Al 1986) Have Been Helpful In The Management Of These Patients By Markedly Increasing The Solubility Of Cystine.
Attempts Have Been Made To **Break Down Cysline Stones By Irrigation** And Although Success Has Been Reported In Vitro, To Date Their Value In Vivo Remains Uncertain.
There Has Been Much Discussion On The Variable Results Achieved With The Use Of Energy In **The Fragmentation Of Cystine Calculii**, Unfortunately, **Ultrasound, Electrohydraulic Lithotripsy, The Laser And And ESWL Are Disappointing.**
The Reason For The Poor Fragmentation Of Cystine Stones Is Not Completely Under Stood, But It May Be Related To The Crystal Structure Of The Stone. The Calculi Having A Uniform Crystal Structure Were Least Fragile And Those With A Smooth External Surface Share The Same Characteristic; Stones With A Rough External Surface Were More Fragile And Responded Better To EDWL (Dretler 1988, Bhatta Et Al 1989).

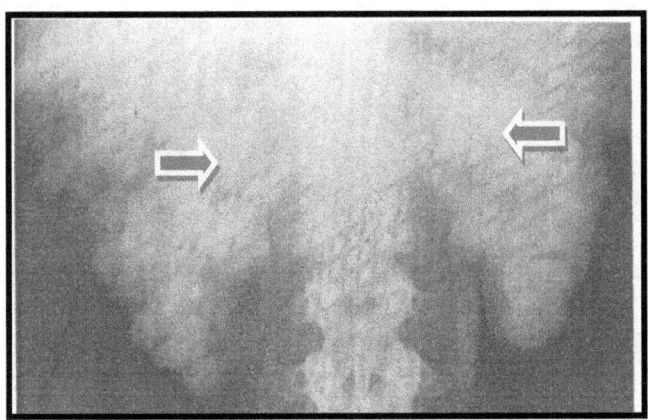

"B/L Renal Cystine Stones"

If There Is A Stone Causing Obstruction, Then It Is Best To Insert A Nephrostomy Tube, Or To Bypass The Stone With A Double Pigtail Stent.

Subsequent Attempts Should Be Made To Disintegrate The Stone With Either Ultrasound, Electro Hydraulic Lithotripsy, The Laser, Or ESWL.
If These Methods Fail To Remove The Stone, Open Surgical Removal May Be Necessary
This Is Particularly Frustrating In The Case Of Single Cytinuria Stone, But In Many Cases Of Cytinuria The Stones Are Multiple And Bilateral And May Be Associated With Deteriorating Renal Function.
All Of These Eventualities May Justify Open Surgery Because Of The Rather Urgent Need To Remove Obstructing Stones
And Thus Improve The Patient's Renal Status.

TRANSPLANTED KIDNEYS CALCULII

Calculi May Developent In A Transplanted Kidney Although Is An Uncommon Occurrence, As May Be Cause Of A Significant Loss Of Function.The Removal Of Such Calculi Needs Removal. In The Past, **Open Surgical Excision** Of The Calculi, Was Not Only Associated With A Significant Morbidity & The Definite Possibility Of Major Loss Of Function In The Transplanted Kidney.

Percutaneous Removal Of Stones In Transplanted Kidneys Has Been Attempted Successfully (Hulbert Et Al 1986).
The Relatively Superficial Location Of The Transplanted Kidney Facilitates Percutaneous Access And Potentially Allow The Possibility For Several Percutaneous Procedures To Be Performed, WithOut Adverse Affects On Renal Function.

STONES IN AUGMENTED BLADDERS & URINARY DIVERSIONS

With The Problem That,The Intra-Abdominal Spillage Of Urine & Irrigation Can Lead To Peritonitis, OtherWise Stone Disease Management Principles, Remain Largely UnChanged For The Stones ManageMent In Augmented Bladders & Urinary Diversions.

The Various TreatMent Modalities Include-
1.TransUrethral Approach(Kronner Et al.Defoor Et Al,2004: Esperance et al.2004).
EndoScopic ManageMent Through A MitroFanoff Catheterizable Conduit Is Not Advised.

2. PerCutaneous Access For Augmented Bladders Stones Has Been Reported, Comparable To OpenCystoLithotomy.

3. Trans-Stromal Approach- SuccessFul In Some Cases, But Not Recommended For Indiana & Penn Pouch Stones, Owing To The Catheterizable Link Or Disruption At The Continence Mechanism.(Patel BelliMan1995:I Esperance et al.2004;Lann et al.2007)

TransUrethral Cystolitholapaxy & Lithotripsy
Electo-Hydraulic Energy Is Associated With A Higher Incidence Of Complications, Includind Mucosal Inury & Haematuria(Teichmann et al.1997;Lipkeet al. 2004).
Other Series Have Reported 1.6% Incidence Of Bladder Perforation,Urethral Injuries Not Recorded By Modern Series.
Holmium Laser LithoTripsy Has Become The Modality Of Choice, Owing To Its Ability To Treat Large Calculii, While Incurring A Minimum Of Collateral Damage.
ESWL Has Not Been SuccessFully Employed For The TreatMent Of Bladder Calculii.
–Patient's Position Being Prone To Eliminate Obfuscation On FluroScopy By Sacral Spine & Pelvis
-Foley's Catheter Is Introduced TO Allow Filling , Drainage Of Bladder, & Providing Fixity Of The Stone During Fragmentation.Although This Method Is Not Adopted By All Authors.(Bhatia & Biyani;1994).
CystoScopic Evacuation Of Stone Fragmentation Is Necessary For Larger Calculii(Bosco & Nich, 1991).
Per Session 1000 To 4800 Shocks Are Generally Required To Produce Adequate Fragmentation & Re-Treatment Is Necessary In 10-25% Cases(Bosco & Nich, 1991).
OverAll Success Rate By ESWL Ranges Between 93-100%(Bosco & Nich;Milan-Rodriguez et al. 2005).
For Subsequent Recurrence Of U.B Stones Treated By Any Method, Bladder OutLet Obstruction Relief Is Imperative.

CONCURRENT RENAL AND URETERIC CALCULI

The Patients With A Calcus In The Ureter And One Or More Calculi Con- Currently In The Kidney, May Present A Therapeutic Dilemma (Fig. 7.4) .
The Basic Principles In The Management Of Ureteric Stones Remains The Same. Evidence Of Infected Urine Proximal To The Stone, Or Pyrexia Or A Tender Palpable Kidney, It Is Preferable To Insert A Percutaneous Nephrostomy Before Contemplating Any Definitive Treatment.
Urine Taken From The Nephrostomy Tube Can Be Sent For Culture And Sensitivity And Appropriate Antibiotic Therapy Instituted. This Is Preferable.To The Attempted Passage Of A Ureteric Catheter As A

Defunctioning Procedure, Requires An Anaesthetic And, If The Stone Is Impacted, May Traumatize The Ureter.
After Insertion Of The Nephrostomy Drainage Tube And Without Any Major Delay, Attention Can Be Directed To The Stones.

If It Is Intended To Treat All Of The Stones With ESWL And A Nephrostomy Tube Is In Place, The Ureteric Stone And Renal Stone Can Be Treated At The Same Session.
If There Is No Clinical Infection And No Requirement For A Nephrostomy Tube, The Stone Burden Must Be Assessed Carefully, For Anticipated Obstruction Developing Following Treatment,
A Double –Pigtail Stent Or DJS Insertion May Be Needed To Overcome This. If A Stent Cannot Be Passed, The Ureteric Stone Should Be Treated In The First Instance By ESWL .
If This Cannot Be Done The Push-Bang'technique Can Be Employed For The Ureteric Stone, And The Renalstone (S) Treated Subsequently.

It Is Also Possible To Treat The Ureteric Stone Ureteroscopically In Situ And The Renal Stone By ESWL At The Same Treatment Session, With The Likelihood Of Excellent Results (Jarowenko Et Al 1989).

THE MANAGEMENT OF THE OBESE PATIENT

Treatment Of The Obese Patient, By Any Type Of Stone Management, May Give Rise To Certain Problems.
Open Surgical Removal The Fatty Addominal Apron Tended To Slide Forwards With The Patient Places Laterally On The Table,
Always A Large Perirenal Fat Collection Under Gerota's Fascia, Which Bled Easily And Made Exposure Of The Kidney Rather Difficult;
This Is Particularly The Case When Trying To Identify The Smaller Vessels At The Upper Or Lower Poles Of The Kidney.
In Addition, The Large Collection Of Fat In The Renal Sinus Made If Difficult To Define The Plane Which Must Be Entered For The Extended Sinus Approach To The Renal Pelvis.
Post Operatively Such Patients Has Difficulty With Chest Complications And, In Some Cases, Deep Venous Thrombosis.

With The Introduction Of **Endourology**,
These Difficulties Did Not Lessen.
Access To The Kidney Through The Loin Was Not As Esay As In The Thinner Person, Because Of Difficulty In Assessing The Depth Of The Kidney. Once Inside The Kidney,
'Cheek-To-Cheek' Problems Arose; That Is To Say, The Cheek Of The Operator Resting Against The Buttock Of The Patient, Preventing The Required Angulation In Order To Reach The Upper Aspects Of The Kidney.

Essentials Of Litho-Tripsy

The Depth Of Insertion Of The Amplatz Sheath Might Also Give Cause For Concern With The Proximal End Of The Sheath Often Being Flush With The Patients Skin.

For **Ureteroscopy** Positioning The Patient In The Lithotomy Position Is Also Difficult.
The Increased Fat In The Patients Thighs Make It Difficult To Enter The Intramural Ureter At The Required Angle,
And This Often Means That The Leg Of The Patient Opposite To The Ureter In Question Must Be Lifted By The Assistant.

By **ESWL** Problems May Also Be Noticed In Managing The Obese Patient Because Of The Increased Thickness Of The Abdominal Wall It May Be Difficult To Position The Patient,
With The Stone Always Being Too High For The Focal Point Of The Shock Wave. It May Be Necessary To Turn The Patient Prone In Order To Perform This Satisfactorily.

Obese Patients Typically Have Poor Outcomes With Lithotripsy, And Treatment Often Fails In Cases In Which The Skin-To-Stone Distance Is Greater Than 9–10 Cm.[29] When The Skin-To-Stone Distance Is Large, The Stone Cannot Be Positioned Precisely At The Focal Point Of The Lithotripter Without Inverting The Cushion Of The Treatment Head—A Situation Almost Certain To Produce Very Poor Coupling. Data On The Trade-Off Between Coupling And Positioning Of The Stone Along The Axis Of A Lithotripter In Obese Patients Have Never Been Reported,
Although Tellingly A Recent Study Found No Effect Of Skin-To-Stone Distance When Using The HM3, A Lithotripter For Which Coupling Is Not An Issue. With Many Lithotripters, However, The Stone Can Be Broken Even If It Is Positioned Distal To The Focal
Point.
Indeed, For Some Lithotripters, Such As The Lithogold LG-380, Breakage Is Actually Best Several Centimeters Distal To The Focus.
Thus, The Obese Patient Presents At Least Two Potential Problems: Overcoming Ineffective Coupling; And Ensuring That The Stone Is Accurately Localized Along The Acoustic Axis. Perhaps A Typical Dry Treatment Head Could Be Fitted With A Partial Water Bath (An Attractive Feature Of The Storz SLX). As For Targeting When The Focal Point Falls Proximal To The Stone, A Positive Step Would Be An Algorithm To Aid Alignment So That The Stone Lies On The Acoustic Axis.
It Is Clear That Even With The Introduction Of New Treatment Modalities For The Management Of Urinary Caluli, Obese Patients May Present Their Own Individual Problems As Outlined Above. Although These May Make The Treatment Difficult, They Do Not Make It Impossible And Can In Virtually Every Case Be Overcome.

References

Pareek G, et al. Extracorporeal shock wave lithotripsy success based on body mass index and Hounsfield units. Urology. 2005;65:33–36. [PubMed]

Jacobs BL, Smaldone MC, Smaldone AM, Ricchiuti DJ, Averch TD. Effect of skin-to-stone distance on shockwave lithotripsy success. J Endourol. 2008;22:1623–1628. [PubMed]

Whelan JP, Finlayson B, Welch J, Newman RC. The blast path: theoretical basis, experimental data and clinical application. J Urol. 1988;140:401–404. [PubMed]

Pishchalnikov YA, et al. Strategies to improve SWL for obese patients: *in vitro* assessment of targeting stones along the distal acoustic axis [abstract #1626] J Urol. 2009;181 (4 Suppl):585.

SPECIAL CONSIDERATIONS

ANTI-MICROBIAL THERAPY-
Patients With Risk Of Endocarditis- The Risk Of EndoCarditis After Urologic Procedures Is Low; HowEver The urinary Tract Is The Second Common Site Of Organisms That Cause EndoCarditis(Dajani et al.1997). NoneTheLess , The 2007 American Heart Associatio's UpDated GuideLines, No Longer Recommend Anti-Microbial Prophylaxis, Solely To Prevent Infectious EndoCarditis
Patients With InDwelling OrthoPaedic HardWare- In General Anti-Microbial Prophylaxis For Urologic Patients With Total Joint Replacements, Pin Plates, Or Screws Is Not Indicated. Prophylaxis Is Advised For Individuals At Higher Risk Of Seeding A Prosthetic Joint, Including These With Recently Inserted Implants.
HowEver American Urological Association & The American Academy Of OrthoPaedic Surgeons & Infectious Disease Specialist,2013 Issued Advisory StateMent- AntiMicrobial Prophylaxis For Urological Patients With Total Joint ReplaceMent.

(2.)(vi.) SUPPORTIVE MEASURES
(A) UROLITHIASIS MEDICAL THERAPY REGIMES

Management
Stone Size Influences The Rate Of Spontaneous Stone Passage.
Up To 98% Of **Small Stones** (Less Than 5 Mm (0.20 In) In Diameter) May Pass Spontaneously Through Urination Within Four Weeks Of The Onset Of Symptoms,
But **For Larger Stones** (5 To 10 Mm (0.20 To 0.39 In) In Diameter), The Rate Of Spontaneous Passage Decreases To Less Than 53%.
Initial Stone Location Also Influences The Likelihood Of Spontaneous Stone Passage. Rates Increase From 48% For Stones Located In The Proximal Ureter To 79% For Stones Located At The Vesicoureteric Junction, Regardless Of Stone Size.
Assuming **No High-Grade Obstruction Or Associated Infection Is Found In The Urinary Tract,** And Symptoms Are Relatively Mild, Various Nonsurgical Measures Can Be Used To Encourage The Passage Of A Stone.
Repeat Stone Formers Benefit From More Intense Management, Including Proper Fluid Intake And Use Of Certain Medications.
In Addition, Careful Surveillance Clearly Is Required To Maximize The Clinical Course For People Who Are Stone Formers.

Analgesia
Management Of Pain Often Requires Intravenous Administration Of Nsaids Or Opioids.
Orally Administered Medications Are Often Effective For Less Severe Discomfort.
Role Of Spasmolytic(Buscopan, Drotaverine) Drugs Alone Or In Combination With NSAIDS.
An Alpha Blocker, Relaxes The Muscles In Ureter, Helping To Pass The Kidney Stone More Quickly And With Less Pain.

MEDICAL THERAPY- **Commonly Used Preparations:**

Zyloric (Allopurinol) - For **Uricemia** (S. Uric Acid ≥7 Mg%) Decreases S. Uric Acid And Thus Disintegrating Uric Acid (Invisible) Component Of Stones,

Various Other Ayurvedic Preparations: Cystone, Neeri, Distone, Calcury, Smash, Expel, Nephrol Etc.
& Commonly Available Urinary Alkalizers.

Tamsulosin (0.4) OD (Breakfast): Relieving Lower Urinary Tract Syndrome, Obstructive Uropathy Symptoms, Thus Facilitating Downward Stone Movement And Passage With Urine, (1-5)

Supported By Mefenamic Acid And Drotaverine
Preparations (Tab. Drotin-M Etc.).
Aminophylline, Nifedipine Deflazacort, And Other Hormonal Preparations Role Have Been Reported.

Medications for Kidney Stones
Medications By Control Of The Level Of Urinary Acidity Or Alkalinity & May Be Helpful In People Who Form Certain Kinds Of Stones.

The Type Of Medication Prescription Depends On The Kidney Stones Variety:
Calcium Stones. To Help Prevent Calcium Stones Formation, **Thiazide Diuretic Or A Phosphate-Containing** Preparation Are Prescribed.

Uric Acid Stones. Administering **Allopurinol (Zyloric, Zyloprim, Aloprim)** To Reduce Uric Acid Levels In Blood And Urine **And A Urine Alkalizer**, Can Dissolve The Uric Acid Stones.

Struvite Stones. Prevention Recommended Strategy Is **To Keep Urine Sterile. Long-Term Use Of Antibiotics In Small Doses** May Be Useful To Achieve This Goal.

Cystine Stones. Can Be Difficult To Treat.
Urine Alkalizer Are Prescribed To **Bind The Cystine In The Urine,** In Addition To Recommending An **Extremely High Urine Output**.

Chelating Agents Are Present In **Normal Urine**,
Such As **Citrate**, That Inhibit The Nucleation, Growth & Aggregation Of **Calcium-Containing Crystals**.

Other Endogenous Inhibitors Include;
Calgranulin (An S-100 Calcium Binding Protein),
Tamm-Horsfall Protein,
Glycosaminoglycans,
Uropontin (A Form Of Osteopontin),
Nephrocalcin (An Acidic Glycoprotein),
Prothrombin F1 Peptide,
And Bikunin (Uronic Acid-Rich Protein).

The Biochemical Mechanisms Of Action Of These Substances Have Not Yet Been Thoroughly Elucidated. However, When These Substances

Essentials Of Litho-Tripsy

Fall Below Their Normal Proportions, Stones Can Form By Aggregation Of Crystals.   (5-10)

Sufficient Dietary Intake Of Magnesium And Citrate, Inhibits Calcium Oxalate And Calcium Phosphate Stones Formation;
In Addition, Magnesium And Citrate Operate Synergistically To Inhibit Kidney Stones. **Magnesium's Efficacy** In Subduing Stone Formation And Growth Is Dose-Dependent.

Drug Treatment   (10-14)
The High Rate Of Renal Stone Disease Recurrences,
Necessitates Medical Preventive Programmes Strategies, Regularly Evaluated By Randomized, Double-Blind, Placebo-Controlled Trials To Validate The Efficacy Of Such Programmes.

The Paucity Of Drug Trials Can Be Ascribed To Several Factors:
(i) Patient Compliance Is Low Because Of The Absence Of Symptoms Between Stone Episodes;
(ii) Stone Disease Is Heterogeneous And The Course Is Unpredictable, Requiring Long Treatment Periods And A Follow-Up Of At Least 5 Years To Show Any Beneficial Effect;
(iii) A Sufficient Sample Size Is Necessary To Compare Treated And Untreated Control Patients; Both Groups Must Have A Similar Risk Profile;
(iv) The Effect Of A Single Drug Has To Be Compared With Placebo Without Associated Dietary Intervention Which Would Be A Potential Confounder.
Despite The Potential Merit Of Conservative Treatment Involving Just Diet And Fluid Intake Modification ie.The So-Called **Stone Clinic Effect** Only Fluid Intake Has Been Validated By A Prospective Study.
For Ethical Purposes, Placebo Groups Of Most Trials Generally Receive Diet And /Or Fluid Recommendations.

Urine Alkalinization

The Mainstay For Medical **Management Of Uric Acid Stones** Is **Alkalinization (Increasing The Ph) Of The Urine**.
Uric Acid Stones Are Among The Few Types Amenable To **'Dissolution Therapy' (Chemolysis)**,
Usually Achieved Through The Use Of Oral Medications, Although In Some Cases, Intravenous Agents Or Even Instillation Of Certain Irrigating Agents Directly Onto The Stone Can Be Performed, Using Antegrade Nephrostomy Or Retrograde Ureteral Catheters.

Acetazolamide (Diamox) Is A Medication That Alkalinizes The Urine.
In Addition To Acetazolamide Or As An Alternative,

Certain Dietary Supplements Are Available That Produce A Similar Alkalinization Of The Urine,
Including Sodium Bicarbonate, Potassium Citrate, Magnesium Citrate, And Bicitra (A Combination Of Citric Acid Monohydrate &Sodium Citrate Dihydrate).
Aside From Alkalinization Of The Urine, These Supplements Have The **Added Advantage Of Increasing The Urinary Citrate Level**,
Which Helps To Reduce The Aggregation Of Calcium Oxalate Stones.[27]

Increasing The Urine Ph To Around 6.5,
Provides Optimal Conditions For **Dissolution Of Uric Acid Stones**.
Increasing The Urine Ph To A Value Higher Than 7.0,
Increases The Risk Of **Calcium Phosphate Stone Formation**.
Testing The Urine Periodically With Nitrazine Paper Can Help To Ensure The Urine Ph Remains In This Optimal Range.
Using This Approach, Stone Dissolution Rate Can Be Expected To Be Around 10 Mm (0.39 In) Of Stone Radius Per Month.

Potassium Citrate
Reduces Urinary Saturation Of Calcium Salts By Complexing Calcium And Reducing Ionic Calcium Concentration.

Due To Its Alkalinizing Effect, It Also Increases The Dissociation Of Uric Acid, Lowers The Amount Of Poorly Soluble Undissociated Uric Acid And **Reduces The Propensity To Form Uric Acid Stones**.

The Decrease Of Urinary Calcium During The Early Period Of Treatment Represents A Promising Additional Advantage Of The Drug.
Potassium Citrate Is Preferable To Sodium Citrate In The Prevention Of Urolithiasis. The Former Has Been Shown To Decrease The Stone Formation Rate In A Randomized Placebo-Controlled Study Involving 18 Patients With Low Citrate Excretion Who Received 45 Meq/Day Of Citrate For 3 Years However, Adverse Effects Of Gastrointestinal Origin Including Epigastric Pain, Abdominal Distention Or Diarrhoea Are Common.
Promising Results With The Use Of **Newer *Citrate Salts* Such As Potassium-Magnesium**, Not Yet Approved By The Food And Drug Administration, Have Also Been Shown In Patients With Idiopathic Calcium Oxalate Nephrolithiasis Irrespective Of Baseline Urinary Biochemistry.

Diuretics
One Of The Recognized Medical Therapies For Prevention Of Stones Is The Thiazide And Thiazide-Like Diuretics, Such As Chlorthalidone Or Indapamide.
These Drugs Inhibit The **Formation Of Calcium-Containing Stones By Reducing Urinary Calcium Excretion**. Sodium Restriction Is Necessary For Clinical Effect Of Thiazides, As Sodium Excess Promotes Calcium

Excretion. Thiazides Work Best For **Renal Leak Hypercalciuria** (High Urine Calcium Levels), A Condition In Which High Urinary Calcium Levels Are Caused By A Primary Kidney Defect. Thiazides Are Useful For Treating **Absorptive Hypercalciuria**, A Condition In Which High Urinary Calcium Is A Result Of Excess Absorption From The Gastrointestinal Tract.

Thiazide

Thiazides Lower Urine Calcium Resulting In A Fall In Calcium Oxalate And Calcium Phosphate Supersaturation.
Two Double-Blind, Randomized, Prospective And Placebo-Controlled Trials, One Involving 25 Patients Given Hydrochlorthiazide, 25 Mg/Day , And Another Involving 42 Patients Given Chlorthalidone, 25 Or 50 Mg/Day Documented A Significantly Lower Rate Of Recurrence After 3 Years (Up To 25%) Compared To Placebo (Up To 55%). Interestingly, These Studies Were Performed In Patients Not Categorized According To Urinary Lithogenic Ions. The Response To Therapy Was Independent Of Baseline Urinary Biochemistry.
We And Others Have Documented The Additional Benefits Of Thiazides On Bone Mass In Small Series.
On The Other Hand, Adverse Effects (Often Dosage Related) Such As Sexual Impotence, Potassium Wasting, Raised Serum Cholesterol And Glucose Tolerance, Are Reported In Almost 23% Of Cases.

Allopurinol

For People With Hyperuricosuria And Calcium Stones, Allopurinol **Is One Of The Few Treatments That Have Been Shown To** Reduce Kidney Stone Recurrences.
Allopurinol Interferes With The Production Of Uric Acid In The Liver. **The Drug Is Also Used In People With** Gout **Or Hyperuricemia (High Serum Uric Acid Levels).**
Dosage Is Adjusted To Maintain A Reduced Urinary Excretion Of Uric Acid. Serum Uric Acid Level At Or Below 6 Mg/100 Ml) Is Often A Therapeutic Goal.
Hyperuricemia Is Not Necessary For The Formation Of Uric Acid Stones; Hyperuricosuria **Can Occur In The Presence Of Normal Or Even** Low Serum Uric Acid. Some Practitioners Advocate Adding Allopurinol Only In People In Whom Hyperuricosuria And Hyperuricemia Persist, **Despite The Use Of A Urine-**Alkalinizing Agent **Such As Sodium Bicarbonate Or Potassium Citrate Inhibitors Of Stone Formation.**
Allopurinol Blocks Uric Acid Production, Reducing Heterogeneous Nucleation **Of Calcium Oxalate By Both Uric Acid And Monosodium Urate. In Addition, Uric Acid And Monosodium Urate Adsorb Normally Occurring Macromolecular Inhibitors Of Calcium Oxalate Crystallization.**
This Stone Promoting Effect Could Be Reversed By The Administration Of Allopurinol.

In The Sole Double-Blind, Placebo-Controlled Study Involving 29 Subjects Receiving Allopurinol 300 Mg Daily For 3 Years, 51% Had Fewer Recurrences Than Those Treated With Placebo. (15-19) Allopurinol Has A Low Incidence Of Side Effects, But The Drug Is Effective In Reducing Stone Recurrence Only In Calcium Oxalate Stone Formers In Whom Hyperuricosuria Is The Only Metabolic Abnormality

Other Drugs

Potassium-Acid Phosphate And Magnesium Hydroxide Were Shown To Have Little Or No Effect On The Prevention Of Stone Formation. A Neutral Potassium Phosphate Preparation Was Shown To Be Better Than Placebo In Reducing Calcium Excretion And Raising Urinary Inhibitors Of Stone Formation, Hence Inhibiting Caox Crystal Agglomeration And Spontaneous Nucleation On Brushite

The Latest Evolution In The Approach To Calcium Oxalate Stone Prevention Is To Abandon Urinary Metabolic Profiling As A Guide To Prophylaxis Both Because This Is Time-Consuming And Expensive. Furthermore Nonselective Therapy Is Effective, As Nicely Reviewed Recently

The Successful Use Of Drugs In Patients Who Have Not Been Categorized According To Different Urinary Derangements Underlines The Usefulness Of Such Approach. Besides, In A Given Subject,

The Stone Formation May Not Be Due To One Single Abnormality. Overall, Potassium Citrate Represents The Most Suitable Drug For Unselective Treatment, Because It Is Indicated For Hypocitraturia, Hypercalciuria, Hyperuricosuria And Renal Tubular Acidosis.

On The Other Hand, Identification Of Abnormal Risk Factors For Urinary Stones Is Still Important To Rule Out Secondary Causes Of Nephrolithiasis, Such As Cystinuria, Hyperoxaluria, Renal Tubular Acidosis And Infection Stones. Among All Of These Examples, Cystinuria, The Most Rare, Represents The Single Entity For Which Specific Therapy With *Tiopronin* Would Be Warranted, In Addition To The Need For Alkalinizing Therapy With Potassium Citrate As Well.

The Dissolution Of Pure Uric Acid Stones By Potassium Citrate Also Takes Place During Treatment, As Suggested In The Present Case. **The Single Contraindication To Potassium Citrate Would Be Urinary Tract Infection Because Of The Alkalinizing Properties Of The Compound.**

In Conclusion, Pain From Renal Colic Provides The Initial Motivation To The Patient To Prevent A Stone Recurrence.
Unfortunately When The Symptoms Subside, The Compliance With Dietary And Pharmacologic Regimens Often Becomes Suboptimal. Well-Designed, Large, Prospective Epidemiological Studies Performed On Healthy Subjects Have Contradicted Some Long-Held Beliefs. Adequate Long-Term Randomized Trials With Dietary

Essentials Of Litho-Tripsy

Interventions Assessing Stone Recurrence And Long-Term Measures Of Urinary Composition As End-Points, Are Difficult, But Must Nevertheless Be Performed.

(B) FORCED DIURESIS(LASIX THERAPY)

Indications-For Stones Size Up To 5-8 Mm,
　　　　　Remnant Post-ESWL Stones
　　　　　SteinaStrasse
　　　　　As Post Lithotripsy Procedure, In Difficult Stones Cases

**Complete Compliance To Following
Recommended Ideal Forced Diuresis Regimen,
Achievement Ensures Promising Good Results:**

5% DNS ≈ 1,500 ml (3 vacs) **(+)** Ringers' Lactate≈ 1,500 ml (3 vacs) (Alternating) In 24 hours.
Inj. Lasix 1 amp. Im, after (II) and (IV) Vac (Regular BP Monitoring). For 1 To 3 Days.

The Role Of Injection Drotaverine (Drotin), Hyoscine (Buscopan), Diclofenac (Voveran) Bd/Tds, Is To Achieve Round The Clock Analgesia And Spasmolytic Effect, As Needed.

The Complete Treatment Schedule Duration Varies From 1 To 4 Days. The Patient Encouraged For High Fluid Intake With Normal Diet, To Ensure About >1.5 To 2 Litres / 24 Hrs Urine Output. Straining Of All Urine Is Done To Filter Passed Stone Particles (Stone Analysis Sampling).

Expulsion therapy (20-24)
The Use Of Medications To Speed The Spontaneous Passage Of Ureteral Calculi Is Referred To As **Medical Expulsive Therapy**. Several Agents, Including Alpha Adrenergic Blockers (Such As Tamsulosin) And Calcium Channel Blockers (Such As Nifedipine), Have Been Found To Be Effective.
A Combination Of Tamsulosin And A Corticosteroid May Be Better Than Tamsulosin Alone.
These Treatments Also Appear To Be A
Useful Adjunct To Lithotripsy.

Source-© 2000 European Renal Association-European Dialysis And Transplant Association

References

1. Preminger, GM (2007). "Chapter 148: Stones in the Urinary Tract". In Cutler, RE. *The Merck Manual of Medical Information Home Edition* (3rd ed.). Whitehouse Station, New Jersey: Merck Sharp and Dohme Corporation.

2. Johri, N; Cooper B, Robertson W, Choong S, Rickards D, Unwin R (2010). "An update and practical guide to renal stone management". *Nephron Clinical Practice* 116 (3): c159–71. doi:10.1159/000317196. PMID 20606476.

3. Riley, J. M.; Kim, H.; Averch, T. D.; Kim, H. J. (Oct 2013). "Effect of Magnesium on Calcium and Oxalate Ion Binding". *J Endourol* 27 (12): 1487–92. doi:10.1089/end.2013.0173. PMID 24127630.

4. Knudsen BE, Beiko DT and Denstedt JD, *Chapter 16: Uric Acid Urolithiasis*, pp. 299–308 in Stoller and Meng (2007)

5. Coe, FL; Evan, A; Worcester, E (2005). "Kidney stone disease". *The Journal of Clinical Investigation* 115 (10): 2598–608. doi:10.1172/JCI26662. PMC 1236703. PMID 16200192.

6. del Valle, E. E.; Spivacow, F. R.; Negri, A. L. (2013). "[Citrate and renal stones]". *Medicina (B Aires)* 73 (4): 363–8. PMID 23924538.

7. Miller, NL; Lingeman, JE (2007). "Management of kidney stones". *BMJ* 334 (7591): 468–72. doi:10.1136/bmj.39113.480185.80. PMC 1808123. PMID 17332586.

8. Cormier, CM; Canzoneri BJ, Lewis DF, Briery C, Knoepp L, Mailhes JB (2006). "Urolithiasis in Pregnancy: Current Diagnosis, Treatment, and Pregnancy Complications". *Obstetrical and Gynecological Survey* 61 (11): 733–41. doi:10.1097/01.ogx.0000243773.05916.7a. PMID 17044950.

9. Cameron, JS; Simmonds, HA (1987). "Use and abuse of allopurinol". *British Medical Journal* 294 (6586): 1504–5. doi:10.1136/bmj.294.6586.1504. PMC 1246665. PMID 3607420.

10. Gettman, MT; Segura, JW (2005). "Management of ureteric stones: issues and controversies". *British Journal of Urology International* 95 (Supplement 2): 85–93. doi:10.1111/j.1464-410X.2005.05206.x. PMID 15720341.

11. Macaluso, JN (1999). "Management of stone disease—bearing the burden". *The Journal of Urology* 156 (5): 1579–80. doi:10.1016/S0022-5347(01)65452-1. PMID 8863542.

12. Seitz, C; Liatsikos, E, Porpiglia, F, Tiselius, HG, Zwergel, U (September 2009). "Medical therapy to facilitate the passage of stones: what is the evidence?". *European Urology* 56 (3): 455–71. doi:10.1016/j.eururo.2009.06.012. PMID 19560860.

13. Laerum E, Larsen S. Thiazide prophylaxis of urolithiasis. *Acta Med Scand* 1984; 215: 383–389 MedlineWeb of Science

14. Ettinger B, Citron JT, Livermore B, Dolman LI. Chlortalidone reduces calcium oxalate calculous recurrence but magnesium hydroxide does not. *J Urol* 1988;139: 679–684
MedlineWeb of Science

15. Heilberg IP, Martini LA, Szejnfeld VL, Schor N. Effect of thiazide diuretics on bone mass of nephrolithiasis patients with idiopathic hypercalciuria and osteopenia. *J Bone Miner Res* 1997; 12: S479 [Abstract]
CrossRefWeb of Science

16. Adams JS, Song CF, Kantorovich V. Rapid recovery of bone mass in hypercalciuric, osteoporotic men treated with hydrochlorthiazide. *Ann Inter Med* 1999; 130: 658–660
MedlineWeb of Science

17. Ettinger B, Tang A, Citron JT, Livermore B, Williams T. Randomized trial of allopurinol in the prevention of calcium oxalate calculi. *N Engl J Med* 1986; 315:1386–1389
MedlineWeb of Science

18. Ettinger B. Hyperuricosuria and calcium oxalate lithiasis: a critical review and future outlook. In: Borghi L, Meschi T, Briganti A, Schianchi T, Novarini A eds, *Kidney Stones (Proceedings of the 8th European Symposium on Urolithiasis)*. Editoriale Bios, Parma, Italy: 1999: 51–57

19. Sakhaee K, Nicar M, Hill K, Pak CYC. Contrasting effects of potassium citrate and sodium citrate therapies on urinary chemistries and crystallization of stone-forming salts. *Kidney Int* 1983; 24: 348–352
CrossRefMedlineWeb of Science

20. Barcelo P, Wuhl O, Servitge E, Rousaud A, Pak CYC. Randomized double-blind study of potassium citrate in idiopathic hypocitraturic calcium nephrolithiasis. *J Urol* 1993; 150: 1761–1764
MedlineWeb of Science

21. Ettinger B, Pak CYC, Citron JT, Thomas C, Adams-Huet B, Van Gessel A. Potassium-magnesium citrate is an effective prophylaxis against recurrent calcium oxalate nephrolithiasis. *J Urol* 1997; 158: 2069–2073
CrossRefMedlineWeb of Science

22. Ettinger B. Recurrent nephrolithiasis: natural history and effect of phosphate therapy; a double-blind controlled study. *Am J Med* 1976; 61: 200–206
CrossRefMedlineWeb of Science

23. Breslau NA, Padalino P, Kok DJ, Kim YG, Pak CYC. Physicochemical effects of a new slow-release potassium phosphate preparation (Urophos-K)* in absorptive hypercalciuria. *J Bone Miner Res* 1995; 10: 1995

24. Pak CYC. Medical prevention of renal stone disease. *Nephron* 1999; 81 [Suppl 1]: 60–65

Further Readings

1. Kidney Stones Natural Therapy And Prevention, Vitamins, Supplements
Www.Raysahelian.Com/Kidneystones... - Kidney Stones Natural Herbs Vitamins. ... The Role Of Calcium Intake And Kidney Stoneformation Seems Rather Difficult To Interpret. In Older Women And Men, Increased Dietaryintake Of Calcium, Potassium, And Total Fluid Reduces .... These Stones Are Analyzed, And Urine Levels Of Substances That Can Form Stones Are Measured.

2. Kidney Stones
Www.Umm.Edu/.../Kidney-Stones-00.. Kidney Stones Are A Painful Disorder Of The Urinary Tract, Affecting About 10% Of Americans. ... Start With Nutritional Guidelines For Prevention Of Recurrence. .... Pasch A. Urine Analyses For Workup Of Kidney Stone Disease -- Interpretation And ...

3. Clinical Practice Calcium Kidney StonesWww.Ncbi.Nlm.Nih.Gov/.../Pmc319...
Em Worcester - 2010 - 47 13-10-2011 – Diagnosis Of A Calcium Stone Requires Analysis After Passage Or ...Hyperuricosuria, Often From High Dietary Intake Of Purines, Is Thought ... Tables 2 And And33 Provide A Suggested Framework For Testing And Interpretation. .... The Guidelinesdo Not Address Evaluation Or Treatment To Prevent Recurrent Stones.

4. Dietary Protein Intake And Renal Function - Nutrition & MetabolismWww.Nutritionandmetabolism.Com/...
   Wf Martin - 2005 - 98 According To The National Kidney Foundation Guidelines, Ckd Is Classified Into ....Using Meta-Analysis To Assess The Efficacy Of Dietary Protein Restriction In .... The Role Of High Protein Diets In Kidney Stone Formation Has Received ... However, Findings In Women Are Difficult To Interpret Due To Conflicting Reports In The Literature.

5. [Pdf]2013 Uapa Annual Meeting Needs And ObjectivesWww.Uapanet.Org/.../Uapa%20201... Pdf/Adobe Acrobat
   Guidelines For Treatment. Other Areas ... Pediatric Urology And Kidney Stones. Additionally ... Explain How To Order Labs And Interpret A 24--Hour Urine. 19. Reviewdietary Management Of Stones Based On Metabolic Evaluation. 20. Describe ...

6. Laboratory Tests InterpretationWww.Nurseslearning.Com/.../Index.H...
   However, The Urine Ph Does Change During The Day Due To Dietary Influences And Water... Some Of The Disease Conditions Which Can Cause Proteinuria Are Renal ... Urinary Calculi (Stones) Are Insoluble Substances Most Commonly Formed Of The ... Explain That There Will Be Certain Food And Fluid Restrictions And Requirements ...

7. [Pdf] Guidelines On Urolithiasis - European Association Of UrologyWww.Uroweb.Org/Fileadmin/User_Upload/Guidelines/Urolithiasis.PdfPdf/Adobe Acrobat
   Hg Tiselius - 2001 – 475 3.3.2 Analysis Of Urine In Search For Risk Factors Of Stone Formation. 14. 3.3.3 Comments On The ... Open And Laparoscopic Surgery For Removal Of Renal Stones. 47 ...

8. HypercalciuriaEmedicine.Medscape.Com/.../43634...
   29-03-2011 – Hypercalciuria Contributes To Kidney Stone Disease And .... Below, Table 2 Provides Simple Test Guidelines For Specific .... The Subjects Were Observed Over A 10-Year Period And Were Assessed With A Thorough History, Dietary Analysis, ... The Need For An Inconvenient Expensive Test That Is Hard To Interpret.

9. Nephrolithiasis Treatment & ManagementEmedicine.Medscape.Com/.../43709... -
   11-02-2013 – Nephrolithiasis Specifically Refers To Calculi In The Kidneys, But Renalcalculi And ... A Stone Chemical Composition Analysis Should Be Performed ..... The Only Other General Dietary Guidelines Are To Avoid Excessive Salt And Protein Intake. ... A Medical Expert In Metabolic Stone Prevention Testing, Interpretation, ...

10. What Is The Underlying Cause Of Kidney Stones?Askville.Amazon.Com/...Kidney-Ston... - 2006
    My Mother Just Got Kidney Stones And Swears That It Is Just "Random" ... Preventive Strategies Include Dietary Modifications And Sometimes .... In Both Analysis,Interpretation Of The Results And Specific Preventive Treatment Recommendations. ... For Example, New Guidelines Are Recomending 800 To 2,000 Ius ...

(C) STONE ANALYSIS

Done With Samples Of Fragmented Stone Particles Passed With Urine Spontaneously Or Otherwise Surgically Extracted. Stone Composition Delineation Rendered By Spectroscopy Techniques, Provides Guidelines For Dietary Regulation And Subsequent Management For Stone Disease, Especially For Recurrence.[23]
The Composition Studies Reveal Either Of The Following Ingredients: Calcium Oxalate Monohydrate Stone, Calcium Oxalate Dihydrate Stone, Uric Acid Stone, Cysteine Stone, Purine Stone, Hydroxyapatite Stone, Carbonate Stone, Struvite Stone (Infection), And Others, e.g., Soft Radiolucent Stone "Indinavir"(A Protease Inhibitor) And Stone Formed During Aids Treatment, Etc.[21,22]

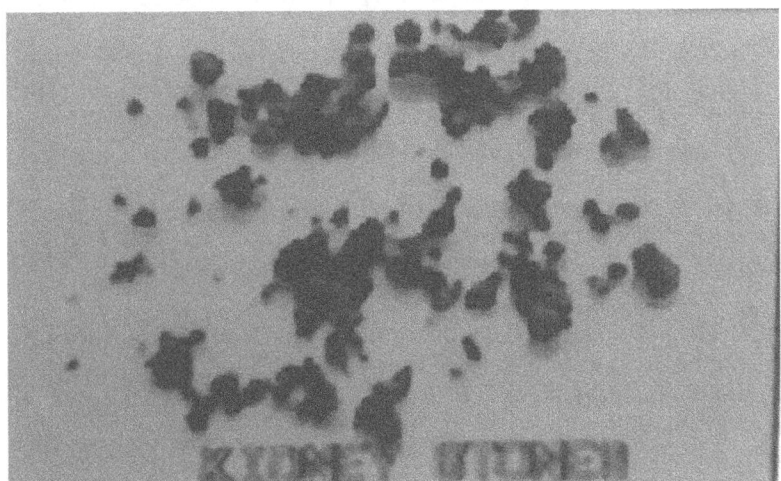

Fragmented Stone Particles Passed With Urine

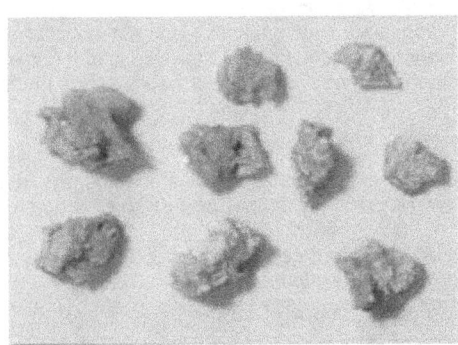

Passed Fragments Of 1-Cm Calcium Oxalate Stone Smashed Using Lithotripsy.

The Various Constituents,
Alone Or In Varying Proportions/Percentages, Provide Directive For
Comprehensive Management Guidelines For Stone Disease.

Stone Components May Be Mineral, Organic, Or Both.
More Than 65 Different Molecules (Including 25 Of
Exogenous Origin) Have Been Found In Urinary Calculi.

Using Such Morphoconstitutional Studies
Leads To A Classification Of Urinary Stones In Seven Distinctive Types
And Twenty-One Subtypes Among Monohydrate (Whewellite)
And Dihydrate (Weddelite) Calcium Oxalates, Phosphates,
Uric Acid, Urates, Protein, And Cystine (Amino Acids) Calculi.

The Same Chemical Component May Crystallize In Different Forms.
Therefore, Proper Stone Analysis Has To Identify Not Only The
Molecular Species Present In The Calculus, But Also The
Crystalline Forms Within Chemical Constituents.

Most Stones Are Of Mixed Composition And, Among Heterogeneous
Calculi, About 80% Are Made Of A Mixture Of Caox And
Calcium Phosphate (CaP) In Various Proportions.
By Contrast, The Presence Of Unique, But Unusual
Compound (E.G. 2,8 Dihydroxyadenine, Xanthine, Cystine, Calcite, Etc.)
Defines A Specific Type Of Urolithiasis.
Quantitative Evaluation Of Components Is Needed To Provide Full
Information.

References

Kidney Stone Analysis: At a Glance
labtestsonline.org/understanding/analytes/kidney-stone-analysis/
27-01-2012 – Overview of kidney stone analysis, used to evaluate the composition of a kidney stone, to help determine the cause of its formation and to guide ...

Louis C. Herring Laboratory
www.herringlab.com/ -
Kidney Stone Analysis Laboratory! Click the stone images! Herring Lab Information · Our Techniques · Interesting Kidney Stone Facts · Kidney Stone References ...

Kidney stone - Wikipedia, the free encyclopedia
en.wikipedia.org/wiki/Kidney_stone -
People with recurrent kidney stones are often screened for these disorders. This is typically done with a 24-hour urine collection that is chemically analyzed for ...

Kidney Stone Analysis - Medical Tests
www.everydayhealth.com/.../kidne...

Essentials Of Litho-Tripsy

20-09-2010 – A kidney stone (renal calculus) forms in the kidney from substances that would normally pass out of the body in the urine. When there are large ...

Kidney Stones - Qmineral: Analysis & Consulting
www.qmineral.com/kidney_stones....
Qmineral analyses kidney stones by X-ray diffraction. Hereby not only the dominant phase in the stone is identified but all minor traces of accessory minerals are ...

Interpretation for 8596 Kidney Stone Analysis
www.mayomedicallaboratories.com...
The composition of urinary stones may vary from a simple crystal to a complex mixture containing several different species of crystals. The composition of the ...
[PDF]

Kidney Stone Analysis by Nicolet FTIR spectrometer
www.ftir.cz/Kidclan2.pdf PDF/Adobe Acrobat F Kesner F.Dominak I. NICODOM s.r.o, Hlavni 2727, CZ-141 00 Praha 4, Czech republic, Europe ftir@ftir.cz ...

How should I interpret the results of a kidney stone analysis ...
www.sharecare.com/.../how-interpr...
How should I interpret the results of a kidney stone analysis? Knowing the type ofkidney stone helps guide the best treatment choice. Your doctor will talk with ...

Chemical and morphological analysis of kidney stones: a ... - SciELO
www.scielo.br/scielo.php?...sci... SFR Silva - 2010 - 9
Chemical and morphological analysis of kidney stones. .... Once the analyses were completed, the results were interpreted according to the instructions of the ...

Kidney Stone Analysis Interpretation
kidneystoneshelp.net/kidney-stone-...
19-08-2012 – Kidney Stones Treatments: Kidney Stone Analysis Interpretation. Kidney Stones Help, %%category_description%%.

Kohan AD, Armenakas NA, Fracchia JA. Indinavir urolithiasis: An emerging cause of renal colic in patients with human immunodeficiency virus. J Urol 1999;161:1765-8.

Reiter WJ, Schön-Pernerstorfer H, Dorfinger K, Hofbauer J, Marberger M. Frequency of urolithiasis in HIV seropositve individuals treatment with indinavir is higher than previously assumed. J Urol 1999;161:1082- 4.

Sakamoto W, Kishimoto T, Takegaki Y, Sugimoto T, Wada S, Yamamoto K, *et al.* Stone fragility –measurement of stone mineral content by dual photon absorptionmetry. Eur Urol 1991;20:150-3.

(D.) DIETARY REGULATIONS

Diet & Stone Diseases

The Association Between Dietary Factors And Stone Formation Is Highlighted By Two Observations-
1. The **`Stone Boom'** Corresponding To The Dramatic Increase In Stone Disease Incidence In Western Industrialized Nations, After World War II, As Compared To The Period During The War When Malnutrition Was The Rule.
2. The **`Stone Clinic Effect'**, A Phenomenon Described By The Mayo Clinic Years Ago To Explain The Reduction Of Stone Recurrence In 2/3 Of The Patients After Basic Dietary Advice.

The Role Of Many Nutrients Evaluation By Their Urinary Excretion, As **Either Promoters Or Inhibitors Of Stone Formation**, Has Been Discussed As Follows-

Calcium

The Fact That Calcium Is A Major Component Of 75% Of Stones, Excessive Calcium Intake Is Very Rarely, The Cause Of Stone Formation,
Clearly Explains Kidney stone formers Frequent Question Regarding Calcium Intake.

In The Past, Calcium Restriction Became A Very Popular Recommendation Based On The High Incidence Of Around 50% Hypercalciuria.
In Calcium Stone Forming Patients, Its Impact On Calcium Oxalate And Phosphate Saturation.
And Also Because Of The Contribution Of Calcium Intake And Intestinal Calcium Hyperabsorption To Hypercalciuria.

Essentials Of Litho-Tripsy

An Acute Oral Calcium Load Test, Described In 1975 By Pak *Et Al.* Was Reported To Clearly **Distinguish Between Absorptive And Renal Hypercalciuria,** In A Previous Evaluation By Our Group.

Conversely, Most Of The **Hypercalciuric** Patients When Challenged To A Higher Calcium Intake Did Not Present A Further **Increase In Their Urinary Calcium,** Showing That Under Conditions Of Low Calcium Intake, As It Is The Case For The Brazilian Population.

As The, With Morning Urinary Fasting Calcium/Creatinine (Ca:Cr) Ratio Seemed To Be The **Single Parameter** Which Would **Distinguish Between Renal And Absorptive Hypercalciuric Patients** A Cutoff Value Of 0.11 Taken Together, These Data Suggest That Absorptive And Renal Hypercalciuria Should Be Considered The Same Rather Than Two Distinct Entities, A Hypothesis Already Raised By Coe *Et Al.* Representing Two Extremes Of A Continuum Behaviour Resulting From An Abnormal Regulation Of 1,25 Vitamin D. In A Large Prospective Epidemiological Study Conducted By Curhan *Et Al.*

Healthy Men With Different Levels Of Calcium Intake Were Followed-Up For 8 Years, And **A Surprising Observation Was Made: The Lower The Calcium Intake, The Higher The Incidence Of Stone Formation.** A Hypothesis To Explain This At First Sight Contraindicative Relationship Was That **Low Calcium Concentrates In The Intestinal Lumen Caused A Secondary Increase In Urinary Oxalate Due To Decreased Binding Of Oxalate To Calcium Within The Gastrointestinal Tract.**
Nevertheless, Bushinsky *Et Al.* Preliminary Results Show A Significant **Decrease Of Urinary Oxalate In Hypercalciuric But Not In Normocalciuric Patients**.
Additional Studies Are Still Needed To Further Clarify Whether The Postulated **Relationship Between Colonic Oxalate Absorption And Colonic Load Of Calcium,** Is Different In Hypercalciuric *Versus* Normocalciuric Subjects.
Focusing On The Bone Issue, Many Investigators Addressed **The Loss Of Bone Mass In Hypercalciuric Patients.** It Was Suggested That **High Animal Protein And Sodium Intake Are Contributory Factors**. The Authors Also Stressed The Role Of A Low Calcium Diet In The Genesis Of Such Loss.
But One Has To Keep In Mind That Calcium Excretion Is Not Solely Affected By The Intake Of Calcium, But That Of Other Nutrients As Well, Such As Animal Protein, Sodium, Oxalate And Potassium.

Today More Experts Advise Higher Calcium Intake. Although Still Hypothetical, This May Even Have Additional Advantages.
The **Substitution Of Meat Protein By Dairy Product-Derived Protein**

Will Provide A **Higher Intake Of Phosphate** Which Co-Precipitates With Calcium In The Intestinal Lumen So That **Urinary Phosphate** Does Not Increase; Since **Calcium And Magnesium Compete For A Common Reabsorptive Mechanism In The Loop Of Henle**, Increases In Urinary Calcium Excretion Are Expected To Induce An Increase In **Urinary Magnesium, A Known Inhibitor Of Crystal Aggregation.**

Nevertheless, One Has To Consider That **The Benefits Of A High Calcium Supply Do Not Apply To Calcium Supplements, Which Usually Are Not Taken With Meals, Hence Losing Their Oxalate Chelating Properties.**
Calcium From Food Does Not Increase The Risk Of Calcium Oxalate Stones. Calcium In The Digestive Tract Binds To Oxalate From Food And Keeps It From Entering The Blood, And Then The Urinary Tract, Where It Can Form Stones.

Stone Formers Are Recommend To **Maintain A Normal Calcium Intake, Preferably From Dietary Sources.**
Female Stone Formers Taking Calcium Supplementation To Prevent **Osteoporosis** Experience A Slightly Increased Risk Of Stones (17%) Which Needs To Be Balanced Against Their Risk Of Osteoporosis.

Calcium Oxalate Stone Formers, Should Include **800 Mg Of Calcium In Diet Every Day,** Not Only For Kidney Stone Prevention But Also To Maintain Bone Density.
A Cup Of Low-Fat Milk Contains 300 Mg Of Calcium.
Other Dairy Products Such As Yogurt Are Also High In Calcium.
In **Lactose Intolerance Persons,** Avoidance Of Dairy Products,
Orange Juice Fortified With Calcium Or Dairy With Reduced Lactose Content May Be Alternatives.
Calcium Supplements May Increase The Risk Of Calcium Oxalate Stones If They Are Not Taken With Food. (1-12)

To Summarize, List Of Many Reasons Why Calcium Restriction Should Be Avoided In Hypercalciuric Patients, Include-
(I) There Is No Clear Distinction Between Absorptive And Renal Hypercalciuria.
(II) No Prospective Studies Are Available To Support The Belief That Calcium Restriction Leads To A Reduction Of Stone Recurrence.
(III) Calcium Restriction Induces Secondary Hyperoxaluria.
(IV) It Predisposes Also To Bone Loss Due To A Negative Calcium Balance.

Essentials Of Litho-Tripsy

(V) In Addition, Chronic Calcium Restriction Might Upregulate Vitamin D Receptors Allowing 1,25 Vitamin D To More Intensely Stimulate Both Intestinal Calcium Absorption And Bone Resorption.

(VI) Other Nutrients Such As Protein, Sodium, Oxalate And Potassium Affect Calcium Excretion As Well.

Oxalate

The Rational Basis For Oxalate Restriction Relies On The Fact That **Calcium Oxalate Is The Main Component Of Most Renal Stones, And That There Is A Lower Molar Urinary Oxalate Concentration Than Calcium (Ca:Ox Ratio Is 5:1).** This Means That Small Changes In Oxalate Concentration Have Much Larger Effects On Caox Crystallyzation Than Large Changes In Calcium Concentration.

While Oxalate Plays An Important Role In The Development Of Calcium Oxalate Stones, Dietary Restriction Does Not Appear To Be Effective In Reducing The Risk Of Stones In The Majority Of Patients. **About 40% Of Urinary Oxalate Comes From Dietary Sources** While The Remainder Is Naturally Made Within The Liver.

Some Of The Oxalate In Urine Is Made By The Body. However, Eating Certain Foods With High Levels Of Oxalate Can Increase The Amount Of Oxalate In The Urine, Where It Combines With Calcium To Form Calcium Oxalate Stones. **Foods That Have Been Shown To Increase The Amount Of Oxalate In Urine Include-**
- Spinach
- Rhubarb
- Nuts
- Wheat Bran

Avoiding These Foods May Help Reduce The Amount Of Oxalate In The Urine.

Stone-Forming Foods Avoidance: Beets, Chocolate, Spinach, Rhubarb, Tea, And Most Nuts Are Rich In Oxalate, And Colas Are Rich In Phosphate, Both Of Which Can Contribute To Kidney Stones.

Aside From **Primary And Enteric Hyperoxaluria**, Most Cases Found In CSF Patients Have `Mild Hyperoxaluria', Defined By Levels Of Urinary Oxalate From 40 To 100 Mg/Day,
With A Reported Frequency Of 12–63%.

Marangella *Et Al*. Have Suggested That `**Mild Hyperoxaluria'** Might Be Secondary To **Calcium Hyperabsorption**.

A Recent Experimental Study By Bushinsky *Et Al.* Results Have Raised The Issue Whether It Is Necessary At All To Limit Dietary Oxalate Intake In Stone Formers. **In Humans, Only 10–15% Of Urinary Oxalate Is Derived From The Diet**.

The Ability Of Oxalate-Rich Food Items To Augment Oxalate Excretion Depends Not Only On The Oxalate Content, But Also On Its Bioavailability, Its Solubility And The Form Of Salt In Which It Is Present. **Only Spinach And Rhubarb Are Considered To Be High Risk Food Items**, For Their High Amounts Of **Bioavailable Oxalate**.
Peanuts, Instant Tea, Almonds, Chocolate And Pecans Are Considered As Moderate Risk Food Items.

The Effect Of Dietary Oxalate On Urine Oxalate Critically Depends Upon Calcium Intake, Since Decreasing The Calcium Load In The Intestinal Lumen Will Increase The Concentration Of Free Oxalate Anions Available For Absorption, As Mentioned Above. In Healthy Subjects,
Hess *Et Al.* Have Recently Shown That The **Hyperoxaluria** Caused By A **20-Fold Increase** In Oxalate Load Can Be Totally Prevented By A Very High Calcium Intake Of About **4Gm/Day**. **The Same Is Being Investigated For** Smaller Amounts Of Both Nutrients In **CSF Patients** (Unpublished Data). Preliminary Results Have Shown No Changes In Oxalate Or Calcium Excretion After A 2-Fold Increase In Oxalate Intake Produced By Consumption Of One Big Milk Chocolate Bar Per Day Containing 95 Mg Of Oxalate And 430 Mg Of Calcium For 3 Days.

Marshall *Et Al.* Have Studied The **Effects Of Either Oxalate Or Calcium Restriction Alone, As Well As This Concomitant Restriction** In Stone Forming Patients And Controls. In Patients, **Oxalate Restriction** Did Not Alter Calcium Excretion To A Major Extent And Produced Only A Very Minor Decrease In Urinary Oxalate. Caox Activity Was Not Altered Much. On The Other Hand, A **Severe Calcium Restrictio**(Down To 250 Mg/Day) Caused An Important Elevation Of Urinary Oxalate Only When The Supply Of Dietary Oxalate Was Normal. **The Combined Restriction Of Calcium And Oxalate** Was The Only Way To Prevent Such An Increase In Urinary Oxalate Excretion, Leading To An Effective Decrease Of Caox Product Activity Far Below The Formation Product.
Bataille *Et Al.* Evaluated The Probability Of Stone Formation After Combined Restriction Of Calcium And Oxalate. He Observed That The Combined Restriction Was Not Able To Decrease
The Probability Of Stone Formation In Dietary-Independent Hypercalciuria Patients, In As Much As A Concomitant Increase In Oxalate Excretion Was Still Noted In These Patients.

Essentials Of Litho-Tripsy

In Summary, The Idea That A Balance Between Calcium And Oxalate Intake Must Be Maintained During Meals Is Unquestionable. Long-Term Controlled Studies Are Needed, However, To Resolve Whether One Should Recommend Restriction Of Both Items Or Recommend No Restriction At All.

Protein

The Nutrient That Clearly Has Universal Effects On Most Of The Urinary Parameters Involved In Stone Formation Is Protein.
High Protein Intake Of Animal Origin Contributes To
Hyperuricosuria Due To The Purine Overload To
Hyperoxaluria Due To The Higher Oxalate Synthesis And To
Hypocitraturia Due To The Higher Tubular Reabsorption Of Citrate.
Protein-Induced Hypercalciuria May Be Caused By
Higher Bone Resorption And Lower Tubular Calcium Reabsorption
To Buffer The Acid Load, And Also By The Elevated Filtered Load Of Calcium And By The Presence Of Non-Reabsorbable Calcium Sulfate In The Tubular Lumen.
An Acute Moderate Protein Restriction Reduces Urinary Oxalate, Phosphate, Hydroxyproline, Calcium, And Uric Acid And Increases Citrate Excretion, As Recently Reported.

Animal Protein In Meat Products **Increase, The Risk Of Stone By Increasing Calcium, Oxalate, And Uric Acid Levels In Urine**.
All Three Of These Changes Increase The Risk Of Stones.
In Comparative Studies High Meat Eaters Were Found To Be At **Increased Risk** Of Forming Stones.

Meats And Other Animal Protein—Such As Eggs And Fish—
Contain Purines, Which Break Down Into **Uric Acid** In The Urine.
Foods Especially Rich In Purines Include Organ Meats, Such As Liver.
So, **Uric Acid Stones Formers** Should Limit Their **Meat Consumption To 6 Ounces Each Day.**

Animal Protein May Also Raise The **Risk Of Calcium Stones** By **Increasing The Excretion Of Calcium And Reducing The Excretion Of Citrate Into The Urine.** Citrate Prevents Kidney Stones,
But The Acid In Animal Protein Reduces The Citrate In Urine

A Randomized Study Of Stone Formers Restricted To A Low Meat Intake Of 52 Grams A Day (Equivalent To 8 0z Of Beef) **In Combination With Sodium Restriction** Found That The Combination Reduced Stone Recurrence By 50% Compared To Calcium Restriction Alone
(Borghi Et Al, Nejm 2002).

Recommendations For Most Stone Formers Is To Try To Reduce Their Meat Intake To 6 Oz A Day(Includes All Types Of Meat: Beef, Pork, Poultry, And Seafood)).

USDA Recommendations Conclude-A **Daily Allowance Of 5-6 Oz Of Protein Intake Among Adults**.
& **Choosing Non-Meat Protein Foods** Such As Nuts And Beans Instead Of Meat Sources.
Protein From Non-Meat Sources Does Not Appear To Increase The Risk Of Stones.
Lowering Animal Protein Intake And Eating More Fruits And Vegetables Also **Benefits Overall Health** By Limiting **Saturated Fats And Cholesterol Levels** In Diet. Thus Reducing The Risk Of Cardiovascular Disease.

Potassium

**An Epidemiological Study Has Reported That The Lower The Potassium Intake, Below 74 Mmol/Day,
The Higher The Relative Risk Of Stone Formation**.
Such An Effect Can Be **Ascribed To An Increase In Urinary Calcium And A Decrease In Urinary Citrate Excretion Induced By A Low Potassium Intake**.
In A Previous Laboratory Study Series A Low-Normal Potassium Intake And A Higher Nacl Intake Observed In Stone Formers When Compared To Healthy Subjects. The Overall Effect Was A Significantly **Higher Urine Na/K Ratio** Increasing The Risk For Stone Formation, As Previously Suggested By Cirillo *Et Al*.

Sodium

The Effect Of Sodium Chloride (Nacl) Intake On Increasing Calcium Excretion Is Well Established. **Every 100 Mmol Increase In Dietary Sodium Increases Urinary Calcium Excretion By 25 Mg**.
The Adverse Effects Of A High Nacl Intake And The Resultant **Higher Calcium Excretion** Have Been Well Documented By Many Investigators.
In A Previous Analysis Group **Multiple Regression** Suggested
That A **High Nacl Intake (≥16 G/Day), Was The Single Variable** That Was Predictive Of Risk Of Low Bone Mineral Density In 85 CSF Patients (Odds Ratio: 3.8) After Adjustments For Age, Weight, Body Mass Index, Duration Of Stone Disease, Calcium And Protein Intakes And Urinary Calcium Citrate And Uric Acid.

Essentials Of Litho-Tripsy

A High Nacl Intake Is Expected To Lower Citrate Excretion As Well.
(13-25)

SALT

A High Sodium Intake Increases The Risk Of Stone Formation By Increasing Calcium Levels And Decreasing Citrate (A Stone Inhibitor) Levels In Urine.
Additionally, High Sodium Intake Will Impair The Ability Of Medications Such As Hydrochlorothiazide To Effectively Reduce Calcium Levels In Urine.
A Study Of Stone Formers Who Were Kept On A Strict Diet With A **Maximum Daily Sodium Intake Of 50 Mmol (1200 Mg)** In Addition To A **Reduced Protein Diet** Demonstrated That The
Low Sodium Diet Was Effective In Reducing Stone Recurrence By 50% As Compared To The Low Calcium Diet.

FDA's Guideline Recommendations Of Limiting Salt Intake
To 2300 mg Of Sodium A Day In The General Population And 1500 mg Of Sodium A Day In Those With Hypertension, African Americans, Or Middle Aged And Older Adults.
2300 Mg Is Equivalent To About 1 Teaspoon Of Table Salt. But Americans' Intake Averages 3,400 Mg, According To The U.S. Department Of Agriculture.[1]
In Addition To Lowering The Risk Of Stones, A Low Sodium Intake Helps To Control Or Prevent High Blood Pressure, Which Can Lead To Heart Disease, Stroke, Heart Failure, And Kidney Disease.

AwareNess About The Sodium Content Of Foods,
Is HelpFul To Control TheSodium Intake.
Following Foods Have Such Large Amounts Of Sodium
(A Single Serving Provides A Major Portion Of The RDA)
Hot Dogs, Canned Soups And Vegetables, Processed Frozen Foods, Luncheon Meats, Fast Food.
For Sodium Intake Limitation Their Should Labels For Ingredients And Hidden Sodium, Checking Follwing Is UseFul-
Monosodium Glutamate, Or MSG
Sodium Bicarbonate, The Chemical Name For Baking Soda
Baking Powder, Which Contains Sodium Bicarbonate & Other Chemicals
Disodium Phosphate
Sodium Alginate
Sodium Nitrate Or Nitrite

Effect Of Sodium Upon Kidney Stone Formation.
Sodium, Often From Salt, Causes The Kidneys To Excrete More Calcium Into The Urine. High Concentrations Of Calcium In The

Urine Combine With Oxalate And Phosphorus To Form Stones.
Reducing Sodium Intake Is Preferred To Reducing Calcium Intake.

Fluid intake

The average daily urine output of normal healthy adults is 1.2 liters a day, ranging from 1 to 2 liters in most individuals and varying with body weight and gender. In stone formers, however, a higher daily urine output is required for stone prevention and achieving a daily volume of at least 2.0 to 2.5 liters a day can significantly reduce the recurrence of future stones.

We recommend that most stone formers increase their daily fluid intake by one liter (an additional two 16 oz water bottles or two tall glasses a day) in order to achieve a urine output of 2.5 liters a day. **A High Fluid Intake Is A Very Important Goal To Reduce Urine Supersaturation.** A Very Well Conducted 5-Year Randomized, Prospective Study Involving First Stone Episode Patients Has Shown Lower Rates Of Recurrence (12%) In Those With A Higher Intake Of Water Compared To Those Without (27%). It Should Be Emphasized That Patients Received No Drug Therapy And Were Not Submitted To Any Dietary Change So That The Effect Was Exclusively Explained By The Selective Increase In Urinary VolumE.
To What Extent The Hardness And Mineral Composition Of Water Affect Stone Risk Remains Controversial.As The Calcium Content Of Drinking Water Increases, Calcium Excretion Increases, But Oxalate Excretion Falls. Water With A Large Amount Of Bicarbonate May Increase Citrate Excretion And Magnesium Content May Favourably Alter Citrate And Magnesium Excretion.
Based On These Findings, There Is Still No Definite Evidence That Hard Water, Rich In Calcium And Magnesium, Is More Lithogenic Than Soft Water. A Very Recent Epidemiological Study Based On Food-Frequency Questionnaires Has Examined The Effects Of Particular Beverages On The Risk Of Symptomatic Kidney Stones In Women. Consumption Of Tea, Caffeinated And Decaffeinated Coffee Was Associated With A Reduction Of Risk Of 8–10%, While Wine Decreased The Risk By 59%. Conversely, Grapefruit Juice Ingestion Was Associated With A 44% Increased Risk For Stone Formation. The Authors Speculated That The Protective Effects Of Coffee, Tea And Wine Were Caused By Urinary Dilution, Determined By The Ability Of Caffeine And Alcohol To Inhibit Antidiuretic Hormone. Therefore, The Decreased Risk For Decaffeinated Coffee Might Have Been Conferred By Another Mechanism. **The Adverse Effects Of Grapefruit Juice Remained Unexplained,**

Essentials Of Litho-Tripsy

Since Other Citrus Juices, Such As Orange And Lemon, Apparently Prevent And At Least Fail To Stimulate Stone Formation Because Of Their High Citrate Content. In Summary, These Results Must Still Be Interpreted With Caution Until Adequate Long-Term Randomized Trials Of Dietary Interventions Are Performed. (25-35)

<u>Type Of Fluid Intake</u>

Preferred Recommendation Because It Is Inexpensive And Contains No Calories, For Stone Patients Who Do Not Enjoy Drinking Water, Any Beverage Will Be Beneficial In Reducing Stone Risk.

Contrary To Popular Belief, Studies Have Found That An Increased Intake Of Tea, Coffee, And Alcoholic Beverage Actually Reduces The Risk Of Stones,
Possibly Because Of An Associated Increase In Urine Output (Curhan Et Al, Am J Of Epidemiology, 1996).
While Tea Contains High Levels Of Oxalate, This Does Not Appear To Result In Increased Stone Formation For The Reasons Discussed Below In Our <u>Discussion On Oxalate</u>.
Soda Intake (Including Colas) And Milk Intake Also Do Not Appear To Increase The Risk Of Stones.

<u>Ctrus Fruit Juices</u>
Including Lemon Juice And Orange Juice, Contain Citrate,
Acts As A Stone Inhibitor For Calcium Based Stones.
Citrate By Binding Calcium, Makie It Unavailable To Combine With Oxalate Or Phosphate: A Necessary First Step In The Formation Of Stones. Citrate Also Seems To Make It More Difficult For Stones To Grow, Once They've Formed.

Citrus Juice In The Form Of Concentrated Lemon Juice Mixed With Water Has Been Shown To Effectively Increase Urinary Citrate Levels And Reduce Urinary Calcium Levels, Both Of Which Will Reduce Stone Risk.

Orange Juice Increase Urinary Citrate Levels But **Appears To Also Increase Urinary Oxalate Levels (A Stone Promoter).**
Amongst Other Sources Of Citrate, Including Grapefruit Juice, Lemon Juice Is Typically Favored Over Other Citrus Juices As A Natural Method To Increase Urinary Citrate Levels.

Stone Formers Are Recommended For, Supplementing Their Daily Fluid Intake With A Mixture Of 60 Ml Of Concentrated Lemon Juice In One Liter Of Water To Increase Their Urinary Citrate Levels.

Increase Daily Fluid Intake By One Liter (An Additional Two 16 Oz Water Bottles Or Two Tall Glasses A Day) In Order To Achieve A Urine Output Of 2.5 Liters A Day.

VITAMIN C

The Effect Of Large Doses Of Vitamin C In Increasing Urinary Oxalate Excretion Is Controversial.

At Least In Part It May Be A Methodological Artifact Accounted For By The Conversion Of Vitamin C To Oxalate During The Analytical Procedure **In A Recent Large Epidemiological Study, The Intake Of Vitamin C Was Not Associated With Risk Of Kidney Stones In Women**.

The Available Research Suggests That **Vitamin D** Replacement With Either Dietary Or Supplements At Standard Normal Doses Is Likely Ok. However, **Overdoses Of Vitamin D, Called "Hypervitaminosis D"** Can Lead To High Calcium Levels In The Blood And Urine And Among Other Adverse Side Effects, Can Promote Stones.

Ref: Leaf, Calcium Kidney Stones, New England Journal Of Medicine 2010

Choose Wholemeal And Wholegrain Foods, Eating Foods Higher In Fibre Can Decrease The Risk Of Stone Formation By Reducing The Amount Of Calcium And Oxalate Absorbed.

Choose Wholemeal And Wholegrain Breads, Flour, Cereals, Pasta, Biscuits And Crackers

DIET PLANS

According To Stone Composition And Availability Of Food Products, Various Scientifically Approved Diet Regulation Regimes Are Available By Different Laboratories And Pharmaceutical Companies, Especially Restricting Oxalate, Calcium, Urate, And Other Mineral-Containing Food Items, While Promoting Intake Of Food Substances With Ingredient Content Known To Be Effectively Helpful For Stone Disease.

Studies Have Shown **The Dietary Approaches To Stop Hypertension (DASH) Diet** Can Reduce The Risk Of Kidney Stones. The DASH Diet Is High In Fruits And Vegetables, Moderate In Low-Fat Dairy Products, And Low In Animal Protein.

(The DASH Diet ,The National Heart, Lung And Blood Institute's Website www.nhlbi.nih.gov/health/health-topics/topics/dash).

Essentials Of Litho-Tripsy

Recommendations Based On The Specific Type Of Kidney Stone Include The Following:

As The Influence Of Diet On Renal Stone Disease Seems To Be Much More Complex Than Thought In The Past,
Because Multiple Interactions Take Place Between The Different Nutrients And Thus Variably Influence Urinary Parameters.

A Specialized Dietitian Guided Supervision For, Kidney Stone Prevention & Or Nutrition For Kidney Problems Patients,
Retains Importance For 'Indivisual Dietary Regime' Plannings,eg The Coincidence Of Kidney Stones, Particularly Uric Acid Stones In Overweight Persons.

Calcium Oxalate Stones
Reducing Sodium
Reducing Animal Protein, Such As Meat, Eggs, And Fish
Getting Enough Calcium From Food Or
Taking Calcium Supplements With Food
Avoiding Foods High In Oxalate Such As,
Spinach, Rhubarb, Nuts, And Wheat Bran

Calcium Phosphate Stones
Reducing Sodium
Reducing Animal Protein
Getting Enough Calcium From Food Or
Taking Calcium Supplements With Food

Uric Acid Stone

- Limiting Animal Protein.
  Meats And Other Animal Protein—Such As Eggs And Fish—Contain **Purines**, Which Break Down Into Uric Acid In The Urine.
- Reducing Sodium Intake Is Preferred To Reducing Calcium Intake.
  Sodium, Often From Salt, Causes The Kidneys To Excrete More Calcium Into The Urine. High Concentrations Of Calcium In The Urine Combine With Oxalate And Phosphorus To Form Stones.

The Recommendations Are That,
Most Stone Formers Should Maintain A Normal Oxalate Intake,
Without The Need For Oxalate Restriction.
High Oxalate Intake Should Be Avoided In Individuals Found To Have **High Urinary Oxalate** Levels On Metabolic Evaluation.

Oxalate Rich Foods

- Tea (black)
- Spinach
- Mustard greens
- Chard
- Beets
- Rhubarb
- Okra
- Berries
- Chocolate
- Nuts
- Sweet potatoes

Lifestyle Changes

Kidney Stones Risk Reduction Measures:

- **Drinking More Water Throughout The Day.** People Who Live In Hot, Dry Climates And Those Who Exercise Frequently May Need To Drink Even More Water To Produce Enough Urine.

  Health Care Providers Recommendations- An Average Person Drinks 2 To 3 Liters Of Fluid A Day. People With Cystine Stones May Need To Drink Even More.
  Though Water Is Best, Other Fluids May Also Help Prevent Kidney Stones, Such As Citrus Drinks.

Drinking Enough Fluids Each Day Is The Best Way To Help Prevent Most Types Of Kidney Stones. As Kidney Stones Can Form When Substances In The Urine—Such As Calcium, Oxalate, And Phosphorus—Become Highly Concentrated. (36-48))

- **Diet** Is One Of Several Factors That Can Promote Or Inhibit Kidney Stone Formation.
  A Dietitian Can Help A Person Plan Meals That Lower The Risk Of Forming Stones Based On The Type Of Stone The Person Formed In The Past,
  With Consideration Of Associated Medical Problems.

References

1. Hosking DH, Erickson SB, Van Den Berg CJ, Wilson DH, Smith LH. The stone clinic effect in patients with idiopathic calcium urolithiasis. *J Urol* 1983; 130:1115–1118
   MedlineWeb of Science

2. Pak CYC. Kidney stones. *Lancet* 1998; 351: 1797–1801
   CrossRefMedlineWeb of Science

3. Coe FL, Parks JH. New insights into the pathophysiology and treatment of nephrolithiasis: new research venues. *J Bone Miner Res* 1997; 12: 522–533
CrossRefMedlineWeb of Science

4. Pak CYC, Kaplan R, Bone H, Townsend J, Waters O. A simple test for the diagnosis of absorptive, resorptive and renal hypercalciuria. *N Engl J Med* 1975;292: 497–500
MedlineWeb of Science

5. Heilberg IP, Martini LA, Draibe SA, Ajzen H, Ramos OL, Schor N. Sensitivity to calcium intake in calcium stone forming patients. *Nephron* 1996; 73: 145–153
CrossRefMedlineWeb of Science

6. Martini LA, Heilberg IP, Cuppari L, Medeiros FAM, Draibe SA, Ajzen H, Schor N. Dietary habits of calcium stone formers. *Brazilian J Med Biol Res* 1993; 26:805–812
MedlineWeb of Science

7. Coe FL, Favus MJ, Crockett T *et al*. Effects of a low calcium diet on urine calcium excretion, parathyroid function and serum 1,25(OH)2D3 levels in patients with idiopathic hypercalciuria and in normal subjects. *Am J Med* 1982;72: 25–32
CrossRefMedlineWeb of Science

8. Curhan GC, Willet WC, Rimm EB, Stampfer MJ. A prospective study of dietary calcium and other nutrients and the risk of symptomatic kidney stones. *N Engl J Med* 1993; 328: 833–838
CrossRefMedlineWeb of Science

9. Bushinsky DA, Kim M, Sessler NE, Nakagawa Y, Coe FL. Increased urinary saturation and kidney calcium content in genetic hypercalciuric rats. *Kidney Int*1994; 45: 58–65
CrossRefMedlineWeb of Science

10. Nishiura JL, Martini LA, Andriolo A, Schor N, Heilberg IP. Effect of calcium intake upon urinary oxalate excretion in calcium stone forming (CSF) patients. In: Borghi L, Meschi T, Briganti A, Schianchi T, Novarini A eds *Kidney Stones (Proceedings of the 8th European Symposium on Urolithiasis)*. Editoriale Bios, Parma, Italy: 1999: 511–512

11. Heilberg IP, Martini LA, Szejnfeld VL *et al*. Bone disease in calcium stone-forming patients. *Clin Nephrol* 1994; 42: 175–182
MedlineWeb of Science

12. Bataille P, Achard JM, Fournier A *et al*. Diet, vitamin D and vertebral mineral density in hypercalciuric calcium stone formers. *Kidney Int* 1991; 39: 1193–1205
MedlineWeb of Science

13. Pietschmann F, Breslau NA, Pak CYC. Reduced vertebral bone density in hypercalciuric nephrolithiasis. *J Bone Miner Res* 1992; 7: 1383–1388
MedlineWeb of Science

14. Heilberg IP, Martini LA, Teixeira SH *et al*. Effect of etidronate treatment on bone mass of male nephrolithiasis patients with idiopathic hypercalciuria and osteopenia. *Nephron* 1998; 79: 430–437
CrossRefMedlineWeb of Science

15. Trinchieri A, Nespoli R, Ostini F, Rovera F, Zanetti G, Pisani E. A study of dietary calcium and other nutrients in idiopathic renal calcium stone formers with low bone mineral content. *J Urol* 1998; 159: 654–657

CrossRefMedlineWeb of Science

16. Massey LK, Roman-Smith H, Sutton RA. Effect of dietary oxalate and calcium on urinary oxalate and risk of formation of calcium oxalate kidney stones. *J Am Diet Assoc* 1993; 93: 901–906
CrossRefMedlineWeb of Science

17. Massey LK, Whiting SJ. Dietary salt, urinary calcium and bone loss. *J Bone Miner Res* 1996; 11: 731–736
MedlineWeb of Science

18. Lemann JJ, Pleuss JÁ, Gray RW, Hoffmann RG. Potassium administration increases and potassium deprivation reduces urinary calcium excretion in healthy adults. *Kidney Int* 1991; 39: 973–983
MedlineWeb of Science

19. Hess B, Jost C, Zipperle L, Takkinen R, Jaeger P. High calcium intake abolishes hyperoxaluria and reduces urinary crystallization during a 20-fold normal oxalate load in humans. *Nephrol Dial Transplant* 1998; 13: 2241–2247
Abstract/FREE Full Text

20. Curhan GC, Willett WC, Speizer FE, Spiegelman D, Stampfer MJ. Comparison of dietary calcium with supplemental calcium and other nutrients as factors affecting the risk for kidney stones in women. *Ann Inter Med* 1997; 126: 497–504
CrossRefMedlineWeb of Science

21. Borsatti A. Calcium oxalate nephrolithiasis: defective oxalate transport.*Kidney Int* 1991; 39: 1283–1298
MedlineWeb of Science

22. Marangella M, Fruttero B, Bruno M, Linari F. Hyperoxaluria in idiopathic calcium stone disease: further evidence of intestinal hyperabsorption of oxalate.*Clin Sci* 1982; 63: 381–385
Medline

23. Bushinsky DA, Bashir MA, Riordon DR, Nakagawa Y, Coe FL, Grynpas MD. Increased dietary oxalate does not increase urinary calcium oxalate saturation in hypercalciuric rats. *Kidney Int* 1999; 55: 602–612
CrossRefMedlineWeb of Science

24. Hess B. Low calcium diet in hypercalciuric calcium nephrolithiasis patients: first do no harm. *Scanning Microsc* 1996; 10: 547–554
Medline

25. Brinkley LJ, Gregory J, Pak CYC. A further study of oxalate bioavailability in foods. *J Urol* 1990; 144: 94–96
MedlineWeb of Science

26. Marshall RW, Cochran M, Hodgkinson A. Relationships between calcium and oxalic acid intake in the diet and their excretion in the urine of normal and renal-stone-forming subjects. *Clin Sci* 1972; 43: 91–99
MedlineWeb of Science

27. Bataille P, Charransol G, Gregoire I *et al.* Effect of calcium restriction on renal excretion of oxalate and the probability of stones in the various pathophysiological groups with calcium stones. *J Urol* 1983; 130: 218–223
MedlineWeb of Science

28. Breslau NA, Brinkley L, Hill KD, Pak CYC. Relationship of animal protein-rich diet to kidney stone formation. *J Clin Endocrinol Metab* 1988; 66: 140–146
CrossRefMedlineWeb of Science

29. Holmes RP, Goodman HO, Hart LJ, Assimos DJ. Relationship of protein intake to urinary oxalate and glycolate excretion. *Kidney Int* 1993; 44: 366–372
CrossRefMedlineWeb of Science

30. Giannini S, Nobile M, Sartori L et al. Acute effects of moderate dietary protein restriction in patients with idiopathic hypercalciuria and calcium nephrolithiasis.*Am J Clin Nutr* 1999; 69: 267–271
Abstract/FREE Full Text

31. Martini LA, Cuppari L, Cunha MA, Schor N, Heilberg. Potassium and sodium intake and excretion in calcium stone forming patients. *J Renal Nutr* 1998; 8:127–131
CrossRefMedline

32. Cirillo M, Laurenzi M, Panarelli W, Stamler J. Urinary sodium to potassium ratio and urinary stone disease. *Kidney Int* 1994; 46: 1133–1139
CrossRefMedlineWeb of Science

33. Lemann JJ, Adams ND, Gray RW. Urinary calcium excretion in human beings.*N Engl J Med* 1979; 301: 535–541
MedlineWeb of Science

34. Muldowney FP, Freaney R, Moloney. Importance of dietary sodium in the hypercalciuria syndrome. *Kidney Int* 1982; 22: 292–296
MedlineWeb of Science

35. Breslau Na, McGuire JL, Zerwekh JE, Pak CYC. The role of dietary sodium on renal excretion and intestinal absorption of calcium and on vitamin D metabolism. *J Clin Endocrinol Metab* 1982; 55: 369–373
CrossRefMedlineWeb of Science

36. Martini LA, Szejnfeld VL, Colugnati AB, Cuppari L, Schor N, Heilberg IP. High sodium chloride intake is associated with low bone density in calcium stone forming patients. *Clin Nephrol* 1999: [in press]

37. Sakhaee K, Harvey JA, Padalino PK, Whitson P, Pak CYC. The potential role of salt abuse on the risk for kidney stone formation. *J Urol* 1993; 150: 310–312
MedlineWeb of Science

38. Borghi L, Meschi T, Amato F, Briganti A, Novarini A, Giannini A. Urinary volume, water and recurrences in idiopathic calcium nephrolithiasis: a 5-year randomized prospective study. *J Urol* 1996; 155: 839–843
CrossRefMedlineWeb of Science

39. Agreste AS, Schor N, Heilberg IP. The effect of hardness of drinking water upon calculi growth in rats. In: Borghi L, Meschi T, Briganti A, Schianchi T, Novarini A eds, *Kidney Stones (Proceedings of the 8th European Symposium on Urolithiasis)*. Editoriale Bios, Parma, Italy: 1999: 487

40. Caudarella R, Rizzoli E, Buffa A, Bottura A, Stefoni S. Comparative study of the influence of 3 types of mineral water in patients with idiopathic calcium lithiasis. *J Urol* 1998; 159: 658–663
CrossRefMedlineWeb of Science

41. Agreste AS, Schor N, Heilberg IP. Mineral composition of natural (NW) and sparkling water (SW) and calculi growth in rats. In: Borghi L, Meschi T, Briganti A, Schianchi T, Novarini A eds, *Kidney Stones (Proceedings of the 8th European Symposium on Urolithiasis)*. Editoriale Bios, Parma, Italy: 1999: 489

42. Marangella M, Vitale C, Petrarulo M, Rovera L, Dutto F. Effects of mineral composition of drinking water on risk for stone formation and bone metabolism in idiopathic calcium nephrolithiasis. *Clin Sci* 1996; 91: 313–318
Medline

43. Rodgers AL. Effect of mineral water containing calcium and magnesium on calcium oxalate urolithiasis risk factors. *Urol Int* 1997; 58: 93–99
CrossRefMedlineWeb of Science

44. Curhan GC, Willett WC, Speizer FE, Stampfer MJ. Beverage use and risk of kidney stones in women. *Ann Inter Med* 1998; 128: 534–540
CrossRefMedlineWeb of Science

45. Seltzer MA, Low RK, McDonald M, Shami GC, Stoller ML. Dietary manipulation with lemonade to treat hypocitraturic nephrolithiasis. *J Urol* 1996; 156: 907–909
CrossRefMedlineWeb of Science

46. Wabner CL, Pak CYC. Effect of orange juice consumption on urinary stone risk factors. *J Urol* 1993; 149: 1405–1408
MedlineWeb of Science

47. Hughes C, Dutton S, Trusell A. High intakes of ascorbic acid and urinary oxalate. *J Hum Nutr* 1981; 35: 274–280
MedlineWeb of Science

48. Wandzilak T, D'Andre S, Davis P, Williams H. Effect of high dose of vitamin C on urinary oxalate levels. *J Urol* 1994; 151: 834–837
MedlineWeb of Science

Essentials Of Litho-Tripsy

(E) METABOLIC EVALUATION RELEVANT INVESTIGATIONS

Consideration Of Metabolic Evaluation Of Patients With Stone Disease Provides Useful Diagnostic And/Or Therapeutic Tool For Medical And Surgical Management Guidelines, More So In Recurrence Cases.
Various Commonly Used Indices: Urine For Crystalluria, Serum

Uric Acid, Serum Calcium, Serum Phosphorous, Serum Magnesium, Parathormone Assay Etc,
Are Utilized For Cauastive Factors Management.

Comprehensive Treatment Plan For Stone Disease Biochemical Evaluation In Renal Stone Disease.

Renal Stone Disease May Ensue From Either Derangements Of Urine Biochemistries Or Anatomic Abnormalities Of Kidneys And Urinary Tract.

An **Adequate Metabolic Evaluation** Should Focus On **The Urinary Excretion Of Promoters And Inhibitors Of Stone Formation** As Well As On The Occurrence Of **Systemic Diseases Potentially Related To Secondary Nephrolithiasis** (i.e., Endocrine Disturbances, Malabsorption, Bone Diseases).

An **Extensive Metabolic Evaluation** Is Recommended In Patients With **Active Stone Disease** (Namely, At Least **One New Stone Within The Last Two Years**), Or In Those Having Had **A Single Stone Episode Occurred In Peculiar Conditions**: Familial History Of Disease, Childhood, Menopause, Pregnancy, Systemic Diseases.

For Non-Active Nephrolithiasis Or In Patients With Single Stone And No Relevant Risk Factors, Simplified Protocols Include-
In Venous Blood: Urea, Creatinine, Uric Acid, Na, K, Total And Ionised Ca, Mg, P, Cl, Alkaline Phosphatase, Gas Analysis.

In 24-Hr Urine Samples: Urea, Creatinine, Uric Acid, Na, K, Ca, Mg, P, Cl, Oxalate, Inorganic Sulphate, Citrate, Ph, Ammonia And Titratable Acidity. Starting From The Main Urine Biochemistries, By Means Of A Dedicated Computer-Based Method, Urine Supersaturations With Calcium Oxalate (Bcaox), Brushite (Bbsh) And Uric Acid (Bua) Are Calculated In Each Patient, To Get An Estimate Of The Propensity Towards The Crystallization Of These Stone-Forming Salts In Urine.[1-8]

In Fasting Urine Samples: Ca, Citrate, Creatinine, Hydroxyproline, Brand's Test For Cistinuria, Urine Sediment, Urine Culture.

Investigations Can Be Used For The Differential Diagnosis Among **Severe Hypercalciuria Syndromes, Or In Case Of Hypercalcemia**.
To This Purpose, **"Second-Level Screening"** Is Focused On The Study Of Both The **Profile Of Calciotropic Hormones And Bone Turnover.**

If The First-Level Evaluation Suggested An Abnormal Bone Turnover, Then Further Determinations Are Warranted, Namely-
Calciotropic Hormones (Blood Vitamin D And PTH), Serum Ionised Calcium, Serum Phosphate And Tubular Resorption Of Phosphate (Tmpo$_4$) Inform On The Biological Activity Of PTH Markers Of Bone Resorption (Urine Pyridinium Crosslinks, Serum Crosslaps) And Formation (Serum Osteocalcin) Bone Mineral Density.

Eventually, **More Sophisticated Investigations** Are Required To Improve The Diagnosis Of Peculiar Diseases: Serum Oxalate And Glycolate, Urine Glycolate And L-Glycerate, Hepatic AGT Activity (Primary Hyperoxalurias); Genetic Tests (Hereditary Nephrolithiasis); Acidification Tests (Renal Tubular Acidosis).

If **Primary Hyperoxaluria** Is Suspected, Oxalate And Glycolate Are Measured In Plasma And Glycolate And Glycerate In Urine As Well.

In Selected Cases Of **Primary Hyperparathyroidism**, Especially When Multiple Endocrine Neoplasia Type I (MEN I) Is Suspected. DNA Assay In Circulating Leukocytes Can Be Used.

If An **Incomplete Form Of Distal Renal Tubular Acidosis (RTA Type I)** Is Suspected, Then The Diagnosis Can Be Confirmed By Means Of Urine Acidification Tests.

The Rationale For The Investigation On The Urinary Composition Of Stone Forming Patients Comes From The Assumption That Derangements Of Urine Biochemistries May Play A Pivotal Role In The Pathogenesis Of Nephrolithiasis. Also, Anatomic Abnormalities Of Kidneys And Urinary Tract, Genetic, Environmental And Dietary Factors May Cooperate In The Pathophysiology Of Renal Stone Disease

The **Urinary Excretions Of Many Substances** (i.e., Water, Electrolytes, Nitrogen, Ash-Acid And Alkali) Depend On Their Glomerular Filtration And The Subsequent Tubular Handling, Which, In Turns, Is Usually Modulated So As To Keep Their External Balance In Equilibrium. (9-15)

In Other Cases (For Example, Fasting Hypercalciuria Syndromes, Renal Tubular Acidosis And Cystinuria) The **Tubular Handling Of Promoters And Inhibitors Of Stone Formation, As Well As Their Urinary Pattern**, Can Be Strongly Influenced By Genetic Factors.

Eventually, Despite Nephrolithiasis Is A Multifactorial Disease, The Study Of The **Propensity Towards The Crystallization Of Stone Forming**

Essentials Of Litho-Tripsy

Salts In Urine Still Remains The Easiest Strategy For The Nephrologist To Estimate The Propensity Towards The Relapses Of Stone Disease In Individual Patients.

In Addition To The Assessment Of The Urinary Pattern Of Promoters And Inhibitors Of Stone Formation, A Suitable Metabolic Evaluation Should Also Focus On The **Occurrence Of Systemic Diseases Potentially Complicating With Secondary Nephrolitiasis**, i.e., Endocrine Disturbances, Intestinal Malabsorption, Bone Diseases.

The Greatest Part Of Both **Sulphate And Urinary Acid Excretion** Comes From The **Metabolism Of Sulphur-Containing Aminoacids**. It Follows That, In This Subset, The Measure Of **Net Acid And Sulphate Excretion Helps In Estimating The Dietary Intake Of Protein Of Animal Origin**, Which Are Believed To Play A Pivotal Role On Calcium Excretion.

As Far As **Vegetable And Fruit Intake** Are Concerned, They Can Be Considered As The **Main Dietary Source Of Alkali**.
It Has Been Demonstrated That The Intestinal Absorption Of Alkali Can Be Reliably Estimated From The **Difference Between Urinary Cations And Anions**.

In Conclusion, **First-Level Biochemical Approach**, By Providing A Reliable Assessment Of Metabolic Profile With The Stone-Forming Patients, Can Be Sufficient For The Nephrologists To Guide Therapeutic Prescriptions In The Majority Of Cases.

On The Other Hand, The **"Second-Level Screening"**, Is Recommended If Urine Biochemistries Or Serum Calcium Levels Are Suggestive For Complex Derangements Of Physiological Bone Turnover, Which Can Develop Either As Primary Or Secondary Disease In Stone-Forming Patients.
In Those Cases, Nephrolithiasis Appears As A Typical Multidisciplinary Disease, Whose Diagnostic And Therapeutic Approaches Take The Best Advantages From The Close Collaboration Among Nephrologist, Endocrinologist, Oncologist, Gynaecologist And General Practitioner.
(16-19)

References
1. Moe OW. Kidney stones: pathophysiology and medical management. Lancet. 2006 Jan 28;367(9507):333–44. [PubMed]
[Review]
2. Taylor EN, Stampfer MJ, Curhan GC. Dietary factors and the risk of incident kidney stones in men: new insights after 14 years of follow-up. J Am Soc Nephrol. 2004 Dec;15(12):3225–32. [PubMed]

3. Ramello A, Vitale C, Marangella M. Epidemiology of nephrolithiasis. J Nephrol. 2000 Nov-Dec;13(3):S45–50. [PubMed] [Review]

4. Vezzoli G, Soldati L, Gambaro G. Update on Primary Hypercalciuria From a Genetic Perspective. J Urol.2008 Mar 14;[Epub ahead of print] [PubMed]

5. Devuyst O, Pirson Y. Genetics of hypercalciuric stone forming diseases. Kidney Int. 2007 Nov;72(9):1065. [PubMed] [72. Epub 2007 Aug 8. Review]

6. Mattoo A, Goldfarb Goldfarb. DS. Cystinuria. Semin Nephrol. 2008 Mar;28(2):181–91. [PubMed]

7. Parks JH, Coward M, Coe FL. Correspondence between stone composition and urine supersaturation in nephrolithiasis. Kidney Int. 1997 Mar;51(3):894–900. [PubMed]

8. Odvina CV, Sakhaee K, Heller HJ, Peterson RD, Poindexter JR, Padalino PK, Pak CY. Biochemical characterization of primary hyperparathyroidism with and without kidney stones. Urol Res. 2007 Jun;35(3):123. [PubMed] [8. Epub 2007 May 3]

9. Worcester EM. Stones from bowel disease. Endocrinol Metab Clin North Am. 2002;31(4):979–99.[PubMed] [Review]

10. Heilberg IP, Weisinger JR. Bone disease in idiopathic hypercalciuria. Curr Opin. Nephrol Hypertens.2006 Jul;15(4):394–402. [PubMed]

11. Marangella M, Daniele PG, Ronzani M, Sonego S, Linari F. Urine saturation with calcium salts in normal subjects and idiopathic calcium stone formers estimated by an improved computer model system.Urol Res. 1985;13:189–93. [PubMed]

12. Marangella M, Petrarulo M, Vitale C, Bagnis C, Berutti S, Ramello A, Amoroso A. The primary hyperoxalurias. Contrib Nephrol. 2001;136:11–32. [PubMed] [Review]

13. Osther PJ, Bollerslev J, Hansen AB, Engel K, Kildeberg P. Pathophysiology of incomplete renal tubular acidosis in recurrent renal stone formers: evidence of disturbed calcium, bone and citrate metabolism. Urol Res. 1993 May;21(3):169–73. [PubMed]

14. Falchetti A, Marini F, Luzi E, Tonelli F, Brandt ML. Multiple endocrine neoplasms. Best Pract Res Clin Rheumatol. 2008 Mar;22(1):149–63. [PubMed]

15. Walsh SB, Shirley DG, Wrong OM, Unwin RJ. Urinary acidification assessed by simultaneous furosemide and fludrocortisone treatment: an alternative to ammonium chloride. Kidney Int. 2007 Jun;71(12):1310–6. [PubMed] [Epub 2007 Apr 4]

16. Kerstetter JE, O'Brien KO, Insogna KL. Low protein intake: the impact on calcium and bone homeostasis in humans. J Nutr. 2003 Mar;133(3):855S–861S. [PubMed] [Review]

17. Marangella M, Vitale C, Bagnis C, Bruno M, Ramello A. Idiopathic calcium nephrolithiasis. Nephron.1999;81(1):38–44. [PubMed]

18. Oh MS. A new method for estimating G-I absorption of alkali. Kidney Int. 1989;36/5:915–7. [PubMed]

19. Pak CY, Odvina CV, Pearle MS, Sakhaee K, Peterson RD, Poindexter JR, Brinkley LJ. Effect of dietary modification on urinary stone risk factors. Kidney Int. 2005 Nov;68(5):2264–73. [PubMed]

Karlin GS, Urivetsky M, Smith AD. Side effect of extracorporeal shock wave lithotripsy: Assessment of urinary excretion of renal enzymes as evidence of tubular injury. In: Lingeman JE, Newman DM, editors.Shock wave lithotripsy 2: Urinary and biliary lithotripsy. New York: Plenum Press; 1989. p. 3-6.

Essentials Of Litho-Tripsy

STONE-PREVENTION STRATEGIES

All Patients Who Undergo Surgery For Stones Should Be Given Information About Kidney-Stone Prevention.

General Measures Include Increased Fluid Intake And Restriction Of Dietary Sodium And Purine. In Patients With Calcium Oxalate Stones, Intake Of Foods High In Oxalate (Eg, Spinach, Nuts, Beer, Chocolate, Rhubarb, Green Leafy Vegetables) Should Be Discouraged. Calcium Intake Should Be Moderated; Extremely High Or Low Levels Of Calcium Can Increase Stone Production.

Blood Work And 24-Hour Urine Collections Measuring For Ph, Urinary Volume, Citrate, Calcium, Oxalate, Uric Acid, Sodium, Magnesium, Phosphates, And Electrolytes Can Assist In Identifying And Alleviating Risk Factors For Future Stone Production.

Following Treatment Of The Initial Stone Event, Testing Should Be Performed In All Children And In Patients With Solitary Kidneys, Chronic Diarrhea, A History Of Bariatric Surgery, Renal Failure, And Nephrocalcinosis,

As Well As In Any Patient With Kidney Stones Who Has Sufficient Motivation **To Follow Long-Term Treatment Recommendations To Prevent Future Stones**.

Twenty-Four–Hour Urine-Testing Protocols Are Available From A Number Of Sources, Including Mission, Dianon, Urocor, Quest, Labcorp, And Litholink.

The National Kidney And Urologic Diseases Information Clearinghouse (NKUDIC), Which Is Part Of The National Institutes Of Health (NIH), Is A Good General Patient Information Web Site.

The NIH Has Also Recommended *The Kidney Stones Handbook* (Savitz And Leslie, 2000). This Award-Winning Patient Guide To Kidney Stones Can Be Ordered Directly From The Publisher (Grant Gibbs) By Email (Gsavitz@Earthlink.Net) Or By Telephone (530-889-1727).

Prevention

Preventative Measures Depend On The Type Of Stones. In Those With Calciums Stone Drinking Lots Of Fluids, Thiazide Diuretics And Citrate Are Effective As Is Allopurinal In Those With High Uric Acid Levels In The Blood Or Urine.[52]

Dietary Measures

Specific Therapy Should Be Tailored To The Type Of Stones Involved. Diet Can Have A Profound Influence On The Development Of Kidney Stones. Preventive Strategies Include Some Combination Of Dietary Modifications And Medications With The Goal Of Reducing The Excretory Load Of Calculogenic Compounds On The Kidneys

Current Dietary Recommendations To Minimize The Formation Of Kidney Stones Include (1-7)

- Increasing Total Fluid Intake, With The Objective Of Increasing Urine Output To More Than Two Liters Per Day

- Increasing Intake Of <u>Citrate</u>-Rich Drinks Such As <u>Lemonade</u> And <u>Orange Juice</u>
- Attempt To Maintain A <u>Calcium</u> Intake Of 1,000–1,200 Mg (1.0–1.2 G) Per Day
- Limiting <u>Sodium</u> Intake To Less Than 2,300 Mg (2.3 G) Per Day
- Limiting <u>Vitamin C</u> Intake To Less Than 1,000 Mg (1.0 G) Per Day
- Limiting Animal Protein Intake To No More Than Two Meals Daily, With Less Than 170–230 G (6.0–8.1 Oz) Per Day. (A Positive Association Between Animal <u>Protein</u> Consumption And Recurrence Of Kidney Stones Has Been Shown In Men.
- Limiting Consumption Of Soft Drinks. Which Contain <u>Phosphoric Acid</u> To Flavor The Soft Drink, Don't Drink More Than A Liter Of Softdrink Per Week.

Maintenance Of Dilute Urine By Means Of Vigorous Fluid Therapy Is Beneficial In All Forms Of Nephrolithiasis, So Increasing Urine Volume Is A Key Principle For The Prevention Of Kidney Stones. Fluid Intake Should Be Sufficient To Maintain A Urine Output Of At Least 2 <u>Litres</u> (68 <u>Us Fl Oz</u>) Per Day. A High Fluid Intake Has Been Associated With A 40% Reduction In Recurrence Risk

Calcium Binds With Available Oxalate In The Gastrointestinal Tract, Thereby Preventing Its Absorption Into The Bloodstream, And Reducing Oxalate Absorption Decreases Kidney Stone Risk In Susceptible People Because Of This, Some <u>Nephrologists</u> And <u>Urologists</u> Recommend Chewing Calcium Tablets During Meals Containing Oxalate Foods. Calcium Citrate Supplements Can Be Taken With Meals If Dietary Calcium Cannot Be Increased By Other Means. The Preferred Calcium Supplement For People At Risk Of Stone Formation Is Calcium Citrate Because It Helps To Increase Urinary Citrate Excretion.

Aside From Vigorous Oral Hydration And Consumption Of More Dietary Calcium, Other Prevention Strategies Include Avoidance Of Large Doses Of Supplemental Vitamin C And Restriction Of Oxalate-Rich Foods Such As <u>Leaf Vegetables</u>, <u>Rhubarb</u>, <u>Soy Products</u> And <u>Chocolate</u>. However, No Randomized, Controlled Trial Of Oxalate Restriction Has Yet Been Performed To Test The Hypothesis That Oxalate Restriction Reduces The Incidence Of Stone Formation. Some Evidence Indicates <u>Magnesium</u> Intake Decreases The Risk Of Symptomatic Nephrolithiasis.

1. "WHAT ARE KIDNEY STONES?". Retrieved August 19, 2013.
2. Heaney, RP (2006). "Nutrition and Chronic Disease". *Mayo Clinic Proceedings* 81 (3): 297–9. doi:<u>10.4065/81.3.297</u>. PMID <u>16529131</u>. Retrieved 2011-07-27.
3. Tiselius, HG (2003). "Epidemiology and medical management of stone disease". *British Journal of Urology International* 91 (8): 758–67. doi:<u>10.1046/j.1464-410X.2003.04208.x</u>. PMID <u>12709088</u>.

Essentials Of Litho-Tripsy

Prognostic factors effecting on recurrence of urinary stone disease: a multivariate analysis of everyday patient parameters.
Unal D, Yeni E, Verit A, Karatas OF.

Research directions

Crystallization of calcium oxalate appears to be inhibited by certain substances in the urine that retard the formation, growth, aggregation, and adherence of crystals to renal cells. By purifying urine using salt precipitation, isoelectric focusing, and size-exclusion chromatography, some researchers have found that calgranulin, a protein formed in the kidney, is a potent inhibitor of the *in vivo* formation of calcium oxalate crystals. Considering its extremely high levels of inhibition of growth and aggregation of calcium oxalate crystals, calgranulin might be an important intrinsic factor in the prevention of nephrolithiasis. (8-13)

References

1. "Tolerable upper intake levels: Calcium and vitamin D". In Committee to Review Dietary Reference Intakes for Vitamin D and Calcium 2011, pp. 403–56.
2. Fang, LST (2009). "Chapter 135: Approach to the Paient with Nephrolithiasis". In Goroll, AH; Mulley, AG. *Primary care medicine: office evaluation and management of the adult patient* (6th ed.). Philadelphia: Lippincott Williams & Wilkins. pp. 962–7. ISBN 978-0-7817-7513-7.
3. Smith-Bindman, R; Aubin, C; Bailitz, J; Bengiamin, RN et al. (18 September 2014). "Ultrasonography versus computed tomography for suspected nephrolithiasis". *The New England Journal of Medicine* 371 (12): 1100–1110.doi:10.1056/NEJMoa1404446. PMID 25229916.
4. Rosenberg, LE; Durant, JL; Elsas, LJ (1968). "Familial iminoglycinuria. An inborn error of renal tubular transport". *The New England Journal of Medicine* 278 (26): 1407–13. doi:10.1056/NEJM196806272782601. PMID 5652624.
5. Coşkun, T; Ozalp, I; Tokatli, A (1993). "Iminoglycinuria: A benign type of inherited aminoaciduria". *The Turkish Journal of Pediatrics* 35 (2): 121–5.PMID 7504361.
6. Merck Sharp & Dohme Corporation (2010). "Patient Information about Crixivan for HIV (Human Immunodeficiency Virus) Infection". *Crixivan® (indinavir sulfate) Capsules*. Whitehouse Station, New Jersey: Merck Sharp & Dohme Corporation. Retrieved 2011-07-27.
7. Schlossberg, D; Samuel, R (2011). "Sulfadiazine". *Antibiotic Manual: A Guide to Commonly Used Antimicrobials* (1st ed.). Shelton, Connecticut: People's Medical Publishing House. pp. 411–12. ISBN 978-1-60795-084-4.
8. Carr, MC; Prien, EL, Jr; Babayan, RK (1990). "Triamterene nephrolithiasis: Renewed attention is warranted". *The Journal of Urology* 144 (6): 1339–40.PMID 2231920.

9. McNutt, WF (1893). "Chapter VII: Vesical Calculi (Cysto-lithiasis)". *Diseases of the Kidneys and Bladder: A Text-book for Students of Medicine*. IV: Diseases of the Bladder. Philadelphia: J.B. Lippincott Company. pp. 185–6.

10. Fink, HA; Wilt, TJ; Eidman, KE; Garimella, PS et al. (2 April 2013). "Medical management to prevent recurrent nephrolithiasis in adults: A systematic review for an American College of Physicians clinical guideline". *Annals of Internal Medicine* 158 (7): 535–43. doi:10.7326/0003-4819-158-7-201304020-00005.PMID 23546565.

11. Qaseem, A; Dallas, P; Forciea, MA; Starkey, M; Denberg, TD; Clinical Guidelines Committee of the American College of, Physicians (4 November 2014). "Dietary and pharmacologic management to prevent recurrent nephrolithiasis in adults: a clinical practice guideline from the American College of Physicians.".*Annals of internal medicine* 161 (9): 659–67. PMID 25364887.

12. Goldfarb, DS; Coe, FL (1999). "Prevention of recurrent nephrolithiasis".*American Family Physician* 60 (8): 2269–76. PMID 10593318.

13. Lam, JS; Gupta, M, Ch. 25: "Ureteral Stents". In Stoller & Meng 2007, pp. 465–83.

Essentials Of Litho-Tripsy
(F) TREATMENT OF CAUSE

Amongst Some **Known Inborn Errors Of Metabolism Aetiologies For Stone Disease e.g Cystinuria, Alkaptonuria**
(Please Note, Cystine & Alkaptonuric Stones-Page- ,).

The Other Metabolic Causes Involving Bio-Chemical Assessment Of Ca, Mg, Phosphorous, Oxalates, Citrates, Uric Acid, Purines Are Managed By Life Style Changes, Diet Regulations, Medications, With Life Long Regular Monitoring Of Involved Bio-Chemical Indices & Management In Accordance.
As Discussed Under Metabolic Evaluation- Strerile Urine, Free Of Crystalluria (Sediments And Casts), AchieveMent By Appropriate AntiMicrobials In Adequate Dosage Duration & Other Medical Therpy, With Life Long Maintainence By Regular Check-Ups,
Helps Drastically For Stone Disease Prone Patients
Clinical Manifestations, Especially In 'Struvite'(Infectious) Stones.

Xanthine Stones- Affliction With Xanthinuria Often Produce Stones Composed Of Xanthine.
2,8-Dihydroxyadenine Stones, In
Adenine Phosphoribosyltransferase Deficiency Affliction.

Alkaptonurics Produce Homogentisic Acid Stones,
Iminoglycinurics Produce Stones Of Glycine, Proline And Hydroxyproline.[4
Urolithiasis Has Also Been Noted To Occur In The Setting Of Therapeutic Drug Use, With Crystals Of Drug Forming Within The Renal Tract In Some People Currently Being Treated With Agents Such As Indinavir, Sulfadiazine[And Triamterene.

While Discussion RegardingThe Most Common Endocrinal Cause- 'ParaTharmone' Has Been Summarized As Follows-

The Parathyroid Glands
The Parathyroid Glands Are Four Tiny Glands Located Within The Thyroid Gland Located In The Neck,. Each Gland Is About The Size Of A Grain Of Rice (Weighs Approximately 30 Milligrams And Is 3-4 Millimeters In Diameter).
They Produce Parathyroid Hormone(PTH),That Regulates,
The Amount Of Calcium In The Blood. By-

1. Breaking Down The Bone (Where Most Of The Body's Calcium Is Stored And Causing Calcium Release
2. Increasing The Body's Ability To Absorb Calcium From Food

3. Increasing The Kidney's Ability To Hold On To Calcium That Would Otherwise Be Lost In The Urine.

Normal Parathyroid Glands Work Like The Thermostat To Keep Blood Calcium Levels In A Very Tightly Controlled Range.

When The Blood Calcium Level Is Too Low, PTH Is Released To Bring The Calcium Level Back Up To Normal.

When The Calcium Level Is Normal Or Gets A Little Too High, Normal Parathyroids Will Stop Releasing PTH.

Proper Calcium Balance Is Crucial To The Normal Functioning Of The Heart, Nervous System, Kidneys, And Bones.

Parathyroid Gland If Enlarged, Can Result In Production Of **Excessive Parathyroid Hormone (Hyperparathyroidism)**. This May Lead To Too Much Calcium In The Urine, With Increased LikelyHood For Calcium Kidney Stones Formation.

Primary Hyperparathyroidism Causes Abnormally High Blood Calcium Levels Mainly Be "Stealing" Calcium From The Bones. Every Cell And Organ In The Body Uses Calcium As A Signal To Regulate Their Normal Function. Therefore, It Is Crucial That Calcium Levels Are Tightly Controlled. Abnormally High Blood Calcium Levels Can Damage Every Organ In The Body Gradually Over Time.

In The Past, Generations Of Doctors Learned The Classic Symptoms Of Primary Hyperparathyroidism Through The Saying **"Bones, Stones, And Groans"** Which Represented Weakened Bones, Kidney Stones, And Abdominal Pain.

In Addition, Many Patients Also Had **"Psychic Moans And Fatigue Overtones"** Which Indicated Mood Disturbances And Fatigue.

In Extreme Cases Of Severe Elevations Of Blood Calcium Levels Called **"Hypercalcemic Crisis"** Patients May Present In Comatose Or Near-Comatose States With Organ Failure. However, Today Most Patients Are Diagnosed Through Routine Blood Testing Or Screening For Osteoporosis And Many Patients Have Only Vague, Non-Specific Symptoms.

Normal Parathyroid Glands Work Like The Thermostat To Keep Blood Calcium Levels In A Very Tightly Controlled Range. When The Blood Calcium Level Is Too Low, PTH Is Released To Bring The Calcium Level Back Up To Normal. When The Calcium Level Is Normal Or Gets A Little Too High, Normal Parathyroids Will Stop Releasing PTH. Proper Calcium Balance Is Crucial To The Normal Functioning Of The Heart, Nervous System, Kidneys, And Bones.

Essentials Of Litho-Tripsy

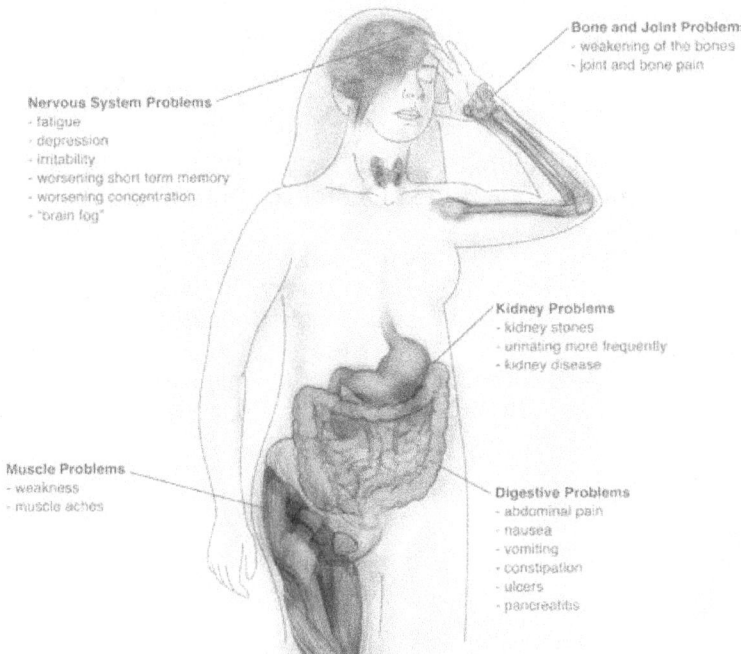

Para-Thyroid Glands:Clinical Manifestations

Kidney Stones
Of All Patients Who Present With Kidney Stones Only 3 To 8% Will Have Primary Hyperparathyroidism. Surgery For Primary Hyperparathyroidism Decreases The Frequency Of Developing New Kidney Stones Among Those Patients With Kidney Stones And Primary Hyperparathyroidism. (2)

Only About 7 To 15% Of People Who Have Primary Hyperparathyroidism Have Kidney Stones.

DIAGNOSIS
Primary Hyperparathyroidism Is Diagnosed Through Blood Tests. Since The Parathyroid Hormone (PTH) Levels Control The Calcium Levels, The Two Levels Normally Move In Opposite Directions. For Example, When The Blood Calcium Level Is High, The PTH Level Should Be Low Or On The Lower End Of Normal. When The Blood Calcium Level Is Low, The PTH Level Should Increase (In Order To Tell The Body To Absorb More Calcium). **In Primary Hyperparathyroidism, Both Levels Are Elevated**.

Ocasionally In Patients With Primary Hyperparathyroidism, One Or Both Of These Levels May Be Normal, But In The Higher End Of Normal (Normocalcemic Hyperparathyroidism).

Additional Tests That May Be Helpful In Making The Diagnosis Of Primary Hyperparathyroidism Include-
The Blood Phosphate Level, The Vitamin D Level, Urine Calcium Levels (A Urine Test Of Calcium Collected Over A 24-Hour Period), And The Blood Creatinine Level (A Measure Of Kidney Function).
The 24 Hour Urine Calcium Level Will Help Determine If The Individual Has Familial **Hypocalciuric Hypercalcemia** (A Benign Condition Not Requiring Surgery).
Vitamin D Levels Should Be Checked Because Low Vitamin D Levels May Be Causing A Problem Called **Secondary Hyperparathyroidism** And Vitamin D Levels Need To Be Cautiously Replaced Before Further Work Up Is Done.
Patients With Elevated Calcium And/Or Parathyroid Hormone Levels Should Also Have Their **Bone Density Tests**, Known As **DEXA-Scan**.

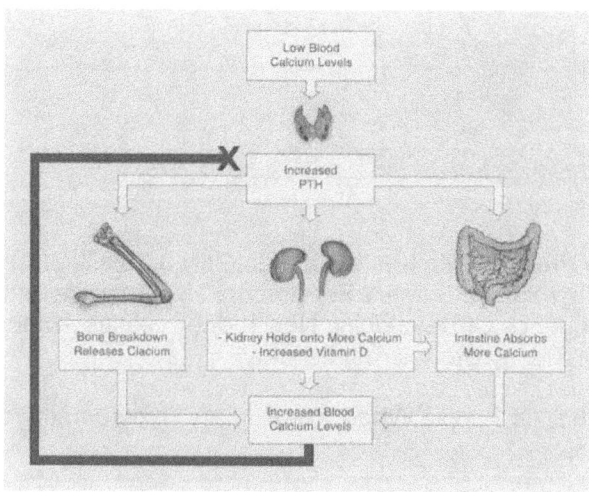

Calcium/ PTH / Vitamin D Regulation

Untreated Primary Hyperparathyroidism Can Cause A Number Of Health Problems Over The Long Term, Such As Kidney Stones And Osteoporosis (Thinning Or Weakening Of The Bones),
But Most Often Does Not Lead To Medical Emergencies.
Once Diagnosed With Primary Hyperparathyroidism,
The Decision For Treatment Should Be Made After Careful Consideration With The Advice Of Primary Care Physician, Endocrinologist, And/Or Endocrine Surgeon.

Essentials Of Litho-Tripsy

Prior To An Operation, A Series Of **"Localizing Tests"** (Radiology Tests To Determine Which Gland(S) Are Abnormal) Are Done.

Treatment Of Primary Hyperparathyroidism

Alternatives To An Operation?

Observation- One Alternative To Have An Operation Is To Observe Closely. Blood Calcium And Parathyroid Hormone (PTH) Levels Will Be Checked On A Routine Basis And Routine Follow-Up Visits To Assess For Development Of Symptoms Will Be Scheduled.

Studies Have Compared The Outcomes Of Those Patients Who Undergo Parathyroidectomy Versus Those Patients Who Do Not Undergo Curative Surgery. Many Patients Who Are Observed Will Go On To Have Increasing Blood Calcium And PTH Levels Or Will Develop One Or More Indications (i.e. Reasons) For Surgery.

Calcimimetics (Sensipar, Cinacalcet, Etc)- Calcimimetics Are Medications That Attach To A Receptor On Parathyroid Cells And Increases The Ability Of Cells To Respond To High Blood Calcium Levels So That Less PTH Is Produced. By Causing Less PTH To Be Made, Calcimimetics Decrease The Amount Of Calcium In The Bloodstream.

Taking Cinacalcet Will Not Cure The Disease Process. It Can Only Decrease Parathyroid Hormone Secretion To A Certain Extent.

Osteoporosis Medications (i.e. Bisphosphonates)- One Of The Main Problems With Primary Hyperparathyroidism Is That High PTH Levels Lead To Lower Bone Density And Potentially Osteoporosis With An Increased Risk For Fractures. Bisphosphonates Are A Type Of Medication That Are Used To Treat Decreased Bone Density. They Inactivate Or Disable The The Bone Cell (i.e. The Osteoclast) That Causes Bone Breakdown In Order To Reduce Bone Turnover. Bisphosphonates Do Not Treat The Underlying Disease But Can Help Improve The Decreased Bone Density Caused By The Disease.

Hormone Replacement Therapy (i.e. Estrogens)- One Of The Main Problems With Primary Hyperparathyroidism Is That High PTH Levels Lead To Lower Bone Density And Potentially Osteoporosis With An Increased Risk For Fractures. Estrogen Replacement Is Well Known To Have Positive Effects On Bone Density And Heart Disease In Women Who Have Gone Through Menopause. Several Studies Have Looked At The Potential Role For Estrogen Replacement Therapy In Postmenopausal Women With Primary Hyperparathyroidism. Estrogen Increases Bone Density By Inactivating Or Disabling The Bone Cell (i.e. The Osteoclast) That Causes Bone Breakdown. Estrogen Does Not Treat The Underlying Disease But Can Help Improve The Decreased Bone Density Caused By The Disease.

Hyperparathyroidism: Localization (i.e. Finding The Abnormal Gland)

In Most Patients With Primary Hyperparathyroidism (80%), Only One Of The Four Parathyroid Glands Is Diseased — These People Have What Is Called A **"Singleadenoma."**
In About 10% Of Affected People, Two Or Three Glands Are Hyperactive- Called "Double Or Triple Adenoma."
Finally, In 10% Of Patients, All Four Glands Are Hyperacitve- Called **"Four Gland Hyperplasia."**

Localizing Tests Are Radiology Tests Designed To Help Identify Which Parathyroid Gland(S) Are Hyperactive.
In The Past, Localization Studies Were Not Routinely Performed Before A First Operation Because A **Bilateral Neck Exploration** (An Operation Where The Surgeon Examines All Four Parathyroid Glands) Was Usually Performed.
However, If A **Focused Parathyroidectomy (**An Operation Where The Surgeon Examines And Removes Just The Hyperactive Gland) Is Going To Be Performed Then Accurate Pre-Operative Localization Is An Essential Component, So Most Patients Undergo Some Form Of Pre-Operative Localization.

If A Bilateral Neck Exploration Is Going To Be Performed, Then Pre-Operative Localization Studies May Not Be Necessary.

The Most Commonly Performed Localizing Tests Are -
Sestamibi Scan And Ultrasound Of The Neck.
Increasingly, High Resolution CT (Computed Tomography Or CAT Scans) And MRI (Magnetic Resonance Imaging) Scans Are Of Significant Help, Depending Upon The Patent, Surgeon Decides The Needed **Localizing Tests.**

Sestamibi Scans Involve Injecting A Small Amount Of Special Radioactive Material Into A Vein And Taking An X-Ray Image Of The Chest, Neck, And Head. Sestamibi Scans Have An Accuracy Rate Of About 80 To 95%. The Accuracy Of The Test Is Very Institution-Specific And Depends On The Quality Of The Equipment Used, The Technique Used To Perform The Test, And The Skill Of The Interpreter. Centers That Perform A Lot Of Parathyroid Surgery Typically Have More Accurate Sestamibi Scans. The Advantages Of Sestamibi Scans Are Its Wide Availability And The Ability To Evaluate For Diseased Glands Outside Of The Neck At The Same Time.

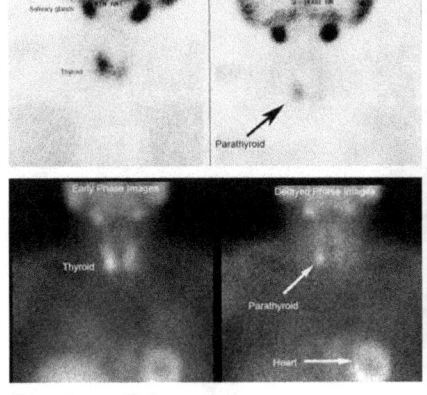 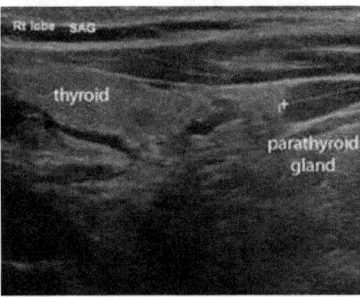

Sestamibi scan   **Ultrasound**

Ultrasound Is Another Commonly Used Localizing Test. Ultrasound Is Noninvasive, Inexpensive, And Requires No Special Preparation. However, USG Also Is Very Dependent On The Skill Of The Person Performing The Test. It Is Very Important That The Person Performing The Ultrasound Knows Where To Look For The Abnormal Glands. Many Parathyroid Surgeons Perform Their Own Ultrasound Exams For This Reason. Ultrasound Is Good For Identifying Glands In The Neck, But Often Cannot See Diseased Glands Located Either Deep In The Neck Or In The Chest. Sometimes It Can Be Difficult To Tell The Difference Between A Parathyroid Gland And A Thyroid Nodule Or A Lymph Node. When The Ultrasound And Sestamibi Scan Agree As To The Location Of The Diseased Gland, There Is A 96% Chance That It Is The Only Diseased Gland.

High Resolution CAT Scan (CT Scan) Of The Neck And Chest Designed Specifically For The Parathyroid Glands Are Available At Select Institutions. While Traditional CT Scans Are Not Very Good At Finding Diseased Parathyroid Glands, Newer Techniques Using Intravenous (IV) Contrast Are Showing Promise In Localizing Parathyroid Glands Both In The Neck And Chest. These Specialized CAT Scans Can Have Accuracy Rates As High As 90 To 95%.

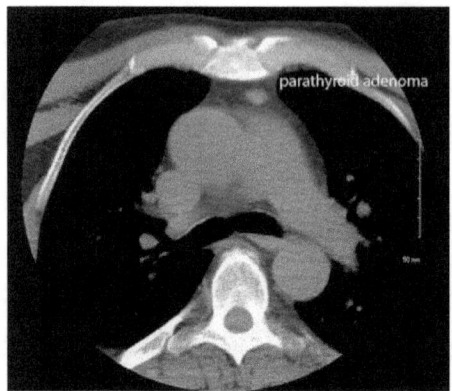

CAT Scan

Parathyroid Biopsy With Parathyroid Hormone (PTH) Testing May Be Used If Patients Are Found To Have A Mass In The Neck On Ultrasound And It Is Unclear If It Is Parathyroid Gland Or Other Structure Like A Thyroid Nodule Or Lymph Node. A Biopsy Can Be Performed In Most Centersand Is Usually Done With Ultrasound Guidance. This Involves Putting A Needle Into The Mass And Removing A Few Cells From It. These Cells Can Be A) Examined Under A Microscope To See If They Resemble Parathyroid Cells Or B) Tested For PTH Levels.

MRI (Magnetic Resonance Imaging) Can Also Be Used To Help Localize Parathyroid Abnormalities But The Accuracy Is Not As Good As The Other Tests And Is Typically Only Used In Cases Of Re-Operative Surgery.
(see Special Cases: Re-operative Parathyroid Surgery)

Parathyroid Venous Sampling (Selective Venous Sampling) Is Another Specialized Test That May Be Performed In Selected Centers. This Test Is Typically Only Used In Cases Of Re-Operative Surgery. It Can Be Done In Two Ways:

1. Jugular Venous Sampling — Your Surgeon Will Pass A Needle Into A Large Vein (The Internal Jugular Vein) On Each Side Of The Neck Under Ultrasound Guidance. A Blood Sample Is Taken And Tested For PTH Levels. Your Surgeon Is Looking To See If One Side Of The Neck Has Higher Levels Which Would Indicate That The Overactive Gland Is On That Side. This Test Does Not Reveal The Exact Location Of The Overactive Parathyroid But Helps To Determine Which Side It Is On.
2. Selective Venous Sampling — A Radiologist Or Vascular Surgeon Inserts A Catheter (A Plastic Tube) Into A Vein In The Groin. It Is Advanced Under Guidance Into Veins In The Neck And Chest To Again Sample Blood For PTH Levels. This Test Is More Invasive And May Take Longer But Allows Your Surgeon To Gain Information About

Blood Levels Of PTH From Both The Neck And Chest To Help Pinpoint The Location Of Your Abnormal Gland.

Surgical Options

<u>Expert Parathyroid Surgeon</u>
<u>Bilateral Neck Exploration</u>
<u>Focused Parathyroidectomy</u>
<u>Radioguided Parathyroidectomy</u>
<u>Video-Assisted Parathyroidectomy</u>
<u>Surgical Options For Four Gland Hyperplasia</u>

For <u>Kidney Stones</u> Due To Enlarged Parathyroid Glands, Surgery To Remove One Or More Of The Glands (Parathyroidectomy), Is Indicated
Performed Under <u>General Anesthesia</u>, With An Incision In The Front Of Neck. Identification Of The Parathyroid Glands Is Done, Determining Their Size, Removal Of Any Enlarged Ones Is Done. In Most People, There Is Only One Enlarged Gland.
Age And General Health Determines The Hospital Stay & Recovery Many People Leave The Hospital A Few Days After Surgery & Typically Can Return To Work With Normal Activities In 1 To 2 Weeks.

REFERENCES

1. Silverberg SJ, Shane E, Jacobs TP, et al. A 10-year prospective study of primary hyperparathyroidism with or without parathyroid surgery. N Engl J Med 1999; 341(17):1249-55.
2. Mollerup CL, Vestergaard P, Frokjaer VG, et al. Risk of renal stone events in primary hyperparathyroidism before and after parathyroid surgery: controlled retrospective follow up study. BMJ 2002; 325(7368):807.
3. Rodman JS, Mahler RJ. Kidney stones as a manifestation of hypercalcemic disorders. Hyperparathyroidism and sarcoidosis. Urol Clin North Am 2000; 27(2):275-85, viii.
4. Giles Y, Baspinar I, Tunca F, et al. Impact of surgical treatment on respiratory muscle dysfunction in symptomatic hyperparathyroidism. Arch Surg 2005; 140(12):1167-71.
5. Kristoffersson A, Bostrom A, Soderberg T. Muscle strength is improved after parathyroidectomy in patients with primary hyperparathyroidism. Br J Surg 1992; 79(2):165-8.
6. Chou FF, Sheen-Chen SM, Leong CP. Neuromuscular recovery after parathyroidectomy in primary hyperparathyroidism. Surgery 1995; 117(1):18-25.
7. Joborn C, Hetta J, Johansson H, et al. Psychiatric morbidity in primary hyperparathyroidism. World J Surg 1988; 12(4):476-81.
8. McAllion SJ, Paterson CR. Psychiatric morbidity in primary hyperparathyroidism. Postgrad Med J 1989; 65(767):628-631.
9. Goyal A, Chumber S, Tandon N, et al. Neuropsychiatric manifestations in patients of primary hyperparathyroidism and outcome following surgery. Indian J Med Sci 2001; 55(12):677-86.

10. Burney RE, Jones KR, Christy B, Thompson NW. Health status improvement after surgical correction of primary hyperparathyroidism in patients with high and low preoperative calcium levels. Surgery 1999; 125(6):608-14.
11. Quiros RM, Alef MJ, Wilhelm SM, et al. Health-related quality of life in hyperparathyroidism measurably improves after parathyroidectomy. Surgery 2003; 134(4):675-81; discussion 681-3.
12. Pasieka JL, Parsons LL. Prospective surgical outcome study of relief of symptoms following surgery in patients with primary hyperparathyroidism. World J Surg 1998; 22(6):513-8; discussion 518-9.
13. Chan AK, Duh QY, Katz MH, et al. Clinical manifestations of primary hyperparathyroidism before and after parathyroidectomy. A case-control study. Ann Surg 1995; 222(3):402-12; discussion 412-4.
14. Rosenblatt S, Faillace LA. Psychiatric manifestations of hyperparathyroidism. Tex Med 1977; 73(2):59-60.
15. Talpos GB, Bone HG, 3rd, Kleerekoper M, et al. Randomized trial of parathyroidectomy in mild asymptomatic primary hyperparathyroidism: patient description and effects on the SF-36 health survey. Surgery 2000; 128(6):1013-20;discussion 1020-1.
16. Vazquez-Diaz O, Castillo-Martinez L, Orea-Tejeda A, et al. Reversible changes of electrocardiographic abnormalities after parathyroidectomy in patients with primary hyperparathyroidism. Cardiol J 2009; 16(3):241-5.
17. Hedback G, Oden A, Tisell LE. The influence of surgery on the risk of death in patients with primary hyperparathyroidism. World J Surg 1991; 15(3):399-405; discussion 406-7.
18. Kebebew E, Hwang J, Reiff E, et al. Predictors of single-gland vs multigland parathyroid disease in primary hyperparathyroidism: a simple and accurate scoring model. Arch Surg 2006; 141(8):777-82; discussion 782.
19. Harari A, Zarnegar R, Lee J, et al. Computed tomography can guide focused exploration in select patients with primary hyperparathyroidism and negative sestamibi scanning. Surgery 2008; 144(6):970-6; discussion 976-9.
20. Vestergaard P, Mollerup CL, Frokjaer VG, et al. Cohort study of risk of fracture before and after surgery for primary hyperparathyroidism. BMJ 2000; 321(7261):598-602.
21. Rubin MR, Bilezikian JP, McMahon DJ, et al. The natural history of primary hyperparathyroidism with or without parathyroid surgery after 15 years. J Clin Endocrinol Metab 2008; 93(9):3462-70.
22. Corlew DS, Bryda SL, Bradley EL, 3rd, DiGirolamo M. Observations on the course of untreated primary hyperparathyroidism. Surgery 1985; 98(6):1064-71.
23. Peacock M, Bilezikian JP, Klassen PS, et al. Cinacalcet hydrochloride maintains long-term normocalcemia in patients with primary hyperparathyroidism. J Clin Endocrinol Metab 2005; 90(1):135-41.
24. Chen H, Parkerson S, Udelsman R. Parathyroidectomy in the elderly: do the benefits outweigh the risks? World J Surg 1998; 22(6):531-5; discussion 535-6.
25. Zanocco K, Angelos P, Sturgeon C. Cost-effectiveness analysis of parathyroidectomy for asymptomatic primary hyperparathyroidism. Surgery 2006; 140(6):874-81; discussion 881-2.
26. Khan AA, Bilezikian JP, Kung AW, et al. Alendronate in primary hyperparathyroidism: a double-blind, randomized, placebo-controlled trial. J Clin Endocrinol Metab 2004; 89(7):3319-25.
27. Guo CY, Thomas WE, al-Dehaimi AW, et al. Longitudinal changes in bone mineral density and bone turnover in postmenopausal women with primary hyperparathyroidism. J Clin Endocrinol Metab 1996; 81(10):3487-91.
28. Orr-Walker BJ, Evans MC, Clearwater JM, et al. Effects of hormone replacement therapy on bone mineral density in postmenopausal women with primary hyperparathyroidism: four-year follow-up and comparison with healthy postmenopausal women. Arch Intern Med 2000; 160(14):2161-6.
29. Sosa JA, Powe NR, Levine MA, et al. Profile of a clinical practice: Thresholds for surgery and surgical outcomes for patients with primary hyperparathyroidism: a

national survey of endocrine surgeons. J Clin Endocrinol Metab 1998; 83(8):2658-65.
30. Bergenfelz A, Lindblom P, Tibblin S, Westerdahl J. Unilateral versus bilateral neck exploration for primary hyperparathyroidism: a prospective randomized controlled trial. Ann Surg 2002; 236(5):543-51.
31. Carneiro DM, Solorzano CC, Irvin GL, 3rd. Recurrent disease after limited parathyroidectomy for sporadic primary hyperparathyroidism. J Am Coll Surg 2004; 199(6):849-53; discussion 853-5.
32. Chen H, Sokoll LJ, Udelsman R. Outpatient minimally invasive parathyroidectomy: a combination of sestamibi-SPECT localization, cervical block anesthesia, and intraoperative parathyroid hormone assay. Surgery 1999; 126(6):1016-21; discussion 1021-2.
33. Barczynski M, Cichon S, Konturek A, Cichon W. Minimally invasive video-assisted parathyroidectomy versus open minimally invasive parathyroidectomy for a solitary parathyroid adenoma: a prospective, randomized, blinded trial. World J Surg 2006; 30(5):721-31.
34. Miccoli P, Berti P. Minimally invasive parathyroid surgery. Best Pract Res Clin Endocrinol Metab 2001; 15(2):139-47.
35. Irvin GL, 3rd, Solorzano CC, Carneiro DM. Quick intraoperative parathyroid hormone assay: surgical adjunct to allow limited parathyroidectomy, improve success rate, and predict outcome. World J Surg 2004; 28(12):1287-92.
36. Bachar G, Gilat H, Mizrachi A, et al. Comparison of perioperative management and outcome of parathyroidectomy between older and younger patients. Head Neck 2008; 30(11):1415-21.
37. Egan KR, Adler JT, Olson JE, Chen H. Parathyroidectomy for primary hyperparathyroidism in octogenarians and nonagenarians: a risk-benefit analysis. J Surg Res 2007; 140(2):194-8.
38. Lowe H, McMahon DJ, Rubin MR, et al. Normocalcemic primary hyperparathyroidism: further characterization of a new clinical phenotype. J Clin Endocrinol Metab 2007; 92(8):3001-5.
39. Gordon W. The consequences of uncontrolled secondary hyperparathyroidism and its treatment in chronic kidney disease. Semin Dial 2004; 17:209-216.
40. Olson JA, Jr., Leight GS, Jr. Surgical management of secondary hyperparathyroidism. Adv Ren Replace Ther 2002; 9(3):209-18.
41. Rothmund M, Wagner PK, Schark C. Subtotal parathyroidectomy versus total parathyroidectomy and autotransplantation in secondary hyperparathyroidism: a randomized trial. World J Surg 1991; 15(6):745-50.
42. Schlosser K, Endres N, Celik I, et al. Surgical treatment of tertiary hyperparathyroidism: the choice of procedure matters! World J Surg 2007; 31(10):1947-53.

Source-
Parathyroid Gland and Kidney Stones - Topic Overview
Parathyroid Gland and Kidney Stones Guide
The American Association Of Endocrine Surgeons

(3.)
(i.) INTRA-CORPOREAL APPLIANCES

By Available 'Flexible' & 'Rigid' Instrumentations,
Produced Shock Waves Are Utilized Within Patients' Body Directly To Stones. SomeTimes Combination Of Ballistic & USG Devices Are Used.

Endoscopic Lithotripsy Refers To The Visualization Of A Calculus, In The Urinary Tract And The Simultaneous Application Of Energy To Fragment The Stone Or Stones Into Either Extractable
Or Passable Pieces.

Depending On **Stone Size And Location And Associated Ureteral Obstruction**, Various Treatments Are In Use.
Most Small (< 5 Mm) Kidney & Ureteral Stones, Pass Spontaneously Without Surgical Intervention.
Many Calculi In The Upper Urinary Tract Are Treated With **Extracorporeal Shockwave Lithotripsy (ESWL)**. Larger Stones (< 1.5 Cm), Not Associated With Complete Ureteral Or Renal Obstruction Can Frequently Be Treated With ESWL In A NonInvasive Manner.
However, For Stones That Are Poor Candidates For This Modality, Endoscopic Therapy Is Indicated. **UreteroScopy** Is The Most Common Means Of Visualizing An Upper Urinary Tract Calculus. In Addition, **Percutaneous Techniques (eg Percutaneous Endourology)** Can Also Be Used.

Most Commonly, **Endoscopic Treatment** Is Used To Manage **Obstructive And / Or Large Stones**. HowEver Most Infectious Calculi Are Large And Usually Located In The Kidney, Are Also Commonly Treated With Endoscopy. In These Scenarios, Retrograde Ureteroscopic Lithotripsy Or Percutaneous Nephrosto-Lithotomy Is Used.

Intracorporeal Devices Have Been Used Over Many Centuries For Removal Of Stones. With No Considerable Change, In The Basic Principles Of Stone Removal Methodology, The Technology Progression To The Modern Devices, In Use NowAdays, Witnessed Drastic Changes In The Last Several Decades.
The First Evidence Of The Endemic Problem Of Stone Formation Provided By Egyptian Mummies, With Several Accounts Of Ancient Egyptian Treatment Methods Including The First Known Method Of Intracorporeal Treatment Of Stones Designed To Treat Bladder Stone (Soft Struvite) Utilizing A Hollow Reed Placed In The Bladder With A Diamond Or Hard Rock Secured To The End With Gum Or Pitch. By Having The Patient Walk Around With The Reed In The Bladder, The

Essentials Of Litho-Tripsy

Struvite Eventually Crumbled And Was Voided. However, For Harder Material Stones(Calcium Oxalate Monohydrate Or Uric Acid),The Treatment Methodology Was Less Successful.

The Historical Alternative To Reed Treatment Was The Method Of Open Cystolithotomy. The Suprapubic Approach Was Attempted And Abandoned Because Of **Frequent Peritoneal Injury And Septic Death**. **The Advent Of General Anesthesia Being Centuries Away**, The Procedures Needed To Be Performed Swiftly With The Assistance Of Several Strong Men To Hold Down The Patient. The Patient Was Invariably Screaming And Performing A Valsalva Maneuver Leading To The Peritoneum Extending Over The Space Of Retzius, Covering The Dome Of The Bladder More Anteriorly Resulting Many Peritoneal Perforations, And The Subsequent Invariably Fatal. Peritonitis.

An Alternative Was Sought. In Ad 30, The Roman Physician Celsus Described The Method Of The Perineal Lithotomy , With 50% Mortality And 50% SuccessFul Stone Removal Rate. The Technique Virtually Remain Unchanged Until The Eighteenth Century, With A Variety Of Forceps,The Stone Grasp,Crush And Extraction Method Was Initiated,

In The Eighteenth Century There Were Many Itinerant Lithotomists Throughout Europe..[26]

In 1782, Colonel Martin, A Physician In India, Developed The First Modern Technique Of Transurethral Treatment Of Bladder Stones By Studies Performed On HimSelf.
For The Bladder Stone, Resistant To Then AvailAble Latest Treatment Of **Intravesical Instillation Of Pigeon Guano And Lye**.
He Devised A File,Capable Of Negotiating ThroughThe Urethra To Bladder & With Supportive Postural Changes(Leaning Forward Against A Wall), By Stone Rubbing Against The File, Three Times A Day The Stone And All Residual Fragments, Were Removed Within 6 Months.

The Next Major Advance In Stone Removal Was A Wire Noose Invented In 1813 By A Munich Physician Named Gruithuisen.
A Hollow Tube Was Inserted Into The Bladder, And The Stone Was Held To The End Of The Tube With The Noose.
By 1824, Civiale, A French Surgeon, Had Made Some Improvements On The Original Techniques Of Gruithuisen, By Using A Three-Prong Grasping Forceps To Grasp The Stone Firmly, And A Screw Was Pressured Into The Stone, Fragmenting Even The Harder Stones. Practicing Tactile Methodolgy To Locate And Fragment Stones.

During The Ensuing Decades, Improvements For Safety & Effectiveness Increase Were In Progress, With The Two-Arm Lithotrite Used To Hold And Grasp Stones.

Bigelow Invented An Evacuator To Remove Stone Fragments. At The Massachusetts General Hospital.
With The Successful **Advent Of General Anesthesia, Suprapubic Stone Removal Procedures Were Able To Be Performed** Without Valsalva. **Radiograph Techniques Also Aided In The Diagnosis And Localization Of Stones**.

In The Early Twentieth Century The Cystoscope Was Invented, Enabling Direct Visualization Of The Stone And Improving Again The Safety And Efficacy Of Stone Removal. The Success Rate, However, Of Removal Of Bladder Stones By Intracorporeal Methods Had Improved Only Marginally During A 100-Year Period..[25]

WithThe Technology Development, Urologists Adopted Change From Nonvisualization Procedures To Direct Visualization Techniques, And Then Indirect Visualization With Extracorporeal Shock Wave Lithothripsy.
Only Recently Has Direct Visualization Of The Ureter And Renal Pelvis Allowed Clinicians Safely To Remove Stones From These Locations, Whereas They Were Removed For The Most Part Via Ureteral Lithotomy Or Pyelolithotomy Only A Decade Ago.
To Remove A Stone, It Must Be Pulled Out Or Broken, And A Stone Can Be Broken With A Hammer. The First Reinvention Of The Hammer Came With The Advent Of The Electrohydraulic Lithotriptor (EHL).

The Lithospec™ Is The Ideal Choice For **Safe And Effective Intracorporeal Lithotripsy Utilizing Electromechanical Energy Source.** It Complements Medispec's ESWL Systems, Offering The Urologist A Highly Affordable Stone Center.

Lithospec Is An **Electromechanical Intracorporeal Lithotripter** For The Treatment Of Urinary Calculi. It Is Indicated For The Fragmentation Of Kidney, Bladder And Ureteral Stones. The Lithospec Is Particularly Effective In Fragmentation Large Stones, Cysteine Stones, Calcium Oxalate Monohydrate Calculi And Other Stones That May Not Respond Well To Extracorporeal Lithotripsy Treatments.

The Electromechanical Technique Ensures That The Lithospec **Delivers High Impact Mechanical Fragmentation Power Tothe Stone**, Therefore **Eliminating The Possibility Of Thermal Injury**. The Lithospec Is User **Friendly, Compact And Portable. The Probes Are Reusable, Which**

Essentials Of Litho-Tripsy

Helps To Reduce The Cost Per Treatment, Providing An Extremely Cost Effective Investment.

BENEFITS
Safe And Effective In Fragmenting Large Stones
- No Compressor Or Air Supply Needed
- Compatible With Any Standard Endoscopes Currently Available In The Market
- Simple To Operate And Maintain
- Portable And Compact

Ultrasonic Lithotripsy
Most Commonly Used Via A Percutaneously Placed Rigid Endoscope. This Form Of Endoscopic Lithotripsy,Requires A Straight Working Channel, As Any Endoscope Deflection Leads To Significant Power Decrease.
Ultrasonic Lithotripsy Is Used Most Commonly To Manage Infectious Calculi In Which The Hollow Core Probe And Suction Can Simultaneously Fragment And Evacuate Stone Particles.
In Addition, A Flexible Nephroscope And Holmium Laser Can Also Be Used For Stone Burden Inaccessible To The Rigid Equipment.

Electrohydraulic Lithotripsy
The Energy Produced, On Sparking An Electrode With A Wire Cable, Conducted To Probes, Placed Through Rigid Or Flexible Endoscopes, Fragment Stones Into Extractable Pieces.
But As Less Efficient Than Holmium:YAG Lasers On Hardest Calculi, In Most Centers,This Endoscopic Lithotrite Variety Has Been Replaced And/Or Supplemented By Holmium Lasers.

Mechanical And Ballistic Lithotripsy
These Powerful Devices, Based On Pneumatically Driven Projectiles Striking A Metallic Probe Placed Endoscopically On A Calculus Methodology. Hence Produced Fragments Need
Extraction With Either An Endoscopic Basket Or Grasper.
The Devices Working Best When Used Through A Rigid Endoscope, And Are Associated With Stone Migration During Treatment.
The Flexible Pneumatic Lithotripsy Probe Developed To Complement Flexible Endoscopes, Has Minimal Clinical Usefulness, Due To Inverse Relation Of Ureteroscope Active Deflection Degree, To Tip Displacement And Fragmentation Ability Of The Probe.

Laser lithotripsy

First Commonly Used Laser Lithotripter Was The **Pulsed-Dye Laser**. Using A Light Energy Of 504 Nm Delivered In A Pulsatile Fashion Through Quartz Fibers, Stone Fragmentation Is Achieved, Along Fracture Planes By **Photo-Acoustic Effect Formation,** In Plasma Between The Tip Of The Fiber And The Calculus.
Limitations Included, The Deliverable Energy Dependance OnFiber Diameter, With The Smallest Fibers Ablity To Deliver Only 80 MJ, Often Insufficient To Fragment The Hardest Stones.
In Addition, This Laser Energy Little EffectiveNess On Cystine Calculi, As 504 Nm Of Light Energy Passes Through Crystal Rather Than Creating The Aforementioned Plasma On The Surface.

References

1. Johnson DE, Cromeens DM, Price RE. Use of the holmium:YAG laser in urology. *Lasers Surg Med.* 1992;12(4):353-63. [Medline].
2. Matsuoka K, Iida S, Nakanami M, et al. Holmium: yttrium-aluminum-garnet laser for endoscopic lithotripsy. *Urology.* Jun 1995;45(6):947-52. [Medline].
3. Dubosq F, Pasqui F, Girard F, et al. Endoscopic lithotripsy and the FREDDY laser: initial experience. *J Endourol.* May 2006;20(5):296-9. [Medline].
4. Kang HW, Lee H, Teichman JM, et al. Comparison of erbium:YAG versus holmium:YAG lithotripsy. *J Urol.* 2006;175 (Suppl 4):574.
5. Marks AJ, Teichman JM. Lasers in clinical urology: state of the art and new horizons. *World J Urol.* Jun 2007;25(3):227-33. [Medline].
6. Auge BK, Sekula JJ, Springhart WP, et al. In vitro comparison of fragmentation efficiency of flexible pneumatic lithotripsy using 2 flexible ureteroscopes. *J Urol.* Sep 2004;172(3):967-70. [Medline].
7. Beaghler M, Poon M, Ruckle H, et al. Complications employing the holmium:YAG laser. *J Endourol.* Dec 1998;12(6):533-5. [Medline].
8. Beiko DT, Denstedt JD. Advances in ureterorenoscopy. *Urol Clin North Am.* Aug 2007;34(3):397-408.[Medline].
9. Bierkens AF, Hendrikx AJ, De La Rosette JJ, et al. Treatment of mid- and lower ureteric calculi: extracorporeal shock-wave lithotripsy vs laser ureteroscopy. A comparison of costs, morbidity and effectiveness. *Br J Urol.* Jan 1998;81(1):31-5. [Medline].
10. Busby JE, Low RK. Ureteroscopic treatment of renal calculi. *Urol Clin North Am.* Feb 2004;31(1):89-98.[Medline].
11. Chaussy C, Fuchs G, Kahn R, et al. Transurethral ultrasonic ureterolithotripsy using a solid-wire probe. *Urology.* May 1987;29(5):531-2. [Medline].
12. Denstedt JD, Clayman RV. Electrohydraulic lithotripsy of renal and ureteral calculi. *J Urol.* Jan 1990;143(1):13-7. [Medline].

Essentials Of Litho-Tripsy

13. Denstedt JD, Eberwein PM, Singh RR. The Swiss Lithoclast: a new device for intracorporeal lithotripsy. *J Urol.* Sep 1992;148(3 Pt 2):1088-90. [Medline].

14. Dretler SP, Watson G, Parrish JA, et al. Pulsed dye laser fragmentation of ureteral calculi: initial clinical experience. *J Urol.* Mar 1987;137(3):386-9. [Medline].

15. Elbahnasy AM, Shalhav AL, Hoenig DM, et al. Lower caliceal stone clearance after shock wave lithotripsy or ureteroscopy: the impact of lower pole radiographic anatomy. *J Urol.* Mar 1998;159(3):676-82. [Medline].

16. Erhard MJ, Bagley DH. Urologic applications of the holmium laser: preliminary experience. *J Endourol.* Oct 1995;9(5):383-6. [Medline].

17. Fabrizio MD, Behari A, Bagley DH. Ureteroscopic management of intrarenal calculi. *J Urol.* Apr 1998;159(4):1139-43. [Medline].

18. Goodfriend R. Disintegration of ureteral calculi by ultrasound. *Urology.* Mar 1973;1(3):260-3. [Medline].

19. Grasso M. Experience with the holmium laser as an endoscopic lithotrite. *Urology.* Aug 1996;48(2):199-206.[Medline].

20. Grasso M. Ureteropyeloscopic treatment of ureteral and intrarenal calculi. *Urol Clin North Am.* Nov 2000;27(4):623-31. [Medline].

21. Grasso M, Beaghler M, Loisides P. The case for primary endoscopic management of upper urinary tract calculi: II. Cost and outcome assessment of 112 primary ureteral calculi. *Urology.* Mar 1995;45(3):372-6.[Medline].

22. Grasso M, Conlin M, Bagley D. Retrograde ureteropyeloscopic treatment of 2 cm. or greater upper urinary tract and minor Staghorn calculi. *J Urol.* Aug 1998;160(2):346-51. [Medline].

23. Grasso M, Ficazzola M. Retrograde ureteropyeloscopy for lower pole caliceal calculi. *J Urol.* Dec 1999;162(6):1904-8. [Medline].

24. Grasso M, Loisides P, Beaghler M, et al. The case for primary endoscopic management of upper urinary tract calculi: I. A critical review of 121 extracorporeal shock-wave lithotripsy failures. *Urology.* Mar 1995;45(3):363-71. [Medline].

25. Hofbauer J, Hobarth K, Marberger M. Lithoclast: new and inexpensive mode of intracorporeal lithotripsy. *J Endourol.* 1992;6:429.

26. Jeon SS, Hyun JH, Lee KS. A comparison of holmium:YAG laser with Lithoclast lithotripsy in ureteral calculi fragmentation. *Int J Urol.* Jun 2005;12(6):544-7. [Medline].

27. Knudsen BE, Glickman RD, Stallman KJ, et al. Performance and safety of holmium: YAG laser optical fibers. *J Endourol.* Nov 2005;19(9):1092-7. [Medline].

28. Leveillee RJ, Lobik L. Intracorporeal lithotripsy: which modality is best?. *Curr Opin Urol.* May 2003;13(3):249-53. [Medline].

29. Raney AM. Electrohydraulic lithotripsy: experimental study and case reports with the stone disintegrator. *J Urol.* Mar 1975;113(3):345-7. [Medline].

30. Weizer AZ, Springhart WP, Ekeruo WO, et al. Ureteroscopic management of renal calculi in anomalous kidneys. *Urology.* Feb 2005;65(2):265-9. [Medline].

(ii.) ROLE OF 'LASERS'

History
To Remove Impacted Stones From The Urinary Tract, In 1980s,
At Wellman Center For Photomedicine **Laser Lithotripsy** Was Invented.
Avoiding Surgery, Pulverization Of The Stone Was Done, Using Laser
Pulses, Delivered Through A Fiber Optic. The Technology Licensed To
Candela Corporation, Which Produced The First Commercial Laser
Lithotripsy System.[1]

Procedure
Urinary Tract Scopy, To Locate The Stone, Is Done, Using **Cystoscope, Ureteroscope, Renoscope Or Nephroscope.**
The Laser Fiber Inserted Through The Working Channel Of The Scope,
Laser Is Directly Emitted To The Stone, Disintegrating
The Stone And The Remaining Pieces Are Washed Out Of The
Urinary Tract. This Procedure, Considered As **Minimally Invasive Surgery,** Is Performed Under Either **Local Or General Anesthesia**.
Gradually Becoming Widely Available In Hospitals Around The World.

Laser Lithotripsy
The First Commonly Used Laser Lithotripter,
Is **'Pulsed-Dye Laser'.**
Fragmentation Of Calculii Is Achieved, Using **Light Energy Of 504 Nm**
Delivered In A Pulsatile Fashion Through Quartz Fibers.
'Photo-Acoustic Effect' Forming Plasma Between Fiber Tip And The
Calculus, Fragments Stones Along Fracture Planes.
The Limitation Of 'Deliverable Energy' Dependant Upon
'Fiber Diameter' (Smallest Fibers Ablity To Deliver Only 80 MJ)
Is Often Insufficient To Fragment The Hardest Stones.
On Cystine Calculii, Such Laser Energy Has Little Effect;
As 504 Nm Of Light Energy Passes Through These Crystal
Rather Than Creating The Above Mentioned Plasma On The Surface.

Various Lasers Used In Lithotripsy Include:

Holmium:YAG Laser
One Of The **Most Commonly Used** Lasers & Achieving **'Universal Acceptance'** As The Standard For **Intracorporeal Lithotripsy.**
Multiple Recent Studies Reported Superiorty Of Holmium:YAG
Laser Lithotripsy As Compared To Electrohydraulic Lithotripsy,
Ultrasonic Lithotripsy & Pneumolithotripsy In Terms Of Stone
Fragmentation And Complications.

Essentials Of Litho-Tripsy

The Thermal Laser variety, Uses 2150-Nm Light Energy In A Pulsatile Fashion, That Produces A **Vaporization Bubble** At The Tip Of Low–Water-Density Quartz Fibers.
Even With The Small 150- To 200-μm Fibers, Sufficient Energy Is Delivered To Fragment All Types Of Urinary Stones Into Fine Dust And Small Pieces, Easily Passable Through The Urinary Tract.
Hard Stones In Difficult Locations (eg, Lower-Pole Calyx) Are Treatable, By Using A Small-Diameter Fiber That Is Easily Deflected With The Ureteroscope.

Rapidly Absorbed By Water, Holmium Laser Energy Created Vaporization Bubble, Has Minimal Effects On Adjacent Tissue (2-3 Mm From The Fiber Tip).The Qualities Rendering
'Minimal Adjacent Tissue Trauma'.
However, **Direct Contact With Tissue Needs Avoidance**, Unless Tissue Resection Is Planned.
Ensuring Sufficient Cooling Irrigant Through The Endoscopic System **Prevents Adjacent Thermal Soft-Tissue Effects.**

For Large And Complex Stone Burdens Composed Of Uric Acid Or Cystine, Holmium Laser Lithotripsy Has Reported Better Efficacy Than Other Endoscopic Lithotrites.

Frequency-Doubled, Double-Pulse Neodymium:YAG (FREDDY) Laser

Recent Comparative Studies, In Europe Demostrated,That The FREDDY Laser Is Inferior To The Holmium:YAG Laser In Lithotripsy.
The Holmium:YAG Laser Controlled Via A Distal Tip Vaporization Bubble That Creates Acoustic Percussion Waves Leading To Stones Destabilization & Fragmentation.
Neodymium:YAG, Even When Pulsed, Is A High-Temperature Laser **With Limited Fragmentation Capabilities For Hard Stones And Causes Significantly Greater Stone Retropulsion.**
Less Versatilityt & Unablity To Treat Urinary-Tissue Lesions[3] Are Additional DrawBacks Of The FREDDY Laser.

Erbium:YAG Laser & Thulium YAG Laser
Are Recent Developments In Laser Technology,
The 'In Clinical' And 'In Vitro' Trials Performance Are In Developmental Phases,To Achive Better Stone Lithotripsy Efficiency In The Future.
While Fiber Delivery For Both Lasers Is Still In Its Infancy.[4, 5]

Laser Lithotripsy

Pre- Procedural Preparations

Patients' Consultation For Urinary Stones Symptoms Include, Medical History, Physical Examination, Laboratory Evaluation And Imaging Tests.
Radio-Diagnosis(X-Rays, Ultrasound CT, CECT) Are Diagnostic Imaging Tools To Determine The Location Of The Calculi.
The Most Common Treatment For Urinary Stones, Extracorporeal Shock Wave Lithotripsy (ESWL) Is Not Ideal For All Stones.
The Dornier *Medilas H20*, A Holmium:YAG Laser, Is A Good Alternative For Very Large Or Difficult To Reach Stones.

Procedural Details

Laser Lithotripsy Procedure Involves, Fragmentation Of Calculi Using The **Holmium Laser.**
The High Absorption Of The Holmium Laser Light (Wavelength: 2.1 μm In The Infrared) By Stone Leads To The Ablation Of The Calculus Material Regardless Of Chemical Composition.
Endoscopic Imaging And Controlled Laser Pulses Ensure Safe Contact Between The Fiber Tip And Calculus.
Thin Fibers With A Core Diameter Of 200 μm Allow Thinner Endoscopes To Be Used For Advancement To The Renal Calyces.
High Success Rate And Low Complication Rates For All Types Of Calculi Are Reported Using Holmium Laser Lithotripsy.

Laser Lithotripsy Is Performed **Under General Anesthesia.**
The Light Energy Of The Laser Is Transported Through A Flexible Light Guide To The Stone. For Ensuring A Safe Procedure The Laser Fiber Is Observed With An Ureterorenoscope.
The Fiber Tip Must Be In Contact With The Stone During The Firing Of The Laser.
The **Stone Breaking Mechanism** Of Laser Lithotripsy Is A **Thermal One.**
The Stone Fragments When Pulses Of Intense Laser Light From The Dornier *Medilas H20* Are Applied.

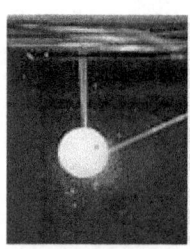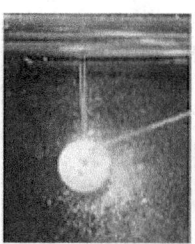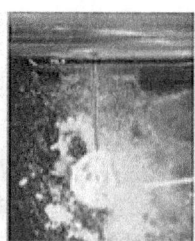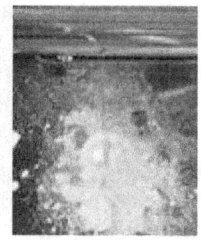

Based Upon The Principle That **Holmium Laser Energy Is Strongly Absorbed By Water,** The Short Laser Pulses **Create A Shockwave** That Causes Fragmentation Of Both Ureteral And Intrarenal Stones.

Essentials Of Litho-Tripsy

Due To The Flexibility And Control Of The System, Different Treatment Techniques Can Be Applied Depending Upon The Location And Shape Of The Stone. For Example, **Smaller Stones Can Be Fragmented Directly**, Whereas **With Larger Concrements**, Holes Are First Made **In The Center, After Which The Edges** Can Then Be Fragmented. Finally, The Stone Residues Can Be Flushed Out Utilizing The Endoscopes Rinsing Fluid.

Lasers In Urology

The Various Applications Include-
Laser Therapy For Benign Prostatic Hyperplasia
Laser Treatment Of Urothelial Malignancies
Lasers For Nephron-Sparing Surgery
Lasers For Urothelial Stricture Disease
Lasers For The Ablation Of Skin Lesions

Tissue Welding

Laser Energy Is Applied In A Constructive Manner To Reapproximate Tissues. Reported Applications Of Tissue Welding Particularly Helpful In Laparoscopic Surgery, In Which Current Methods Of Reapproximation Are Clumsy And Time Consuming.
Vasovasotomy For Vasectomy Reversal Using A Tissue Welding Technique Has A Reported Patency Rate Near 95% And A Subsequent Pregnancy Rate Of 35%,
Comparable To Current Microsurgical Techniques To
Tissue-Welding Repair In Urology Include **Hypospadias Repair Pyeloplasty, Augmentation Cystoplasty,**
And Continent Urinary Diversion.
Autofluorescence

The Ability To Ablate And Weld Increases The Laser's Use As A Diagnostic Tool. In This Capacity, Light Of A Specific Wavelength Is Used To Differentiate Healthy From Dysplastic Or Malignant Tissue.
Source-Lasers in Urology Treatment & Management
Author: Michael Grasso III, MD; Chief Editor: Bradley Fields Schwartz, DO, FACS

References

1. Anderholm, N.C. **Laser generated stress waves.** *Applied Physics Letters.* 1970;16:113.z
2. Begun, F.P., Jacobs, S.C., Lawson, R.F. **Use of a prototype 3F electrohydraulic electrode with ureteroscopy for treatment of ureteral calculus disease.** *J Urol.* 1988;139:1188.
3. Chaussy, C., Fuchs, G., Kahn, R. et al, **Transurethral ultrasonic ureterolithotripsy using a solid wire probe.***Urology.* 1987;29:531.
4. Denstedt, J.D., Clayman, R.V. **Electrohydraulic lithotripsy of renal and ureteral calculi.** *J Urol.* 1990;143:13.

5. Denstedt, J.D., Eberwein, P.M., Singh, R.R. **The Swiss lithoclast: A new device for endoscopic stone disintegration.** *J Urol.* 1992;148:1088.
6. Dretler, S.P. **Special article: Calculus breakability— fragility and durility.** *J Endourol.* 1994;8:1.
7. Dretler, S.P., Bhatta, K.M. **Clinical experience with high power (140 mJ), large fiber (320 microns) pulsed dye laser lithotripsy.** *J Urol.* 1991;146:1228.
8. Eaton, J.M. Jr, Malin, J.M. Jr, Glenn, J.F. **Electrohydraulic lithotripsy.** *J Urol.* 1972;108:865.
9. Fair, H.D. **In-vitro destruction of urinary calculi by laser-induced stress waves.** *Med Instrum.* 1978;12:100.
10. Goodfriend, R. **Disintegration of ureteral calculi by ultrasound.** *Urology.* 1973;1:260.
11. Green, D.F., Lytton, B. **Early experience with direct vision electrohydraulic lithotripsy of ureteral calculi.** *J Urol.*1985;133:767.
12. Loisides, P., Grasso, M., Bagley, D.H. **Mechanical impactor employing nitinol probes to fragment human calculi: Fragmentation efficiency with flexible endoscope deflection.** *J Endourol.* 1995;9:371.
13. Marburger, M. **Presentation at the 11th World Congress of Endourology and ESWL.** Florence, Italy; 1993.
14. Mitchell, Kerr, Kerr, W.S. Jr. **Experience with the electrohydraulic disintegrator.** *J Urol.* 1977;117:159.
15. Mulvaney, W. **Attempted disintegration of calculi by ultrasonic vibration.** *J Urol.* 1953;70:704.
16. Mulvaney, W.P., Beck, C.W. **The laser beam in urology.** *J Urol.* 1968;99:112.
17. Raney, A.M. **Electrohydraulic cystolithotripsy.** *Urology.* 1976;8:379.
18. Raney, A.M. **Electrohydraulic ureterolithotripsy.** *Urology.* 1978;12:284.Ronvalis, P. **Electronic lithotripsy for vesical calculus with Urat-1.** *Br J Urol.* 1970;42:486.
19. Schulze, H., Haupt, G., Piergiovanni, M. et al, **The Swiss lithoclast: A new device for intracorporeal lithotripsy.** *J Urol.* 1993;149:15.
20. Spindell, M., Molem, A., Bhatia, K. et al, **Comparison of Holmium and flashlamp pumped dye lasers for use in lithotripsy and biliary calculi.** *Lasers Surg Med.* 1992;12:482.
21. Strunge, C., Brinkman, R., Flemming, G., Englehardt, R. **Interspersion of fragmented fiber's splinters into tissue during pulsed Alexandrite laser lithotripsy.** *Lasers Surg Med.* 1991;11:183.
22. Tasca, A., Cecchetti, W., Zattoni, F., Pagano, F. **Photosensitization of cystine stones to induce laser lithotripsy.** *J Urol.* 1993;149:709.
23. Tessler, A.M., Kossow, J. **Electrohydraulic stone disintegration.** *Urology.* 1975;5:470.
24. Thornwald, J. **The Century of the Surgeon.** Pantheon Books, New York; 1957.
25. Urquhart-Hay, D. **Samuel Pepys and his bladder stone.** *Br J Urol.* 1992;70:509.
26. Watson, G.M., Murray, S., Dretler, S.P., Parrish, J.A. **The pulsed dye laser for fragmentation of urinary calculi.** *J Urol.* 1987;138:195.
27. Watson, G.M., Wickham, J.E.A., Mills, T.N. et al, **Laser fragmentation of renal calculi.** *Br J Urol.* 1983;55:613.
28. Yutkin L: Electrohydraulic lithotripsy. English translation for US Department of Commerce, Office of Technical services, DOC 62-15184, MDL 1207/1-2, 1955.

Further Readings-

1. Holmium **Laser Lithotripsy** - YourUrologyhealth.com
www.yoururologyhealth.com/holmi... **Laser lithotripsy** carries a slightly greater risk of **complications** than extracorporeal shock wave lithotripsy. However, lithotripsy using the holmium laser is ...

Essentials Of Litho-Tripsy

2. **Laser** Kidney Stone Surgery : Learn About the Procedure and ...
   www.healthguideinfo.com/.../p136... 03-11-2008 – **Laser Lithotripsy** is able to dissolve 100% of kidney stones of all compositions. Read about procedure and **complications**.

3. **Laser Lithotripsy Complications** - Doctor insights on HealthTap
   https://www.healthtap.com/topics/**laser-lithotripsy-complications**

   Doctors give unbiased, helpful information on indications, contra-indications, benefits, and **complications**: Dr. Khanna and others: The pain you are having is ...

4. Ureteroscopic Holmium **Laser Lithotripsy** Post Procedure Symptoms ...
   www.livestrong.com/.../35079-uret... 26-04-2011 – Uteroscopic **laser lithotripsy** is a surgical procedure to remove kidney stones, ... the procedure during a study experienced no **complications**.

5. Holmium **laser lithotripsy** for ureteral calculi: predictive factors for ...
   www.ncbi.nlm.nih.gov/.../1829403.. JA Leijte - 2008 -
   PURPOSE: To define possible predictive factors for success and **complications** for ureteroscopic holmium **laser lithotripsy** procedures. PATIENTS AND ...

6. **Laser lithotripsy** for ureteric calculi: results in 250 patients.
   www.ncbi.nlm.nih.gov/.../PMC244 JD Kelly - 1995 -
   This procedure is a safe and effective treatment for ureteric calculi and is associated with a low **complication** rate and a high clearance rate. **Laser lithotripsy** is ...

7. **complications** related to urologic applications of **lasers** - ExpertConsult
   www.expertconsultbook.com/.../lin... COMPLICATIONS RELATED TO UROLOGIC APPLICATIONS OF LASERS. **Laser Lithotripsy**. The surgical management of nephrolithiasis has undergone ...

8. Holmium **Laser Lithotripsy** for Ureteral Calculi: Predictive Factors for ...
   online.liebertpub.com/.../end.2007... JAP Leijte - 2008 -
   22-02-2008 – Conclusion: Surgeon experience is a predictive factor for **complications** and success for ureteroscopic holmium **laser lithotripsy** for ureteric ...

9. [PDF] PP-119 Holmium **laser lithotripsy** for ureteral calculi - ESD
   2012 www.esd2012.org/pdf/.../PP-119.p... PDF/Adobe Acrobat
   Introduction: Ureteroscopic holmium **laser lithotripsy** is a safe and effective ... However, little is known about the changes in success and **complication** rate over ...

10. International braz j urol - Flexible ureteroscopy and Holmium:YAG ...
    www.scielo.br/scielo.php?pid... OM Aboumarzouk - 2012 -
    Flexible ureteroscopy and Holmium:YAG **laser lithotripsy** for stone disease in ... There were no major **complications** and only 11% of the patients developed ...
    11.complication laser ... **LASCAD** ww.las-cad.com/lascad.php**LASer** Cavity Analysis & Design Optimize Your **Laser** Design!
    12.**Lithotripsy Kidney Stones**www.ask.com/**Lithotripsy+Kidney+Stones**

CHAPTER(4.)
(i)ESWL:BILIARY STONE DISEASES

Surgical Anatomy, Physiology & Pathology Of The Gallbladder

The gallbladder is. It is a small, pear-shaped organ
The body can function without the gallbladder. If doctors need to remove it because of disease, there are no serious long-term effects and the body can still digest food.

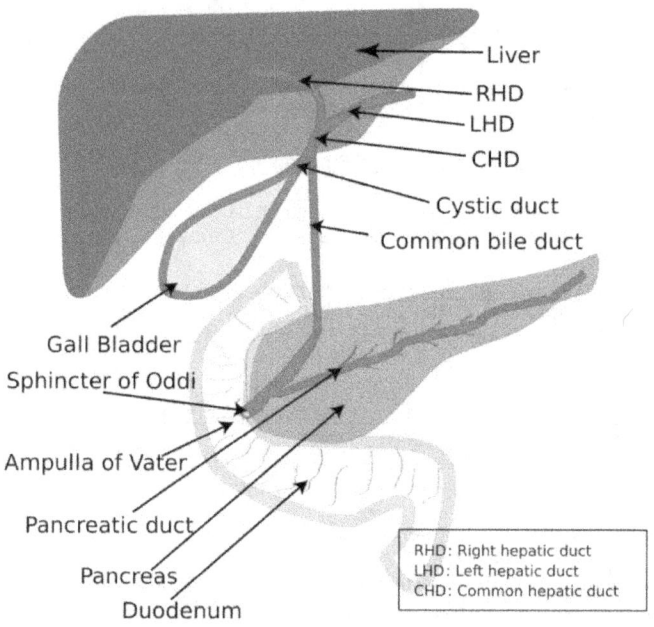

RHD: Right hepatic duct
LHD: Left hepatic duct
CHD: Common hepatic duct

The Gallbladder

Is A Part Of The Digestive System , A Hollow, Pear-Shaped Organ, Present On The Right Side Of The Body, Under The Right Lobe Of The Liver, Lying In **'Gallbladder Fossa'**, Along The Visceral Surface Of The Liver.Normally 7-10 Cm In Length And About A 2.5 Cm (1 Inch) Wide, With About 50ml Capacity.

Conventionally, Divided Into Three Parts-
Fundus - Blind, Wide End Of Gallbladder,
Body - Constituting Majority Of The Organ
Neck - Narrow,Tapered End Contiguous With The Cystic Duct & Draining Through The Spiral Valve.

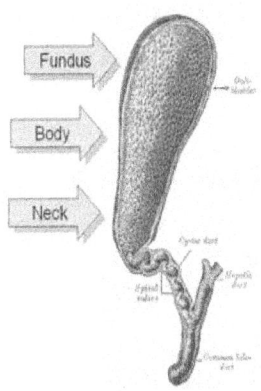

The Cystic Duct
Is The Outflow Tract Of The Gallbladder, Connecting The Neck Of The Gallbladder To The **Common Hepatic Duct**, That Becomes The **Common Bile Duct.**
Cystic Duct Is Typically **About 4cm In Length**(Short Cystic Ducts Presence Is Quite Common). It Courses Between The Layers Of The Lesser Omentum, Usually Parallel To The Common Hepatic Duct, Before Joining To Form The **Common Bile Duct**,That Eventually Meet **The Pancreatic Duct** To Drain Into Second Part Of Duodenum, At **The Ampulla Of Vater**.
The Gallbladder And Bile Ducts Ts Named As,
The Biliary System Or Biliary Tract,
Collectively, Along WithThe **Common Hepatic Duct** Draining Bile From The Liver Through The Left And Right Hepatic Ducts, They Constitute**'Hepato-Biliary System'**.

Histology
The Gallbladder Is Made Up Of Layers Of Tissue:
Mucosa-The Inner Layer Of Epithelial Cells (Epithelium) And Lamina Propria (Loose Connective Tissue)
A Muscular Layer
A Layer Of Smooth Muscle
Perimuscular Layer-Connective Tissue That Covers The Muscular Layer
Serosa- The Outer Covering Of The Gallbladder.

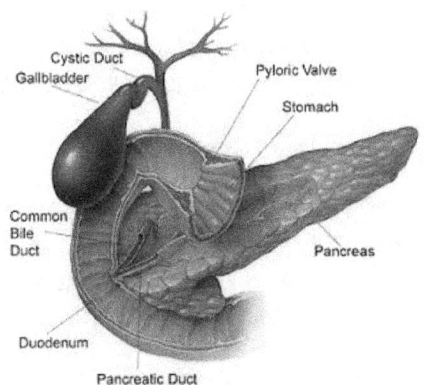

Functions

The Gallbladder Stores And Concentrates Bile, A Yellowish-Green Fluid Produced By The Liver.
Bile Helps The Body Digest Fats.
Bile Is Mainly Made Up Of:
Bile Salts
Bile Pigments (Such As Bilirubin)
Cholesterol
Water
The Liver Releases Bile Into The Hepatic Duct.
If The Bile Is Not Needed For Digestion, It Flows Into The Cystic Duct And Then Into The Gallbladder, Where It Is Stored.
The Gallbladder Can **Store About 40–70 Ml Of Bile**.
The Gallbladder Absorbs Water From The Bile, Making It More Concentrated. When Bile Is Needed For Digestion After A Meal, The Gallbladder Contracts And Releases It Into The Cystic Duct. The Bile Then Flows Into The Common Bile Duct And Is Emptied Into The Small Intestine, Where It Breaks Down Fats.

Any Obstruction In The Hepato-Biliary System- GallBladder & Connecting Ductal System, Due To Infection, Stone, Stricture,Tumour Etc, Leads To Stagnation Of Bile, Clinically Manifesting As **'Obstructive Jaundice'** & Or **MucoCele, Empyema, Gangrene**, When Only GallBladder & Cystic Duct Is Involved.

Blood Supply And Nerves

The Gallbladder And Cystic Duct Are Supplied Principally By The **Cystic Artery, Branch Of Right Hepatic Artery** (75% Of The Time).
Variations In The Origin And Course Of The Cystic Artery Occur In Approximately 25% Of Individuals eg **Accessory Cystic Artery** & Is Of Important Clinical Significance During Gallbladder Surgeries.

The Veins Of The Gallbladder Neck (**Cystic Veins**) Communicate With Veins Along The Cystic And Bile Ducts.
Draining Through The **Portal Vein To The Liver**, Or After Joining The Veins Of The Hepatic Ducts And Upper Bile Duct. In Addition, Small **Cystic Veins From The Fundus And Body** Of The Gallbladder May Pass Directly Into The Liver.

Lymphatic Drainage Of The Gallbladder Courses To The **Hepatic Nodes Through The Cystic Lymph Nodes**, That Are Typically Located Near The Neck Of The Gallbladder.

The Gallbladder And Cystic Duct Are Supplied By **3 Types Of Innervation**, Which Course With The Cystic Artery.

Essentials Of Litho-Tripsy

The **Celiac Plexus** Supplies Sympathetic Innervation,
The **Vagus Nerve** Supplies Parasympathetic Innervation,
The **Right Phrenic Nerve** Conveys Sensory Information.

Gall Stones

A **Gallstone** Is A Crystalline Concretion Formed Within The Gallbladder By Accretion Of Bile Components.
These Calculi Are Formed In The Gallbladder But May Distally Pass Into Other Parts Of The Biliary Tract Such As The Cystic Duct, Common Bile Duct, Pancreatic Duct, Or The Ampulla Of Vater. Rarely,

TYPES OF GALL STONES
Cholesterol Stones - 10% Cases
        Pure Cholesterol Stones
        Are Dark Yellowish, Small To Large Size,
        May Be Solitary

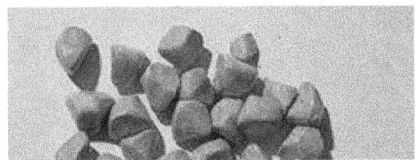

Pigment Stones - 5-10% Cases
        Bilirubin Pigment - Green / Black Colour
        Pure Pigment Stones

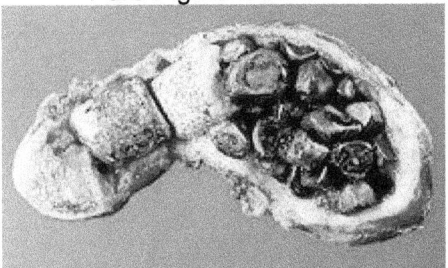

Gallbladder Opened To Show Numerous Gallstones. The Large, Yellow Calculus Probably Comprises Cholesterol, While The Green-To-Brown Stones Suggest Bile Pigments, Such As Biliverdin And Stercobilin.

Mixed Stones –
80% Of Gallstone Dis.

Composition;
Chloresterol
CA Bilirubinae, Bile Pigment

Calcium, Proteins, Carbohydrates, Mucus
And Cellular Debris.

RISK FACTORS
Obscured Aetiology
(4)Fs - Fat. Forty, Fertile, Female With Susceptibility
Female Sex
Obesity
Pregnancy
Age
Oral Contraception
Clofibrate Therapy
Thiazide Diuretics
Genetic & Ethnic Factors
High Fat & ↓ Fibre Diet
Diabetes Mellitus
Iliac Disesase & Resection
Haemolytic Anaemia
Parasitic Infestations Of Biliary System

PATHOGENSIS
Disturbances In Cholesterol Phospholipids & Bile Salts Stable Equilibrium
Phospholipids (Lecithin) - Dissolved In Bile Salts As 'Micelle'.
Cholesterol Insoluble In Aq. Solution- Solubile In Lithogenic Bile -
Patient Tendency ⟶ Stasis Infection

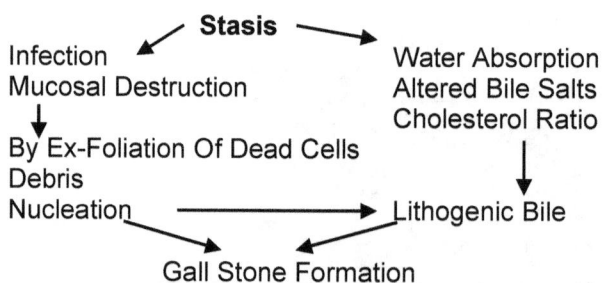

CLINICAL MANIFESTATIONS
Presence Of Gallstones In The Gallbladder May Lead To
Acute *Cholecystitis*, An *Inflammatory* Condition Characterized
By *Retention Of Bile In The Gallbladder* And Often
Secondary *Infection* By *Intestinal Microorganisms*,
Predominantly *Escherichia Coli* And *Bacteroides* Species.

Essentials Of Litho-Tripsy

Presence Of Gallstones In Other Parts Of The Biliary Tract Can Cause Obstruction Of The <u>Bile Ducts</u>, Which Can Lead To Serious Conditions Such As <u>Ascending Cholangitis</u> Or <u>Pancreatitis</u>. Either Of These Two Conditions Can Be Life-Threatening And Are Therefore Considered To Be<u>medical Emergencies</u>.

In Cases Of Severe Inflammation, Gallstones May Erode Through The Gallbladder Into Adherent Bowel Potentially Causing An Obstruction Termed <u>Gallstone Ileus</u>

<u>The Common Cl. Presentations Are</u>-
- Ac, Chr, SubAc Cholecystitis
- A Calculus Cholecystitis
- Gall Bladder Lump Formation
- Mucocele – Due To Impacted Stone At The Neck GB, Mucus Filled G.B & Subsequently White Bile due To Absorption Of Bile Pigments Of The Stored Bile By G.B Mucosa & No Hepatic Secreyions Entering G.B
- Empyema G.B.
- Gangrenous G.B.

<u>Clinical Signs</u>

Murphys' Sign ,Boas Sign,Kehr's Sign, Charcoat Biliary Triad

Courvoisier's Law

<u>Investigations</u>
(A)   Routine
(B)   Specific- Radiology,USG Whole ABD (Full Bladder)
        CT Scan MRI
         Hepatic Scans
           Lab. Investigations- LFT, Pancreatic Profile
              Tumour Markers

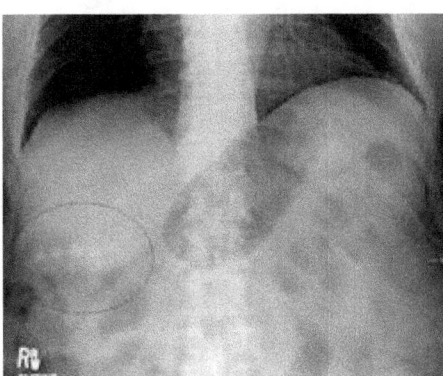

<u>Gallstones As Seen On Plain Xray</u>.

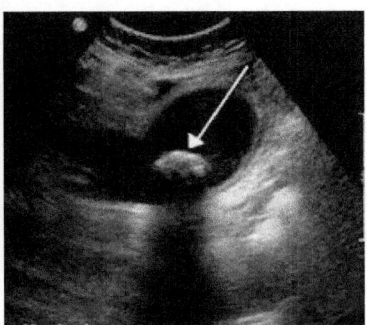

A 1.9 Cm Gallstone Impacted In The Neck Of The Gallbladder

And Leading To Cholecystitis As Seen On <u>Ultrasound</u>. Note The 4 Mm Gall Bladder Wall Thickening.

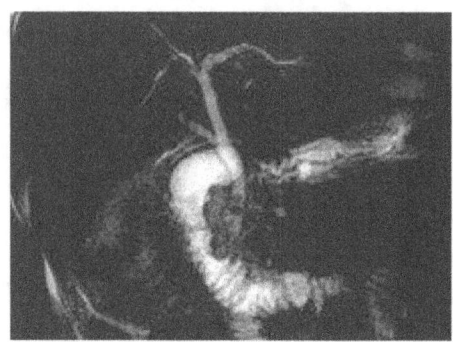

MRCP Image Of Two Stones In The Distal Common Bile Duct

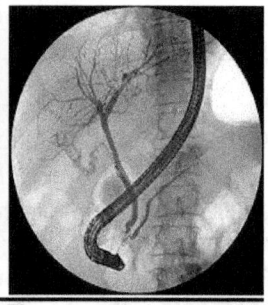

Fluoroscopic Image - ERCP;. Multiple Gallstones In The Gallbladder & Cystic Duct. The CBD, Pancreatic Duct Appear To Be Patent.

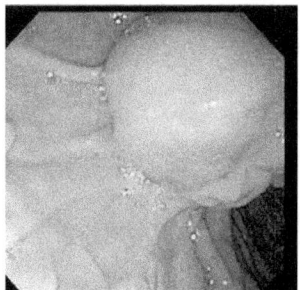

<u>ERCP</u> - Common Bile Duct Stone Impacted At <u>Ampulla Of Vater</u>

Essentials Of Litho-Tripsy

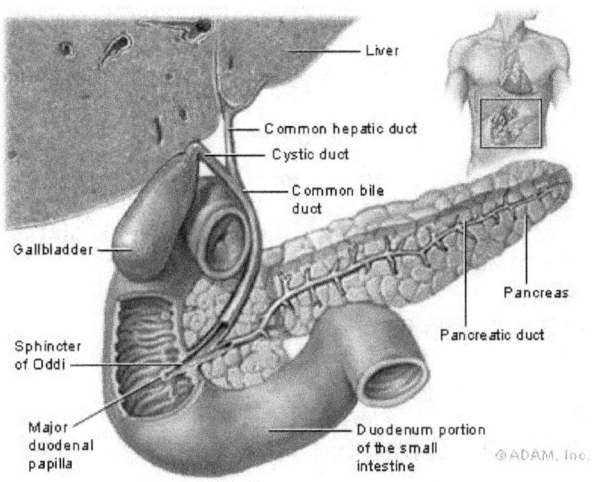

Sources – Goggle, Wikipedia, A.D.A.M., Inc.

Biliary Stone Diseases"
(A.) Gall Stone Disease – 'CHOLELITHIASIS'
(B.) Gall Stone Disease With/WithOut
  BileDuctStone Diseases- 'CHOLEDOCHOLITHIASIS'

'MANAGEMENT MODALITIES'
i. **SURGICAL TREATMENT**

- Classical Open Cholecystectomy
- Mini – Cholecystectomy
- Laparoscopic Cholecystectomy
- Open Cholecystectomy, Choledochotomy (+-) T- Tube Drainage
- Laparoscopic Cholecystectomy (+) ERCP/MRCP For CBD Stones / Other Endoscopic Procedures ?Sphinterotomy Etc.

ii. **MEDICAL TREATMENT : BILIARY STONE DISEASES**

(A) **DISSOLUTION THERAPY**
(1.) **ORAL DISSOLUTION THERAPY(ODT):**
Supersaturation Of Bile With Cholesterol Lead To The Formation Of Cholesterol Gall Stones,

Reversal Of These Conditions Result Into Dissolution Of These Stones. Cholesterol Stones Are Dissolved In The Presence Of Sourounding Medium Capable Of Solubilizing The Cholesterol In The Stones.

<u>Therapeutic Agents</u>;
Both Cheno-DeoxyCholic Acid(CDA) & Urso-DeoxyCholic Acid (UDA)Dissolve Gall Stones By Decreasing Biliary Cholesterol Secretion & DeSaturation Of Bile.

Pharmaco-Kinetics; By Encouraging The Removal Of Cholesterol From Stones Via-Micellar Slubilization, Formation Of Liquid Crystalline Phase, Or Both.

Rate Of Stone Dissolution; Depends Upon-
1. <u>Thermo-Dynamic Forces</u>- Degree Of Bile De-Saturation & Concentration Of 'UDA' In Bile.
2. <u>KineticForces</u> – Stirring Of Bile
3. <u>Surface To Volume Ratio Of Stones</u> – Determines ODT Efficay By Influence Upon Thermo-Dynamic Forces.
   Hence, Patient Selection Criterion Recommends-
   Stone Diametre<6mm(Optimal) & 6-10mm(Acceptable) For ODT.
4. Studies Regarding **Role Of Pro-Kinetic Agents** Including Alpha-Adrenergic Antagonists & Clarithromycin, By Increasing G.B Motility Thus Improving Gall Bladder Stasis & Hence Preventing & Or Treating Gall Stones Are Reported.

Cheno-DeoxyCholic Acid(CDA): First Bile Acid, Used For Gall Stones Dissolution, But Abandoned Due To Side-Effects- Including Diarrhoea & Increased Serum Amino-Transferase & Cholesterol Levels.

Urso-DeoxyCholic Acid(UDA): Is Well Tolerated & Is The Recent Drug Of Choice.
The Radomized Comparative Control Studies Report Suggest That, Urso-DeoxyCholic Acid , Is As Effective When Used Alone Or In Combination With Cheno-DeoxyCholic Acid.

<u>Therapeutic Regimes</u>;
'ODT' Drug Of Choice- 'UDA'(Ursodiol), Due To Better Tolerance
                         & No Important Side-Effects.
Dose; 10-15 mgm/kg Body Wt./Day
Night Time Dosing- More Effective With Better Patient Compliance, As Compared To Meal Time Dosing.

<u>Duration</u>;
- **Continuance Of Tt.;** (1.)Till Stone Dissolution, Documented By,
                         (2.) Consecutve Negative USGs One Month Apart.
- **Stoppage Of TreatMent;**
  - In-Tolerance To Drug
  - Gall Stone Complication Occurs
  - Failure Of Stone Dissolution After (6) Months Or Dissolve Partially After (6) Months, With Lack Of Progression To Complete Dissolution By (2) Years.

Essentials Of Litho-Tripsy

Therapeutic Regimes Efficay;
- Complete Dissolution Achieved In 20% -70% Cases.
- The Variability Of Response Rates Due To Patient Selection Criterion, Doses Of Bile Acid, Treatment Time & Diagnostic Tools Used To Document Stone Dissolution.
- A Meta-Analysis Of All Radomized Trials Of 'ODT' Reveals-
  -Stone Dissolution In 37% Patients
  -Frequency For Stone Dissolution-29% For Stones >10mm
                                -49% For Stones >5mm
                                -Time Of Dissolution
                                Variations With Median
                                Rate Of 0.7 mm/Month
- Long Term Tt. Decreaes Biliary Pain & Ac.Cholecystitis, Independent Of Gall Stone Dissolution.
- **Recurrence-** In Properly Selected Patients, Despite Initial Dissolution Of Stones, Recurrence Rate In 'ODT' Pts Is 50% After (5) Years, While Most Recurrences Occuring Within The First (2) Years, With Lower Risk Rates In Solitary Stone Than In Multiple Stones Cases.

PATIENT SELECTION:
For Oral Dissolution Therapy Is Based Upon-
1. **Stage Of Gall Stone Disease;** UnComplicated Gall Stone Disease Including Mild, Infrequent Biliary Colics,
   While Complications Of Cholelithiasis-Cholecystitis, Pancreatitis & Cholangitis Are ContraIndications For ODT.
2. **Gall Stone Function;** Proper Functioning G.B With Patent Cystic Duct, Allowing Passage Of UnSaturated Bile & Stones From Gall Bladder.
   As Assessed By Diagnostic Tools- Oral CholeCystoGraphy, Stimulated Cholescintigraphy & Functional USG.
3. **Stone Characterstics;** Important ParaMetre For Efficay, As ODT Is Effective Only For Cholesterol Stones.
   An Idea About The Composition Of Gall Stones, By
   Radio-Diagnosis- Radio-Lucent On Conventional RadioGraphy
         -Iso-Dense Or Hypo-Dense To Bile & Lack Stone
           Calcification On CT Scan
         -During OCG;Buoyancy Of Cholesterol Stones Is
Demonstrable, Due To Their Less Than Or Equal Sp. Gravity, To That Of Sourounding Contrast Enriched Bile.
- Small Stones Have Smaller **'Surface To Volume Ratio'**,
  Have Effective & Reliable 'ODT' Result Outcomes.
  Effective Upto 10 mm DiaMetre Stones,
  Best Results In Less Than 5 mm Size Stones.
- **Number Of Stones** Does Not Influence'ODT' Efficay, However Only

Patients Where Stones Are Occupying Less Than Half Gall Bladder Volume Should Be Subjected To 'ODT'.

(2.) CONTACT CHEMICAL DISSOLUTION THERAPY;
i. **For 'CBD Stones'**
Adminstration Of Chemical Solvents Via-
- Indwelling Naso-Biliary Tube
- Per-Cutaneous Trans Hepatic Catheter
- Chole-Cystostomy Tube
- Existing T-Tube

Contact Chemical Agents Used-
- **A Semi-Synthetic Vegetable Oil**, Mono-Ocatanoin Composed Of 70% Glycerol-1-mono-octanoate & 30%Glycerol-1, 2-dioctanoate – Beginning 1977
- **Organic Solvents**-DiPhasic Ether, Methyl-teret-Butyl Ether (Allen et al,1985)

Results- Complete & Or Partial Success Rate Variations Ranged Between 25% -35% In 1980s ,While 30-45% As Reported In 1990s With Use Of Ether Base Solvents.

Complications
- By Semi-Synthetic Vegetable Oil, Serious Adverse-Effects Leading To DisContinuation Of Tt. Occurred In 50% Cases Including Duodenal Haemorrhage, Ulceration, Ac.Pancreatitis,Jaundice, Pulmonary Oedema, Acidosis, Anaphylaxis, Septicaemia, Leukopenia, But No Reported Mortality.
- Un Aceptable Complication Rate Due To Systemic Absorption Of Organic Ether Based Solvent Spill Over Into Duodenum & Intra-Hepatic Biliary System, Reported In 1990s.

Future Prospects-
- Advent Of Sophisticated Computerized **Two Way Pump System** Devices,Can Be Of Definite Help In Minimizing Complications & Improving Efficay.
- But For OverAll Success Of Large CBD Stones, Composed Mainly By Bile-Pigments & Small Concentrations Of Bile Salts,

The Needed Development Of **Solvent Chelating Agent** Like, Ethylene Diamine TetraAcetic Acid, For Pigment Stones, Is Awaited.

Essentials Of Litho-Tripsy

ii. Per–Cutaneous Ablation Of Gall-Bladder

Gall Blader Preserving TreatMent, Does Not Eliminate The Risk Of Recurrence & Gall Bladder Carcinoma Due To Persisting In-Situ Presence Of AbNormal Lithogenic Gall Bladder, Despite Sucessful Gall Stones Removal By Per-Cutaneous Tehniques.

Non-Surgical Ablation Of Gall Bladder Is The Technique Of Fibrotic Obliteration Of The Gall Bladder Lumen, By Eradication Of G.B Mucosa Completely, Thus Eliminating The Possibility Of Gall Stones Recurrence & Risk Of GallBladder Adeno-Carcinoma.

Technique; Tested Experimentally & Clinically, Involves Elimination Of Functioning GallBladder Through 'Chole-Cystostomy'.

Developed Two Step Approach Includes-
1. **Preliminary Obliteration Of 'Cystic Duct'** By Bi-Polar Radio-Frequency Electro-Cauterization
1. **Subsequent Gall Bladder Sclero-Therapy** Using Concentrated Ethanol & Sodium TetraDecyl Sulfate, WithOut Toxic Effects.

Histological Studies- In The **Animal Experimental Models** Revealed Necrosis Of Gall Bladder Wall Within (2)Weeks & Fibrotic Obliteration Of G.B LumenWithin (8)Weeks.

The FollwUp USGs Studies- No Mucocele Formation, Gall Stone Recurrence, But Persistence Of GB Lumina Indicating Incomplete Mucosal Ablation, Have Been Reported.

The Methodology Of Per–Cutaneous Ablation Of Gall-Bladder, Is In The Developmental Phases, Needing Further Technical Improvements Before Its Wider Clinical Applications.

EXTRA-CORPOREAL SHOCK WAVE LITHOTRIPSY

ESWL , A Non-Invasive Form Of Treatment In Selected Gall Stone Patients With Symptomatic, UnComplicated Chole-Cystolitiasis, Was Developed In 1980s(Sauerbruch et al,1986; Burhenne1989; Sackmann et al.1991).

Most Treatment Protocols Suggest The Rationale For Shock Wave Litho-Tripsy As To;
- Diminish The Surface To Volume Ratio Of Stone ThereBy Increasing Efficacy Of 'ODT'
- Decrease Stone Size Facilitating The Passage Of Small Stone Fragments & Debris From GallBladder To GIT WithOut Causing Symptoms.

While The- ESWL RestrictionTo Cholesterol Stones

(Radio-Lucent Or Faintly Calcified Calculii On Plain X-Rays), ESWLCombination With Adjuvant Oral Bile Acid Therapy, & Its Extended Role For 'Bile Duct Stones' Is Available Resources Circumstances Dependant.

Mechanisms; (2) Competing Mechanisms Lead To Clearance Of Gall Bladder Stones-
1. Spontaneous Passage Of Stone Fragments Through Cystic Duct
2. Stone Fragment Dissolution By Oral Bile Acids(ODT)
ESWL Alone Can Be Efficacious In SuccessFul ManageMent Of Gall Bladder Stones, Irrespective Of Stone Composition, By Increased No. Of Shock Wave Deliveries & Multiple TreatMent Sessions.

BIO-MECHANICS; The Techniques Involves The Focussed Delivery OF High Pressure Sound Waves To Gall Stones.
Shock Wave Generators : (3) Principal Types Are Available
- Under Water Spark Gap, Piezo-Electric Crystals & Electro-Magnetic Membrane Lithotripters.
- All Of Them Effective In Stone Fragmention & Achieve 'ESWL' As A Successful 'OPD Procedure'.
- RegardLess Of The Energy Source Shock Waves From Lithotripters Are Delivered From An UnderWater Source To Soft Tissues.

- The Passage Of Shock Waves WithOut Significant Dimininuition Of Energy Wave, On Passing Through The Anterior & Posterior Surface Walls Of Stone Liberates Compressive & Tensile Forces Causing Cavitation At The Anterior Surface Of Stones With Resultant Stone Fragmentation.
Factors Influencing Stone Fragmentation Include Size, Micr-Crystalline Structure & Architecture Of Stone.

LITHO-TRIPSY & BILE DUCT STONES

Indications For Different Litho-Tripsy Modalities-
Large Impacted CBD Stones Not Amenable To Endo-Scopic Extraction, Intra-Heatic Stones, Stones Above Biliary Strictures, Cystic Duct Remnant Stones & Bile Stones Associated With Mirizzi's Syndrome (Compression Of Common Hepatic Duct).

Selection Criteria For 'Shock Wave Litho-Tripsy, Are Similar To That Of Uncomplicated Gall Stones.
Reported Success Rates Are 70-90%, Most Patients Needing Endoscopic Extraction Of Stone Fragments.

Complications; Being Similar That Of **Uncomplicated Gall Stones,** Occurrence Of Mild Transient HaematoBilia(10%),

Essentials Of Litho-Tripsy

Biliary Sepsis(4%) Is In Reports.
To Prevent The Potential Of Biliary Sepsis Complications, Pre-Procedure Naso-Biliary, Endoscopic Or Per-Cutaneous Biliary Drainages Are Performed, With The Administration Of Proper Antibiotics.

LITHO-TRIPSY MODALITIES:
The Differently Available Appliances Include-

i.Mechanical LithoTripsy; Remains The Best Initial Option For Difficult Large CBD Stones, That Can Not Be Removed By Conventional Methods, Due To Its Safe, Effective Application,
As Initial Endoscopic Procdures.
Mechanical Litho-Tripters Are Modifications Of Standard Dormia Baskets, With The Available Standard Type Litho-Tripsy Compatible & Litho-Tripsy Covertible ManiFold Baskets, With Great Tensile Strength, Facilitate Holding, Fragmenting & Retrieval Of Larger Stones Endoscopically.
Studies In Experienced Centres Reported, >90% Success Rates For Difficult CBD Stones, Refractory To Standard Extraction Techniques,By Mechanical Lithotripsy Modality.

For 5% Of Biliary Stones Cases Resistant To Endoscopic Sphincterotomy & Mechanical Lithotripsy,Other Available Modalities Include-

Intra-Corporeal Tehniques (Laser Or Electr-Hydraulic Probes)

Laser LithoTripsy;

First Generation Devices eg Nd:YAG; ReportedInEffective Stone Fragmentation & High Risk Of Thermal Bile Duct Injuries.
Second Generation Devices; That Gained Acceptance Have High Energy, Flash Lamp, Pulled-Dye LaserTechnology.
The Application Of laser Pulse Leads To Rapid Expansion & Collapse Of Plasma On The Stone Surface, With Resultant Shock Wave.
Mother & Baby Dual Endoscope Systems, Previously,
Were The Only Means To Ensure Laser Stone Apposition , But Recently, Under Fluro-Scopic Guidance,Laser Litho-Tripsy Has Been Rendered More Efficaious, By The Use Of Devices Capable Of Differentiation Between Stone &Tissue.
Xenon Flash Lamp Pulsed Rhodamine 6G Laser With Integrated Stone Tissue Detection System, Is The Latest Availability.
IntraDuctal LithoTripsy Devices
Recent Devices With Recognition Of Stone & Tissue.

ElectroHydraulic LithoTripsy;
From Its Development In Former Soviet Union, During 1950s,

For Stone Fragmentations In Mining, The Method Has Been Adapted For Medical Use In The Tt. Of Nephro-Calcinosis & More Recently For Biliary Tract Calculii.

With The Advent Availability Of Gradually Improved,
Modified Electro-Hydraulic Probes, Working Under Direct Vision, Through Working Channel Of A Daughter EndoScope, Minimizing CBD Injuries & Perforations Etc, With About 85% Stone Clearance Rates,
Electro-Hydraulic Lithotripsy Has Low Costs & Increased Portability, As Main Advantages Over Laser Litho-Tripsy.

Extra- Corporeal Shock Wave LithoTripsy;

PATIENT SELECTION; Original & Most Subsequent Workers Advocated Adherence To -
Comparatively Strict Selection Criteria Including
-UltraSonoGraphy;A Normal GallBladder
-Oral Chole-Cystography;Opacification Of GB
-Limited Number Of Stones(One To Three)
  Stone Size(0.5 To 3 Cms)

As 'Shock Wave Litho-Tripsy' Is Usually Administered In Combination With ODT, Hence Patient Selection Criterion Being Almost Similar To That Of Oral Dissolution Therapy, As Summarized-

i. Stage Of Gall Stone Disease; SymtoMatic(Biliary Pain),
   WithOut Complications.
ii. Gall Stone Function;
   (Monitored By As Available Oral Chole-Cystography, Stimulated Cholescintigraphy, Functional Ultra-Sonography)
   - Opacified Gall Bladder With Patent Cystic Duct- Oral Chole-Cystography
   - Normal Gall Bladder Emptying On Stimulated Cholescintigraphy
   - Normal Gall Bladder Emptying After A Test On Functional Ultra-Sonography
iii. Stone Characterstics; -Radio-Lucent On Radio-Graphy
                -IsoDense Or HypoDense To Bile
                 & On CT Scan-Absence Of Calification
                -Single
                -DiaMetre<20mm

Procedural Details;
For Transmission Of Shock Waves, All Recent Generation Devices Utilize Water Cushions With Coupling Membranes, While Stone Targeting Is Accomplished With Real Time Ultra Sound.
i. Sedation, Analgesia & Or Anaesthesia
ii. Prone Position -To Minimize Distance Between Energy Source
                & Stone

Essentials Of Litho-Tripsy

-For Elimination Of Interference By Intestinal Gases & Costal Margins
iii. Targetting & Monitoring For Fragmentation- By USG,
? Contrast Delineated Integrated C-Arm Monitoring

Contra-Indications;-Cholestasis
-Pancreatitis
-Severe Hepatic Dysfunction Disease
-Haemorrhagic Diasthesis
-Abdominal Aortic Aneurysm
-Pregnancy

OverAll Result OutCome Of 'Shock Wave TreatMent' :
Depends Significantly Upon-
i. Degree Of Fragmentation
 - 'Shock Power', 'Shock No.', No. Of Sessions/Settings ParaMetres.
 - Stone CharacterStics
   Total Stone Volume, Stone Size
   Stone Composition
   Surface Distance
   Density- (CT Scan Density Of >84 HounsField Units
         Is Relative Limitation)
   Calcification Etc.

- Consideration Of ESWL Success Is Decided By Largest Remnant StoneFragment Size. Upto (4) mm Stone Fragments Are Acceptable, As They Can Be Managed SuccessFully With 1-2 Susequent Treatment Sessions.

ii. Gall Bladder Emptying

Results; After SuccessFul 'ESWL',
Reported Stone Free Patients Are About 70% After One Year,
While With 'ESWL' & Adjuvant Bile Acid Therapy ,
About 80% Within One And A Half Year.
In Solitary Gall Stone Of About 2 Cms Size,
The Reported Stone Clearance Success Rate Is 80-90%
Within 6-18 Months.

Side-Effects; Are **Minor** Including-
Cutaneous Petichial Haemorrhage(8%), Haematuria(4%),
Liver Haematoma(<1%), No Long Term Hepatic Bio-Chemical Abnormalities,

One Or More Episodes Of Biliary Pain Attributable To Stone Fragments Passage Till Complete Gall Bladder Clearance Are Observed, In About One Third Of Patients.
Others Include- Cystic Duct Obstruction(5%)
- Mild Transient Biliary Pancreatitis (About 2% Of Patients)
- Cholestasis & Ac. Chlecystitis, Less Frequently.

ESWL With Oral Bile Acid Therapy(Stone Dissolution Tt.);
Offers EffectiveSucceessFul Treatment In Symptomatic Patients With Single Radio-Lucent Gall Stone In Functioning Gall Bladder(Contraction >60% Of The Fasting Volume).
The Applicability Of This 'TreatMent Modality' In Such Group Of Patients, Is Supported By About 50% Success Rate WithOut Hazrds Of General Anaesthesia, Invasive Surgical Proceure,Risk Of Bile Duct Injuries & That Failure Of It Doesnot Preclude Surgery At A Later Date.

Recurrences: Of Gall Stones **Remain UnResolved Problem**.
Studies Indicate Development Of Stones Within 6 Years,
In More Than Two Thirds Of Patients.
While The FollowUp Data Reveal 27%,41% &54%
Cumulative Recurrence Rates At 3,5 &10 Years Respectively.

Attributable Causes Of Recurrence Include, Lithogenic Bile & Gall Bladder DysMotility Rather Than Patient Variables Of Gender, Age & Weight.
BeSides Various Different Available Statistical Studies Regarding Cost EffectiveNess In Different Age Groups, Categories Of Patients.
Comparative Evaluation Indicates CholeCystectomy(Open, Laproscopic) As The TreatMent Of Choice,
Till Further Future Developments To Control Recurrences.Comparatively Better Result OutComes ? Stone Chemistry.

Essentials Of Litho-Tripsy

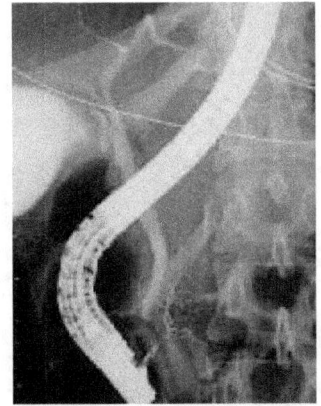

Pancreas Divisum Imaging
Emedicine.Medscape.Com150 × 200Search By Image
Endoscopic Retrograde Cholangiopancreatography.

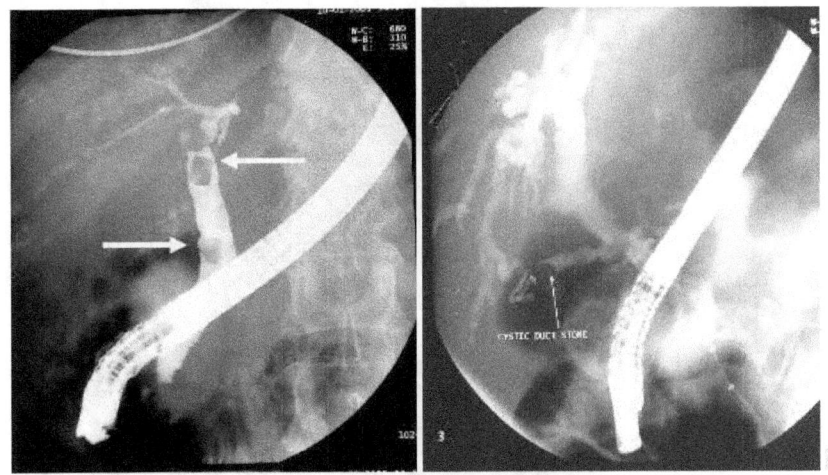

Stone Removal
Pixshark.Com574 × 331Search By Image
ERCP Stone Removal ERCP Demonstrates Stones.

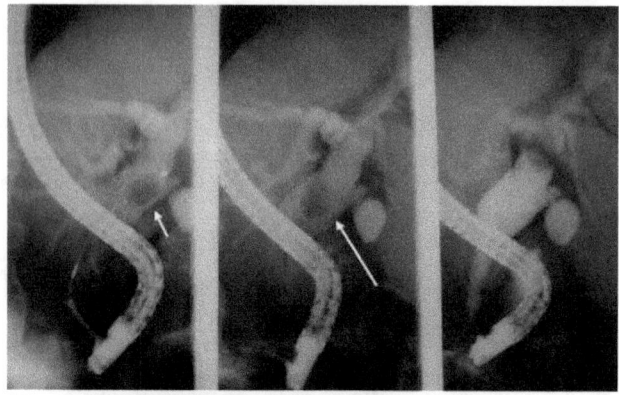

Www.Gastrores.Org485 × 306Search By Image.

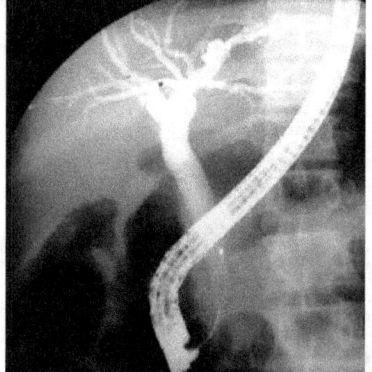

Www.Ceessentials.Net271 × 290Search By ImageDuring ERCP Stones And Sludge Are Removed And The Biliary Tree Checked Fo NeedFul.

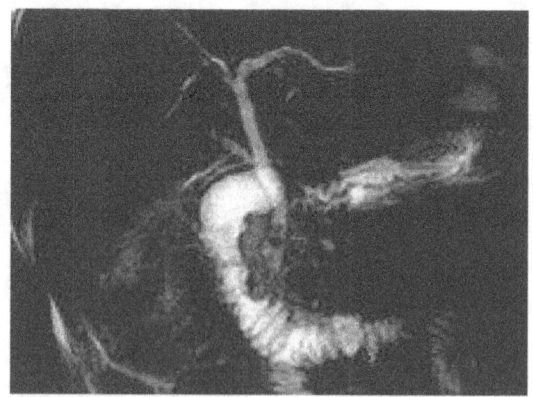

MRCP Image Of Two Stones
In The Distal Common Bile Duct

Essentials Of Litho-Tripsy
Biliary Laser lithotripsy

Laser Lithotripsy Of Bile Duct Stones Has Become A Widely Accepted Endoscopic Treatment Modality For Giant, Impacted, Or Very Hard Stones. The Procedure Is Usually Carried Out Under Direct Endoscopic Control In View Of The Potential Risk Of Bile Duct Injuries In "Blind" Laser Application.

Evaluation Of The Use Of A Rhodamine 6G Laser Lithotriptor With An Integrated Optical Stone Tissue Detection System (Ostds).

Reported Completely Stone-Clearance. The Only Major Complications Included Transient Haemobilia, Cholangitis, And Pancreatitis In Few Patients, Were Successfully Treated By Conservative Methods.

Concludes That Laser Lithotripsy Using The Described Rhodamine 6G Dye Laser With Ostds Seems To Be Safe And Effective And Allows "Blind" Fragmentation Of Difficult Common Bile Duct Stones Under Radiological Control Only.

LASER SYSTEM

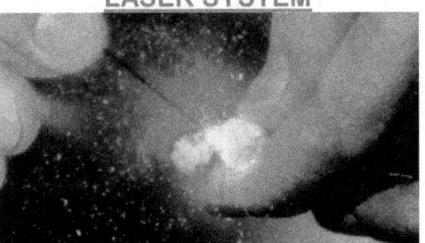

Figure 1
Laser Fragmentation Of A Biliary Concrement Using The Rhodamine 6G Dye Laser In Vitro.

OPTICAL STONE TISSUE DETECTION SYSTEM

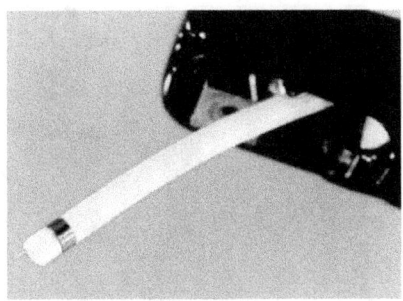

Figure 2
Standard Duodenoscope With Metal Marked 7F Plastic Catheter, Distal Metal Marking, And Central Laser Fibre.

ENDOSCOPIC EQUIPMENT AND APPLICATION TECHNIQUE

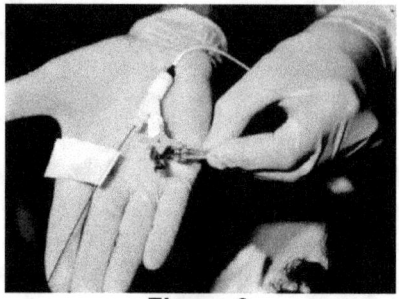

Figure 3
Side Flushing System (Tuohy-Borst Adapter, William-Cook, Europe) For Coaxial Irrigation Of The Laser Fibre Via A Standard 7f ERCP Catheter.

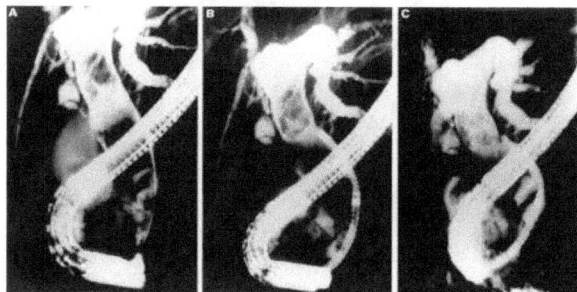

Figure 4
Laser Lithotripsy Under Direct Cholangioscopic Vision Using A Mother And Babyscope System Before (A), During (B), And After (C) Treatment (See Ell Et Al[16]; Reprinted With Permission).

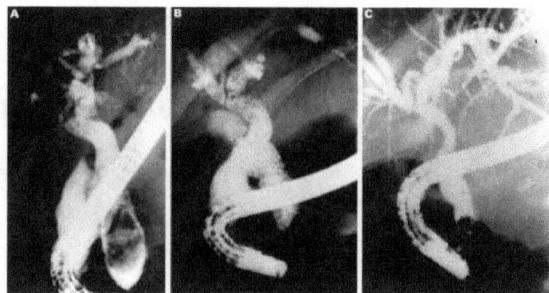

Figure 5
Blind Laser Application Of Giant Common Bile Duct Stones Before (A), During (B), And After (C) Treatment Using The Standard ERCP Catheter With Distal Metal Marking Under Control Of The Ostds And Intermittent Fluoroscopic Control.

Essentials Of Litho-Tripsy

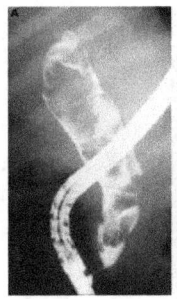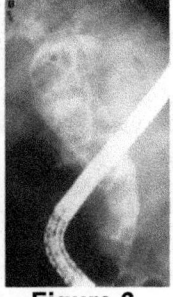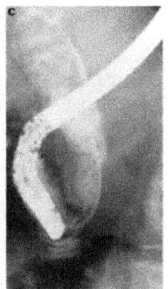

Figure 6
Blind Laser Application Of Giant Common Bile Duct Stones Before (A), During (B), And After (C) Treatment Using The Standard ERCP Catheter With Distal Metal Marking Under Control Of The Ostds And Intermittent Fluoroscopic Control.

Source-
Laser Lithotripsy Of Difficult Bile Duct Stones: Results In 60 Patients Using A Rhodamine 6g Dye Laser With Optical Stone Tissue Detection System.
J Hochberger[a], J Bayer[a], A May[a], S Mühldorfer[a], J Maiss[a], E G Hahn[a], C Ell[b] *Department Of Medicine I, Friedrich Alexander University, Erlangen, Germany, Department Of Medicine Ii, Hsk Wiesbaden, Germany* J Hochberger, Medizinische Klinik I Mit Poliklinik, Friedrich Alexander Universität, Krankenhausstrasse 12, D-91054 Erlangen, Germany.
Gut **1998;43:823-829 Doi:10.1136/Gut.43.6.823.**

Anil K. Sahni

CHOICE OF TREATMENT
ROLE IN GALL STONE DISEASES

In Cholelithiasis (Solitary Gallstone), Choledocholithiasis, T-Tube Drainage Or Otherwise, Contrast Delineated Stones Are Fragmented Into Minute Particles, Pass Away Down The Gastrointestinal Tract, Leaving Stone-Free Patient.
In The Nonavailability Of ERCP And Related Procedures, It Has Shown Good Results In CBD Stone Patients And May Be Suggestive Of Alternative To ERCP (MRCP), As Adjunct To Open/Laparoscopic Cholecystectomy Etc.
Pancreatic Duct Calculi In Association With Ductal Stricture And/Or Otherwise: ERCP And Lithotripsy.

The Present Discussed Study, Advocates The Role Of ESWL As An Adjuctive Methodology, For CholedoCholithiasisEspecially In The Non Availability Of Endoscopic ERCP/MRCP Facilities.

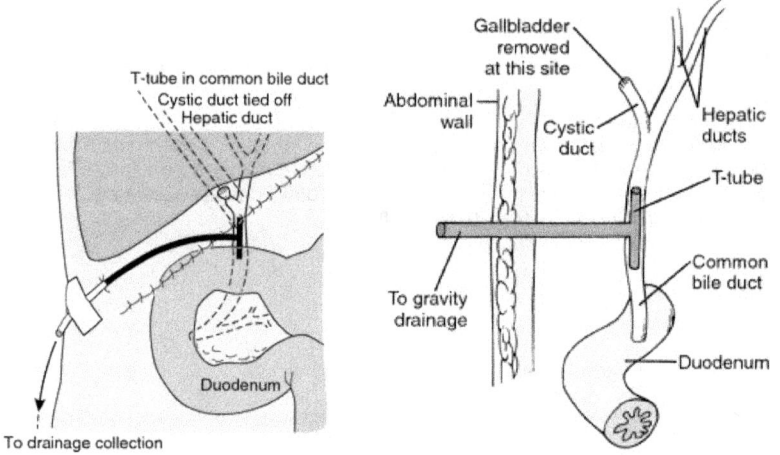

Post-Cholecystectomy With T-Tube Drainage
Source-Medical-Dictionary.Thefreedictionary.Com

The Important Adjacent Anatomical Structures-Hepatic artery, Portal Vein, Vena Cava, Aorta, Pancreas & Others, Have To Be Taken Into Consideration, For Post-Cholecystectomy With T-Tube Drainage, CBD Stones Delineated By T-Tube Contrast Radiology & Broken By ESWL, As An Alternative To Open Chole-Dochotomy/ ERCP Etc.

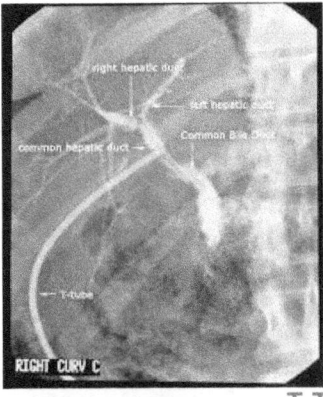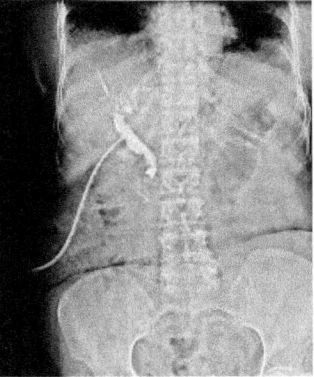

T-Tube Cholangiography

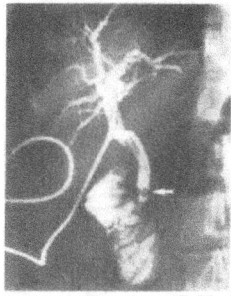

Postoperative T-TubeCholangiogram Enhancement Following Showing Free Entry Of Contrast Into Duodenum Despite A Residual Non-Opaque Calculus At The Lower End Of The Common Bile Duct.

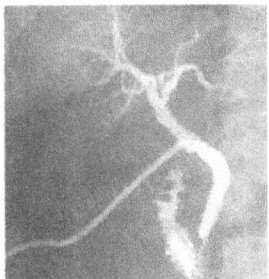

Intravenous Injection Is Frequently Undertaken To Highlight Focal Lesions.Dynamic Scans Involving Rapid Serial Images After Contrast Injection May Assist In Diagnosing Vascular Lesions Such As Haemangiomas And Some Tumours.

Source-RADIOLOGICAL EXAMINATION OF THE LIVER, BILIARY TRACT AND PANCREAS Intranet.Tdmu.Edu.Ua382 × 420Search By Image

Patient Selection Criterion

Inclusion Criteria
- Patient's informed consent.
- Bile duct stones that are not extractable endoscopically or percutaneously based on the experience of the individual investigator are treated. The presumed risk of ESWL must be below that of surgery.
- Successful test-positioning of the patient and localization of the stone.
- Preoperative anesthesia risk assignment (ASA) group I–IV.
- The focal axis of the shockwave must avoid lung, bodies of vertebra, aneurysms of aorta or renal artery and large bone areas with the exception of ribs.
- Absence of disturbance of coagulation.

Exclusion Criteria
- Informed consent not obtained.
- All inclusion criteria not fulfilled.
- Pregnancy; all premenopausal female patients have laboratory tests to exclude pregnancy.
- Failure to localize stone.
- Disturbance of coagulation.
- Presence of pacemaker and arrythmia.
- Vascular aneurysms or large bone areas in the path of the shockwaves.
- Upper abdominal surgery within 6 weeks prior to ESWL.

Adverse Effects and Complications

Biliary Pain
Abdominal Pain
Liver Hematoma
Gallbladder Empyema
Pancreatitis
Rupture Of A Juxtapapillary
Diverticulum
Hemobilia
Hematoma Of The Skin
Macrohematuria
Fever
Significant Drop In The Hemoglobin Levels

Essentials Of Litho-Tripsy

Procedural Details

During The Present Discussed Study Methodology,
In Post-Cholecystectomy With T-Tube Drainage Patients,
For CBD Stones, **Patient's Position Supine**,
Available Contrast Material(Usually GastroGraffin),After Sensitivity Test
Instilled Through T-Tube Gradually, Under Continuous CT Monitoring
Surveillance, CBD Stones Revealed As SOLs In Contrast Filled CBD,
Are Focussed For CareFully Conducted Shock Wave Deliveries &
Achieving Stone/ Stones Shattering Into Minute Particles, Passing Down
The GIT, Through Duodenum, WithOut Further Obstructive Complications.

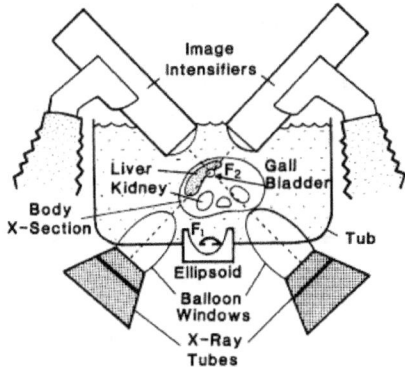

A Cross-Sectional View Of The Dornier HM-3 Lithotriptor Bath Tub,
With Positioning Of Biliary Tract To Focus At F_2.
Mostly Shock Waves Enter The Abdomen Posteriorly,
Under Appropriate Anaesthesia Or Analgesia, With Real Time
RadioGraphic Contrast Media Surveillance, Shock Wave Discharges
Triggered By An ElectroCardioGram, Are Delivered To Bile Duct Calculi
With Shock Wave Focus At F_2.

HowEver,Fragmentation Of Bile Duct Stones By Extracorporeal Shock
Waves A New Approach To Biliary Calculi After Failure Of Routine
Endoscopic Measures T. SAUERBRUCH, M. STERN, And The Study Group For
Shock-Wave Lithotripsy Of Bile Duct Stones.
Methodology Description Is As Follows-
 Extracorporeal Shock-Wave Lithotripsy Of Bile Duct Stones,
The Patient Is In **Supine Position** And The Shock Waves. Enter The
Body From The Rear.

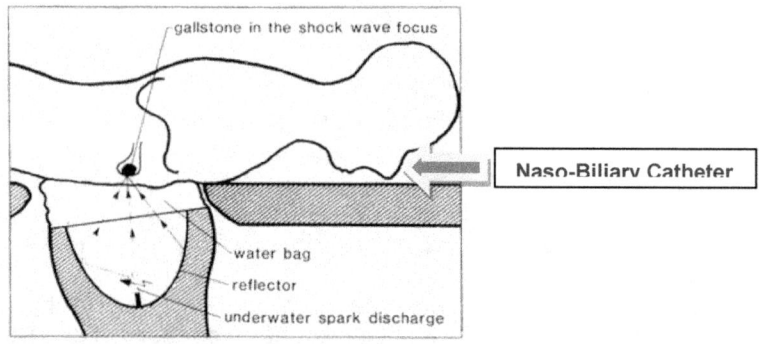

An Endoscopically Placed Nasohiliary Catheter Permits Injection Of Contrast Medium For Visualization Of The Stone By Fluoroscopy, Allowing Positioning And Disintegration Of The Stone.

A Large Stone In The Common Bile Duct After ESWL , By Visualization Of The Bile Duct Via A Nasobiliary Tube Shows Optimal Disintegration Of The Stone.

A Large Stone In The Left Hepatic Duct In A Study, Was Successfully Extracted After Fragmentation By ESWL

AVAILABLE FURTHER STUDIES-

Ann Surg. 1989 Jun; 209(6): 743–755.

PMCID: PMC1494134

Extracorporeal Shock-Wave Lithotripsy Of Bile Duct Calculi. An Interim Report Of The Dornier U.S. Bile Duct Lithotripsy Prospective Study.

K I Bland, R S Jones, J W Maher, P B Cotton, T C Pennell, J R Amerson, J L Munson, G Berci, G J Fuchs, L W Way

Extracorporeal Shock Wave Lithotripsy

Gallstone Fragmentation By Extracorporeal Shock Wave Lithotripsy (ESWL) **May Be An Appropriate Therapy For Some Patients Who Cannot Undergo Surgery**,
But It Is No Longer Widely Used. The Treatment Works Best On **Solitary Stones That Are Less Than 2 Centimeters In Diameter**.
Less Than 15% Of Patients Are Good Candidates For Lithotripsy.
The Typical Procedure Is Performed As Follows:
- The Patient Sits In A Tub Of Water.

Essentials Of Litho-Tripsy

- High-Energy, Ultrasound Shock Waves Are Directed Through The Abdominal Wall Toward The Stones.
- The Shock Waves Travel Through The Soft Tissues Of The Body And Break Up The Stones.
- The Stone Fragments Are Then Usually Small Enough To Be Passed Through The Bile Duct And Into The Intestines.
- **Lithotripsy Is Generally Combined With Oral Dissolution Treatment** To Help Dissolve The Fragmented Pieces Of The Original Gallstone.

Complications- Include Pain In The Gallbladder Area And Pancreatitis, Usually Occurring Within A Month Of Treatment.
In Addition, Not All Of The Fragments May Clear The Bile Duct. Adding Erythromycin To The Treatment Regimen May Help Remove These Fragments. About 35% Of Patients Who Are Left With Fragments Are At Risk For Further Problems, Which Can Be Severe.
The Chance Of Recurrence Is High With This Procedure, And In One Study, 45% Of Patients Eventually Required Surgery. Elderly People May Have A Lower Risk For Recurrence Than Younger Adults.

Other Procedures

Percutaneous Cholecystostomy Is A Procedure That May Be Used In **Seriously ill Patients With Severe Gallbladder Infection Who Cannot Tolerate Immediate Surgery**.
It Is Also The Standard Treatment For Patients With **Acalculous Cholecystitis (Gallbladder Inflammation Without Stones)**. This Procedure Uses A Needle To Withdraw Fluid From (Aspirate) The Gallbladder. A Drainage Catheter Is Inserted Through The Skin And Into The Gallbladder While The Fluid Drains Out. In Some Cases, The Catheter May Be Left In Place For Up To 8 Weeks. After That Time,
If Possible, **Laparoscopy Or An Open Cholecystectomy** May Be Performed. Without A Laparoscopy, Recurrence Rates With This Procedure Are High.

Gallbladder Aspiration- With This Procedure, Fluid Is Removed While The Gallbladder Is Viewed Using Ultrasound. It Does **Not Require Leaving A Catheter** In The Abdomen Afterward, And May Have **Fewer Complications Than Percutaneous Cholecystostomy.**

Mini-Laparotomy Cholecystostomy- Uses Small Abdominal Incisions But, Unlike Laparoscopy, It Is An "Open" Procedure, And The Surgeon Does Not Operate Through A Scope. The Surgical Instruments Used Are Very Small (2 - 3 Mm In Diameter, Or About A Tenth Of An Inch).

Eventually, This Technique May Reduce Operative Time And Enable Surgeons To Obtain Better Results Than With Laparoscopy.

Natural Orifice Translumenal Endoscopic Surgery (Notes)- A New Procedure May Enable Surgeons To Remove The Gallbladder With Less Pain And A Faster Recovery Time Than Conventional Laparoscopic Surgery. In The Notes Procedure, Doctors Pass An Endoscope Through A Natural Opening In The Body (Such As The Vagina In The Case Of The Gallbladder), And Then Through An Internal Incision In The Stomach, Vagina, Bladder, Or Colon. **There Are No External Incisions. This Procedure Is Still Considered Investigational.**

The place of lithotripsy and surgery in the management of gallstone disease.
Heberer G, Sackmann M, Krämling HJ, Sauerbruch T, Paumgartner G.
Source
Department of Surgery, Ludwig-Maximilians University, Munich, Federal Republic of Germany.
Abstract
Surgery of the gallbladder remains the "gold standard" of curative therapy of gallbladder stones, against which ESWL and other nonsurgical techniques have to be evaluated. For the therapy of bile duct stones, ESWL is a helpful and effective nonsurgical adjunct.
     2403461 [PubMed - indexed for MEDLINE]
Ann Surg. 1989 Jun;209(6):743-53; discussion 753-5.

Gallstone lithotripsy.
www.ncbi.nlm.nih.gov/pubmed/1998151
by BD Schirmer - 1991 - Cited by 1 - Related articles
Gallstone lithotripsy. Schirmer BD. ESWL, in its present state of technology, is unlikely to displace endoscopy as the treatment of first choice for common duct ...
Surg Annu. 1991;23 Pt 1:91-114.
Gallstone lithotripsy.
Schirmer BD.
Abstract
ESWL, In Its Present State Of Technology, Is Unlikely To Displace Endoscopy As The Treatment Of First Choice For Common Duct Stones Present After Cholecystectomy, Since Endoscopic Sphincterotomy Is Necessary To Enhance Passage Of Stones From The Ductal System. However, When Endoscopy Fails, ESWL May Prove A Useful Adjunctive Treatment For Both Choledocholithiasis And Intrahepatic Stones. ESWL for gallstones is currently an evolving treatment option for patients with symptomatic gallstones. ESWL in its present state may be treatment for only a few patients with gallstones, but advancing technology could

increase its applicability. Surgeons should therefore continue to lead by knowing how to use lithotripsy to treat cholelithiasis.
PMID:1998151 [PubMed - indexed for MEDLINE]
Adv Surg. 1990;23:291-314.

Extracorporeal shockwave lithotripsy of gallstones. Possibilities and limitations.
Vergunst H, Terpstra OT, Brakel K, Laméris JS, van Blankenstein M, Schröder FH.
Source
Department of Surgery, University Hospital Dijkzigt, Rotterdam, The Netherlands.
Abstract
Recently extracorporeal shockwave lithotripsy (ESWL) has been introduced as a nonoperative treatment for gallstone disease. Except for lung damage, no significant adverse effects of ESWL of gallbladder stones have been observed in animals. In clinical use ESWL of gallbladder stones is now confined to 15% to 30% of symptomatic patients. To achieve complete stone clearance, ESWL of gallbladder stones must be supplemented by an adjuvant therapy. ESWL of bile duct stones is highly effective and can be considered in patients in whom primary endoscopic or surgical stone removal fails.
ESWL for cholelithiasis is a promising treatment modality with good short-term and unknown long-term results.
PMID:2684058[PubMed - indexed for MEDLINE]
PMCID:PMC1357788
 Free PMC Article
Scand J Gastroenterol. 1996 Sep;31(9):934-9.

Gallstones Extracorporeal Shock Wave **Lithotripsy** - Health - The ...
health.nytimes.com › Times Health Guide › g › Gallstones
Jul 19, 2011 – In-Depth From A.D.A.M. Extracorporeal Shock Wave **Lithotripsy**.**Gallstone** fragmentation by extracorporeal shock wave **lithotripsy** (ESWL) may ...

Gallstones
www.uptodate.com/contents/**gallstones**-beyond-the-basics
Oct 26, 2012 – The success of **lithotripsy** for **gallstones** varies, with experienced centers successfully treating 90 to 100 percent of people with one stone and ...

Extracorporeal shockwave lithotripsy of common bile duct stones without preliminary endoscopic sphincterotomy.
Yasuda I, Tomita E.Source
Dept. of Gastroenterology, Gifu Municipal Hospital, Japan.

This treatment offers several advantages because it is less invasive, has few complications, and can preserve the papilla of Vater. This method is especially suitable for patients with smaller, floating stones.
Background: Endoscopic sphincterotomy (EST) is now a standard procedure for common bile duct stones. It is less invasive than surgical treatment and is well established, but complications such as bleeding and perforation occasionally occur. We have been investigating the safest and most useful method of preserving the papilla of Vater. In the present study we evaluated the effectiveness and safety of extracorporeal shock wave lithotripsy (ESWL) for common bile duct stones without preliminary EST. *Methods:* From May 1992 to May 1995 ESWL was performed on 52 patients with common bile duct stones at our hospital. In all 52 patients a nasobiliary tube was inserted endoscopically, without preliminary EST, and ESWL was performed. *Results:* Fragmentation and subsequent complete clearance of stones was achieved in 35 patients (67.3%), and no additional treatment was necessary. In 17 patients (25.0%) fragmentation was not achieved, so EST and endoscopic extraction were performed, and the stones were cleared completely. None of the patients had major complications with clinical sequelae. We compared the completely cleared group and the failed group, to assess the influence of various factors. Our findings indicated that smaller, 'floating' stones responded more favorably to ESWL. When the largest stone was <15 mm in diameter and the stone index (diameter of common bile duct/diameter of stone) was >1.0, the success rate was very high 25 of 27 = 92.6%). *Conclusions:* This treatment offers several advantages because it is less invasive, has few complications, and can preserve the papilla of Vater. This method is especially suitable for patients with smaller, floating stones.
ReadMore: http://informahealthcare.com/doi/abs/10.3109/0036552960905 2005?journalCode=gas
Endoscopy. 2002 Aug;34(8):624-7.

Impact of gallbladder status on the outcome in patients with retained bile duct stones treated with extracorporeal shockwave lithotripsy.
Adamek HE, Kudis V, Jakobs R, Buttmann A, Adamek MU, Riemann JF.
Source
Department of Medicine C, Klinikum Ludwigshafen, Academic Hospital of the University of Mainz, Ludwigshafen, Germany. MedCLu@t-online.de
The Use Of Endoscopic Therapy In Combination With Lithotripsy Techniques Has Become Increasingly Common In Patients With Complicated Common Bile Duct Stones. In Many Units, Although This Is Controversial, Cholecystectomy Is Then Performed, Because Of Possible Subsequent Cholecystitis And Recurrence Of Choledocholithiasis. The Aim Of This Study Was To Investigate Whether Gallbladder Status Influences The Long-Term Outcome In Patients After Extracorporeal Shockwave Lithotripsy (ESWL) Of Common Bile Duct Stones.

Essentials Of Litho-Tripsy

The Intact Gallbladder Is Not A Risk Factor For Recurrent Biliary Complications After ESWL Of Common Bile Duct Stones; Therefore, As Far As Patients With Complicated Bile Duct Stones Which Require Additional Lithotripsy Techniques Are Concerned, Elective Cholecystectomy After Endoscopic Clearance Of The Bile Duct No Longer Seems Appropriate.[Pubmed - Indexed For MEDLINE]

Other Readings-

1. **Gallstones** Non-Surgical Treatment: **Lithotripsy**, Contact Dissolution **...**
   www.webmd.com/digestive-disorders/tc/**gallstones**-other-treatment
   Jul 15, 2011 – Other treatment options for **gallstones** are not widely available. Less is known about their effectiveness and long - term impact compared with **...**
2. **Gallstones** and gallbladder disease - Extracorporeal Shock Wave **...**
   www.umm.edu › Medical Reference › Patient Education
   Gallstone fragmentation by extracorporeal shock wave **lithotripsy** (ESWL) may be an appropriate therapy for some patients who cannot undergo surgery, but it is **...**
3. **Gallstones** - Treatment - NHS Choices
   www.nhs.uk/Conditions/**Gallstones**/Pages/Treatment.aspx
   Lithotripsy is a method of concentrating ultrasonic shock waves on to the **gallstones** to break them up into tiny pieces. Once the **gallstones** have been broken up, **...**

Endoscopic retrograde cholangiopancreatology (ERCP)
Endoscopic retrograde cholangiopancreatology (ERCP) is a procedure that aims to remove bile duct stones. In some patients this is the only treatment required. However, the gallbladder and stones in the gallbladder remain.
An ERCP is usually carried out under sedation, which means that you will be awake throughout the procedure but will not experience any pain.
ERCP is similar to a diagnostic cholangiography, except that an electrically heated wire is passed through the endoscope and is used to widen the opening to your bile duct. The bile duct stones are then removed or left to pass into your intestine. Sometimes a small narrow tube called a stent is placed in the bile duct to help the bile and stones pass.

Alternative treatments
A number of alternative treatments have been tried but they are not very successful, have problems of their own and gallstones can reoccur very quickly once treatment is stopped.

Tablets to dissolve the gallstones (ursodeoxycholic acid)
A few patients' small non-calcified gallstones made of cholesterol in a normally functioning gallbladder can be dissolved by taking a medication called ursodeoxycholic acid for up to two years. To make treatment more effective, you may be advised to eat a low-cholesterol diet.
Side effects of ursodeoxycholic acid are uncommon and are usually mild. The most commonly reported side effects are feeling sick, being sick and

itchy skin. The use of ursodeoxycholic acid is not usually recommended for pregnant or breastfeeding women.

Sexually active women should use either a barrier method of contraception, such as a condom, or a low-dose oestrogen contraceptive pill while taking ursodeoxycholic acid, as it may affect other types of oral contraceptive pills.

Once the treatment is stopped the gallstones usually reoccur. Ursodeoxycholic acid can also be prescribed as a precaution against gallstones if it is thought that you are at risk of developing them. For example, you may be prescribed ursodeoxycholic acid if you have recently had weight loss surgery.

Lithotripsy

Lithotripsy is a method of concentrating ultrasonic shock waves on to the gallstones to break them up into tiny pieces. Once the gallstones have been broken up, they can pass out of your body in your stools (poo). Unfortunately, in some patients the gallstones remain and grow, and in others the debris causes acute pancreatitis or jaundice.

It is rarely used when other treatments are possible as there can be up to a 50% chance of symptoms returning within five years of treatment.

The healthcare professional carrying out the lithotripsy procedure will first use an <u>ultrasound scan</u> to determine the location of the gallstones.

They will press a sensor against your abdomen, next to the gallstones, which will then deliver the ultrasonic waves on to the gallstones.

4. Recently-Approved Devices > Medstone STS™ **Lithotripter** - P970042
   www.fda.gov/MedicalDevices/.../Recently.../ucm089770.htm
   Nov 29, 2012 – The Medstone STS™ **Lithotripter** uses high energy shock waves to fragment **gallstones**. These shock waves are generated by the deviceand ...
5. Extracorporeal Shock Wave **Lithotripsy** for **Gallstones**
   https://www.bcidaho.com/providers/.../mp_70135.asp - United States
   Extracorporeal shock wave **lithotripsy** (ESWL) for **gallstones** is a non-invasive procedure for disintegrating **gallstones**. High-intensity shock.
6. **Gallstones** and Gallbladder Removal and Surgery | Healthhype.com
   www.healthhype.com › Liver and Gallbladder
   Jump to **Lithotripsy**: **Lithotripsy**. **Lithotripsy** is the fragmentation of a **gallstone**, within the gallbladder or bile duct, by the use of sound shock waves.
7. **Lithotripsy** for the Treatment of **Gallstones** - Full Text View ...
   clinicaltrials.gov/ct2/show/NCT00042549
   Lithotripsy for the Treatment of **Gallstones**. This study has been terminated. Sponsor: Medstone International. Information provided by: Medstone International ...

Essentials Of Litho-Tripsy
References

1. ^ Fitzgerald JEF, Fitzgerald LA, Maxwell-Armstrong CA, Brooks AJ (2009). "Recurrent gallstone ileus: time to change our surgery?". *Journal of Digestive Diseases* **10**: 149–151. PMID 19426399.
2. ^ Gallstones - Cholelithiasis; Gallbladder attack; Biliary colic; Gallstone attack; Bile calculus; Biliary calculus Last reviewed: July 6, 2009. Reviewed by: George F. Longstreth. Also reviewed by David Zieve
3. ^ Channa, Naseem A.; Khand, Fateh D.; Khand, Tayab U.; Leghari, Mhhammad H.; Memon, Allah N. (2007). "Analysis of human gallstones by Fourier Transform Infrared (FTIR)".*Pakistan Journal of Medical Sciences* **23** (4): 546–50. ISSN 1682-024X. Retrieved 2010-11-06.
4. ^ a b c Kim IS, Myung SJ, Lee SS, Lee SK, Kim MH (2003). "Classification and nomenclature of gallstones revisited". *Yonsei Medical Journal* **44** (4): 561–70. ISSN 0513-5796.PMID 12950109. Retrieved 2010-11-06.
5. ^ a b c d National Institute of Diabetes and Digestive and Kidney Diseases (2007). "Gallstones". Bethesda, Maryland: National Digestive Diseases Information Clearinghouse,National Institutes of Health, United States Department of Health and Human Services. Retrieved 2010-11-06.
6. ^ Heuman DM, Mihas AA, Allen J (2010). "Cholelithiasis". Omaha, Nebraska: Medscape (WebMD). Retrieved 2010-11-06.
7. ^ National Library of Medicine (2010). "Gallstones". Bethesda, Maryland: United States National Library of Medicine, National Institutes of Health, United States Department of Health and Human Services. Retrieved 2010-11-06.
8. ^ Roizen MF and Oz MC, *Gut Feelings: Your Digestive System*, pp. 175–206 in Roizen and Oz (2005)
9. ^ Koppisetti, Sreedevi; Jenigiri, Bharat; Terron, M. Pilar; Tengattini, Sandra; Tamura, Hiroshi; Flores, Luis J.; Tan, Dun-Xian; Reiter, Russel J. (2008). "Reactive Oxygen Species and the Hypomotility of the Gall Bladder as Targets for the Treatment of Gallstones with Melatonin: A Review". *Digestive Diseases and Sciences* **53** (10): 2592–603. doi:10.1007/s10620-007-0195-5. PMID 18338264.
10. ^ Ortega RM, Fernández-Azuela M, Encinas-Sotillos A, Andrés P, López-Sobaler AM (1997). "Differences in diet and food habits between patients with gallstones and controls".*Journal of the American College of Nutrition* **16** (1): 88–95. PMID 9013440. Retrieved 2010-11-06.
11. ^ Misciagna, Giovanni; Leoci, Claudio; Guerra, Vito; Chiloiro, Marisa; Elba, Silvana; Petruzzi, José; Mossa, Ascanio; Noviello, Maria R. et al. (1996). "Epidemiology of cholelithiasis in southern Italy. Part II". *European Journal of Gastroenterology & Hepatology* **8**: 585–93. doi:10.1097/00042737-199606000-00017.
12. ^ Trotman, Bruce W.; Bernstein, Seldon E.; Bove, Kevin E.; Wirt, Gary D. (1980). "Studies on the Pathogenesis of Pigment Gallstones in Hemolytic Anemia". *Journal of Clinical Investigation* **65** (6): 1301–8. doi:10.1172/JCI109793. PMC 371467. PMID 7410545.
13. ^ *Endocrine and Metabolic Disorders: Cutaneous Porphyrias*, pp. 63–220 in Beers, Porter and Jones (2006)
14. ^ Thunell S (2008). "Endocrine and Metabolic Disorders: Cutaneous Porphyrias". Whitehouse Station, New Jersey: Merck Sharp & Dohme Corporation. Retrieved 2010-11-07.
15. ^ M. A. Cahan; L. Balduf, K. Colton, B. Palacioz, W. McCartney and T. M. Farrell. "Proton pump inhibitors reduce gallbladder function". *Surgical Endoscopy* **20** (9): 1364–1367.doi:10.1007/s00464-005-0247-x. PMID 16858534.
16. ^ Experimental investigation of the flow of bile in patient specific cystic duct models M Al-Atabi, SB Chin... - Journal of biomechanical engineering, 2010
17. ^ a b National Health Service (2010). "Gallstones — Treatment". *NHS Choices: Health A-Z - Conditions and treatments*. London: National Health Service. Retrieved 2010-11-06.
18. ^ Jensen (2010). "Postcholecystectomy syndrome". Omaha, Nebraska: Medscape (WebMD). Retrieved 2011-01-20.

19. ^ Marks, Janet; Shuster, Sam; Watson, A. J. (1966). "Small-bowel changes in dermatitis herpetiformis". *The Lancet* **288** (7476): 1280–2. doi:10.1016/S0140-6736(66)91692-8.PMID 4163419.
20. ^ Keus, Frederik; de Jong, Jeroen; Gooszen, H G; Laarhoven, C JHM; Keus, Frederik (2006). "Laparoscopic versus open cholecystectomy for patients with symptomatic cholecystolithiasis". *Cochrane Database of Systematic Reviews* (4): CD006231. doi:10.1002/14651858.CD006231. PMID 17054285.
21. ^ Moritz, Andreas (1998). *The Amazing Liver/Gallbladder Flush*.
22. ^ Ross JK & Leklem JE "The effect of dietary citrus pectin on the excretion and the activity of 7-alfa-dehydroxylase and beta-glucuronidase." *The American Journal of Clinical Nutrition* Oct 1981; 34: pp 2068-2077 [1]
23. ^ "Apple juice and the chemical-contact softening of gallstones", THE LANCET • Vol 354 • December 18/25, 1999, p2171 [2]
24. ^ "Adjuvant herbal treatment for gallstones", *British Journal of Surgery* 1992, Vol. 79, February, 168 [3]
25. ^ Alan R. Gaby. "The gallstone cure that wasn't". Townsend Letter for Doctors and Patients. Retrieved 2007-02-10.
26. ^ "Could these be Gallstones?", *The Lancet*, Vol 365 April 16, 2005, p1388 [4]
27. ^ Vivian McAlister, Eric Davenport, and Elizabeth Renouf. "Cholecystectomy Deferral in Patients with Endoscopic Sphincterotomy. *Cochrane Database of Systematic Reviews* .4 (2007): CD006233. Available at: [5]
28. ^ "Interview with Darren Wise. Transcrip". Omaha, Nebraska: Medscape (WebMD). Retrieved 2010-11-06.

(4.)(ii.)ESWL: OTHER INDICATIONS

Beside Established Role In Urolithiasis & Biliary Stones, The Other Scopes Of Application Include-

Pancreatic Calculii

Pancreatic Duct Stones Are One Of The Commenst Manifestations In **Chronic Obstructive Pancreatitis.**
They Are Commonly Formed Proximal To A **Pancreatic Duct Stricture,** And Are Usually Firmly Impacted.
Stone ManageMent Standard Modalities Include-

A. **Mechanical LithoTripsy-** The Simplest & Most Effective Methodology With 80-90% Success Rates(Schneider et al,1988),
Involves Stone EntrapMent & Forcible Crushing In The Arms Of 'Dormia Basket', Achieved By Either Of (2)Techniques-
   i. **Non-EndoScopic Method-** WithIn A 'Standard Dormia Basket' Sone Is Grasped & EndoScope Is Removed After Cutting Basket Handle.
   Mechanical LithoTripsy Is Performed By A Coil Metal Sheath Inserted Over Gide Wire, In Contact With Stone.
   ii. **EndoScopic Method** – By A Special LithTripsy Basket Contained Within The Metal Sheath, Inserted Using The EndosCope Working Channel, Stone Is Captured & Mechanical LithoTripsy Performed.
   With The Advantage Of Endosopist Anticipation Regarding Need For Mechanical LithoTripsy Before Attempting Stone Extraction.
B. **IntraDuctal Short Wave LithoTripsy** – In Cases Of Mechanical LithoTripsy Failures Due To Large Size, Firmly Impacted Stones, Fragmentation Is Achieved By 'Shock Waves' Delivered IntraDuctally Or ExtraCorporeally.
The Principles & Technique Of IntraDuctal LithoTripsy Are Similar To Bile Duct Calculii.
C. **ExtraCorporeal Shock Wave LithoTripsy** – Has Been Demonstrated As A Safe,Effective Method For Bile & Pancreatic Ductal Calculii, Defying Endoscopic Extraction.
For **Bile Duct Stone Fragmentation** 95% Success Rates With 50% Pts. Requiring **Adjunctive TreatMents**, For Complete Ductal Clearance Have Been Reported In U.S Multi-Institutional Study (Bland et al. 1989).
IntraDuctal SWL Has Been Reported To Be Better Than ESWL For Complete CBD Stone Clearance (NeuHaus et al.,1998).

High Success Rates Reported For Pancreatic Ductal Stones Fragmentation & Pain Relief In Most Pts. While 50% Of Them Needing Subsequent Stenting For Associated Strictures (Delhaye et al. 1992;Smith et al.1996b).
While ESWL – For Bile & Pancreatic Ductal Stone Fragmentation, Successfully Used In Several Countries, Is Not Appoved In US For These Indications.

D. **Dissolution Therapy** – Despite Initial Encouraging Results, Reported Use Of MonocTanoin & Ters-Butyl Ether Via NasoBiliary Drainage & T-Tube Catheters (Allen et al.1985: Palmer & HoffMann 1986), Abandoned Due To Poor OverAll Results,CumberSome, Time Consuming Technique & Adverse Effects Due To Leakage Of Solvent Into Duodenum.
The Adjunctive Technique Involving UDA Administration & EndoScopic Stenting Demonstrated Softening & Decrease Size Of CBDStones, In One Study(JohnSon et al.1993). The Approach Is Appealing In The Non-Availability Of High Technology LitoTripsy Methods.

E. **Pancreatic Ductal Stricture Dilatation** – Is Done By 'Push Type Dilators Catheters(Bougies) Or High Pressure HydroStatic Balloons, With / WithOut Stenting For Variable Duration & Intervals, Depending Upon The Aetio-Pathogenesis & Extent Of Disease Process.

Peyronie's Disease

First Reported By Fallopius, 1561, Known By Peyronie's Disease (Peyronie,1743), Also Known As 'Induratio Plastica Of Penis',
Is Usually Associated With Dupytren Disease & Other Fibrotic Conditions Like Contracture Of Plantar Fascia (Ledder Hose Disease) & TypanacoSclerosis.
Medical ManageMent Being The First Line Treatment, Most Of The Patients DoesNot Require Surgery Except For Palliating Mechanical Effects Of Disease & Erectile Dysfunction.

With Different AvailAble Medical ManageMent Modalities Studies -
Oral Medications-Vitamin E, Colchicine, Tamoxifen, Intalesional Verapamil, Radiation Therapy, Vaccum Erection, Penile Traction Devices,
**Placement Of ESWL Role For Peyronie's Disease
Is Not Adequately Determined**.

Erectile Dysfunction-Low Intensity ESWL May Promote Neovascularization And Improve Erectile Function
Vardi Y, Appel B, Jacob G, Et Al: **Can Low Intensity Extracorporeal Shockwave Therapy Improve Erectile Function? A 6-Month Follow-Up Pilot Study In Patients With Organic Erectile Dysfunction**.
Euro Urol 2010; 58:243-248.

"ESWL" Other Scope Applicabilities-

Available Study Reports-

Salivary Stones Management
http://www.nlm.nih.gov/medlineplus/ency/article/001039.htm

Impact Of Extracorporeal Shock Waves On The Human Skin With Cellulite: A Case Study Of An Unique Instance
F Angehrn, C Kuhn, O Sonnabend, A Voss - Clinical Interventions in Ageing, 2008

Effects Of Shock Wave Therapy In The Skin Of Patients With Progressive Systemic Sclerosis: A Pilot Study
E Tinazzi, E Amelio, E Marangoni, C Guerra... - Rheumatology ..., 2011 - Springer
Abstract Vasculopathy, immunological abnormalities, and excessive tissue fibrosis are key elements in the pathogenesis of progressive systemic sclerosis (SSC). Extracorporeal shock waves (ESW) have anti-inflammatory and regenerative effects on different tissues.

Aspects Of Current Management Extracorporeal Shock-Wave Therapy In The Management Of Chronic Soft-Tissue Conditions C. A. Speed C. A. Speed, Honorary Consultant Rheumatology, Sports & Exercise Medicine, Addenbrooke's Hospital, Hills Road, Cambridge CB2 2QQ, UK. ©2004 British Editorial Society of Bone and Joint Surgery doi:10.1302/0301-620X.86B2. 14253 $2.00 J Bone Joint Surg [Br] 2004;86-B:165-71.

An Overview Of Shock Wave Therapy In Musculoskeletal Disorders
Ching-Jen Wang, MD Additional information including the cellular and molecular changes after shock wave therapy are needed for further clarification on the mechanism of shock wave therapy in musculoskeletal system. *(Chang Gung Med J 2003;26:220-32)*

Extracorporeal Shockwave Therapy (ESWT), An Option For Chronic Tendinopathy Management: A Clinical Perspective
K Craig, A Miller - New Zealand Pain Society Publication, 2011

Medical Shockwaves For The Treatment Of Peripheral Neuropathic Pain In A Type Ii Diabetic: A Case Report
K Craig, M Walker - New Zealand Pain Society Publication, Winter Issue, 2012.

(4.)(iii.) EXTRACORPOREAL TISSUE LITHOTRIPSY

Recent Rapid Technology Development, Appears To Nearly Achieve Realize, Mankind's ForeSeen Ambition Of,
'Within Body, Targeted Tissue Destruction',
By Extra Corporeal Energy Source,
Using No Touch Technique
& No Collateral(Surrounding Tissue) Damage.

The Relevant Examples Include-

RADIOSURGERY

Comparative Clinical Appraisals Of Available Modalities, Can Be Summarized As-
High Energy External Beam Irradiation Use- Has Limitation For Focal Lesions In Radio-Senstive Organs,
Due To Sourrounding Tissue Affection.
BrachyTherapy(Internal Beam Irradiation) Use- Achieves Sharply Defined Tissue Ablation,
But Need Radio-Active Material Placement Within Target,
SteroTactic Technology Use- Has OverAll Enormous Contribution, To Achieve Highly Focussed Radiation Application EitherWise,
Recent Advent Includes **CyberKnife**-Frame Less Image Guided Radio-Surgical Device.[1]

MECHANICAL TISSUE LITHOTRIPSY

IntraCorporeal Approach Tissue Ablation
Forcing Of Water Through A Small Nozzle, Under High Pressure At 10-15 Kgm/Cm^2, Parenchymatous Tissue Can Be Ahieved, While Vessels>200µm Diametre Remain UnDamaged.
The Tissue Skeletonization Thus Achieved By Water Jet Facilitates Subsequent HaemoStasis By Electro-Cautery & Suturing & Is Being Utilized Clinically e.g Partial Hepatectomy & Nephrectomy.

By Using Probes Generated Transverse & Longitudinal Oscillations Of 200-300µm By UltraSound In 20-50kHz Range, Structures UpTo DiaMetre Of About 500µm Are Dissectable.
Combining Mechanical Tissue Fragmentation & Larger Vessels Thermal Sealing, By The Heat Generated During Tissue Fragmentation Process, Blood Free Dissection Of Even Heavily Vascularized Structures Rendered Standarized Surgical Equipment Status To
UltraSound Dissectors.
HowEver, Both Techniques Utilization Need Direct Tissue Contact & Hence Can Not Be Included Under ExtraCorporeal Approach. [2-10]

Essentials Of Litho-Tripsy

ExtraCorporeal Approach Tissue Ablation

The SuccessFul Applicability Of ExtraCorporeal Shock Wave LithoTripsy & Particularly Its Soft Tissue SideEffects Analysis,
Led To Innovation Of Shock Wave Energy Use For ExtraCorporeal Tissue Ablation.

The Relatively Weak Acoustic Shock Waves Used For LithoTripsy, Exert Both Positive & Negative Pressures Upto 100 & 10 Mpa, Respectively. Especially, The Latter Are Sufficient To Cause Cavitation From Liquid Failure At Numerous Sites Near The Focus.

With The Liquid Failure, Initially Developed Vapour Filled Cavities Collapse With Enormous Force.(11-14)

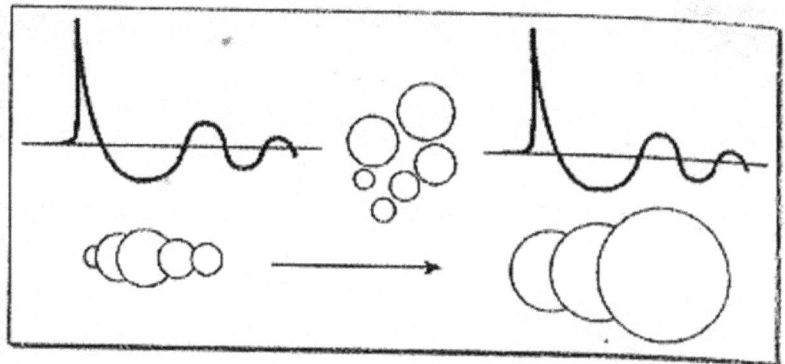

Figure-1: Profile -Extra-Corporeal Shock Wave Used For LithoTripsy: Negative Pressure Phase Resultant Cavitation Bubble Formation.
Source - MadersBacher S, Marberger M. Therapeutic Applications Of UltraSound In Urology.In Marberger M.edApplication OF Newer Form Of Energy In UroLogy.OxFord:ISIS,1995:115-136

Asymmetric High Speed Liquid Micro-Jets With Velocities Of 130-170m/sec Are Generated At Their Surface, That Are Considered To Be PriMary Mechanisms For Stone DisIntegration & Also For Trauma To Sourrounding Soft Tissue.

High Speed Of Bubble BreakDown, Results In Virtually No Temperature Rise Within The Focus. **Free Radical Formation**, May Also Occur Due To Homolytic Clevage & Has Been Speculated To Result In Additional Tumoricidal Effect.

A Number Of In Vitro And In Vivo Experimental Studies With The Electromagnetic And Electrohydraulic Shock-Wave Sources Used For Lithotripsy Have Documented Shock- Wave-Induced Cellular Damage In The Focal Area.. (15-16)

But The Microenvironments Of The Cells Treated Impact Significantly On The Shock-Wave Effect. If Tumor Cell In Suspension Are Treated, The Effect Is Significantly More Pronounced Than When The Same Type And Number Of Cells Are Immobilized In Gelatin. (17-18)

In Vivo Studies On More Complex In Vivo Models With Implanted Tumors Have Yet Failed To Define Structures Effects Of Shock Waves As Used In Lithotripsy Other Then Hemorrhage And Signs Of Mechanical Tissue Dissipation. (16,20)

Augmentation Of Tissue Cavitation Within The Focal Zone, By Increasing The Negative Pressure Of Shock Waves Or More Effectively By Increasing The Frequency Of Shock Waves To More Than 10 Exposures/Second(i.e >10 Hz). Figure-2

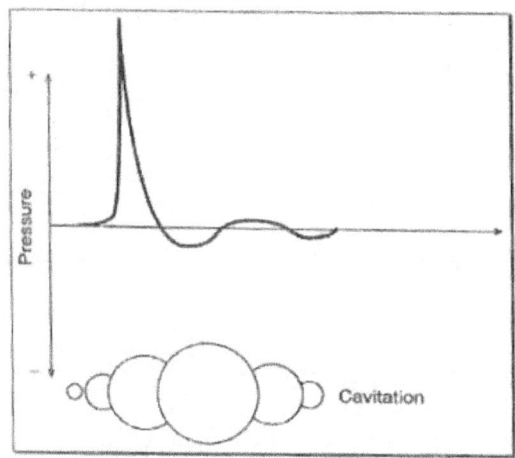

Figure-2: By Increasing The Negative Pressure Of Shock Wave & Shock Wave Generation Beyond 10 HA,
Augmentation Of Cavitation Process Within The Focal Zone, Results In Focal Zone Hitting Of Next Shock Wave, Before The Collapse Of Cavtation Bubble Formed By Previous Wave.
Source - MadersBacher S, Marberger M. Therapeutic Applications Of UltraSound In Urology.In Marberger M.edApplication OF Newer Form Of Energy In UroLogy.OxFord:ISIS,1995:115-136

By Using UltraSound Shock Waves Generated From Piezo-Ceramic Elements, Using Concave Disk, Focussed To A Joint Focus, Both High Intensities & Site Intensities Can Be Obtainedm Which Results In Immediate Cellular Disruption, Within The Focus. Figure-3.

Essentials Of Litho-Tripsy

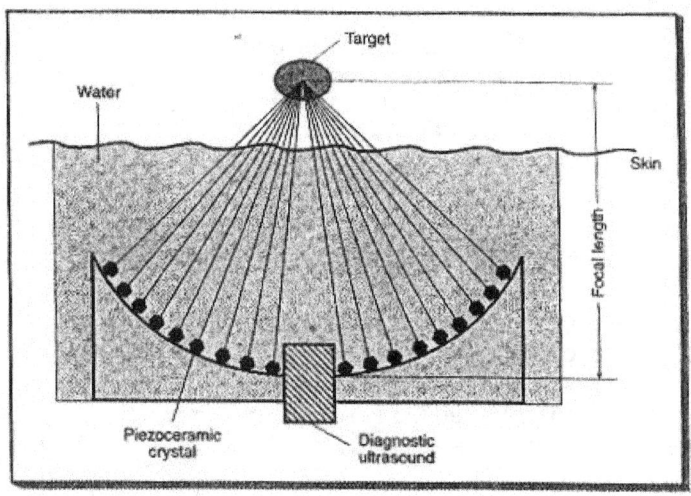

Figure-3: ExtraCorporeal High Energy Tissue LithoTripsy System Schematic Depiction

UltraSound Shock Waves Generated At High Frequency From Multiple PiezoCeramic Elements Focussed To A Giant Focus.
A Gas Free Water Filled Cushion Serves For Air Free Coupling Of Shock Waves To The Skin.

Source – VallanCien G, Chartier-Kastler E, Chopin D, Veillon B, Brisset JM, Andre-Bougran J. Focussed ExtraCorporeal PyroTherapy: Experimental Results. Eur Urol 1991; 20:21-219.

TheTechnique Has Been Defined As "High-Energy Shock Wave" Tissue Tripsy Or **"Pyrotherapy"** And Has Received Considerable Experimental And Phase II Clinical Attention. [21]

Although The Majority Of These Studies Yielded Encouraging Data, High-Energy Shock Wave Has Not Been Introduced Into Broader Clinical Use For Oncologic Indications To Data. This Is Mainly Attributable To Insufficient Tumor Targeting And The Fact That Cell Damage From High-Energy Shock Wave Is Mediated Primarily Via The Mechanical Effects Of Ultrasound (i.e., Tissue Cavitation), Which Is Difficult To Target, Control, And Predict. Reliable Destruction Of Deep Lying Tissues (A Prerequisite For Use In Oncologic Indications) Is Hard To Achive With Current High-Energy Shock Wave Devices.

THERMAL TISSUE ABLATION –
Protein Degradation Of Tissue Of Tissues Occur By Heating Above 47°C, Extent Of Tissue Damage Depending Upon Extent Of Heat Exposure & To A Lesser Degree, Upon Type Of Tissue & Its Structure.
Heating >60°c, Results In Instantaneous Protien Defradation Of All Biological Tissue, With Irreversible Coagulation Necrosis Of The Targeted Structures Occur.
Temperatures Beyond This Range Can Be Achieved By In Vivo, Using Extra-Corporeal High Intensity Focussed UltraSound.

High Intensity Foccused UltraSound(HIFU)
As An Ultrasound Wave Propagates Though Biologics Tissues, Or Any Medium That Is Not Ideally Viscoelastic, It Is Progressively Absorbed And The Energy Is Converted To Heat, If The Ultrasound Beam Is Brought To A Tight Focus At A Selected Depth Within The Body, The High Energy Density Produced In This Region Results In Temperatures Exceeding The Threshold Level Of Protein Denaturation. As A Consequence Coagulative Necrosis Occurs.

The Antineoplastic Effect Of High-Intensity Focused Ultrasound Has Been Clearly Demonstrated In Vivo In A Number Of Experimental Settings. (23)

These Data Demonstrate That High-Intensity Focused Ultrasound Applied Extracorporeally Is Capable Of Inducing Precise, Well-Controlled Contact- And Irradiation-Free In-Depth Tissue Destruction. Howener, It Needs To Be Emphasized That None Of These Experimental Studies Were 100% Successful.

Prostate Diseases-Gelet Et Al. Pioneered The Use Of Transrectal High-Intensity Focused Ultrasound For The Treatment Of **Localized Prostate Cancer**.

Testis Tumour-A Clinical Phase II Study In Patients With Tumors In The Solitary Testis In Whom The Contralateral Testis Had Been Removed For A Malignant Tumor Demonstrated The Possibility Of Cure With High-Intensity Focused Ultrasound And Postoperative Irradiation. (29)

Renal Tumors-Percutaneous Techniques Using Either Cryoablation Or Thermal Coagulation Are Widely Employed For This Today But The Need To Puncture The Tumor With The Potential Risk Of Hemorrhage And Tumor Spillage Raises Some Caveats. Transrectal High-Intensity Focused Ultrasound Systems Operating In The 4mhz Range Have Been Modified For Laparoscopic Use.

Essentials Of Litho-Tripsy

In A Curative Attempt In Vivo In A Patient With Three Tumors In A Solitary Kidney, Two Were Completely Ablated By Extracorporeal High-Intensity Focused Ultrasound, With A Follow-Up Of Six Months.

Storz™ System For Extra-Corporeal High Intensity Foccused UltraSound(HIFU)

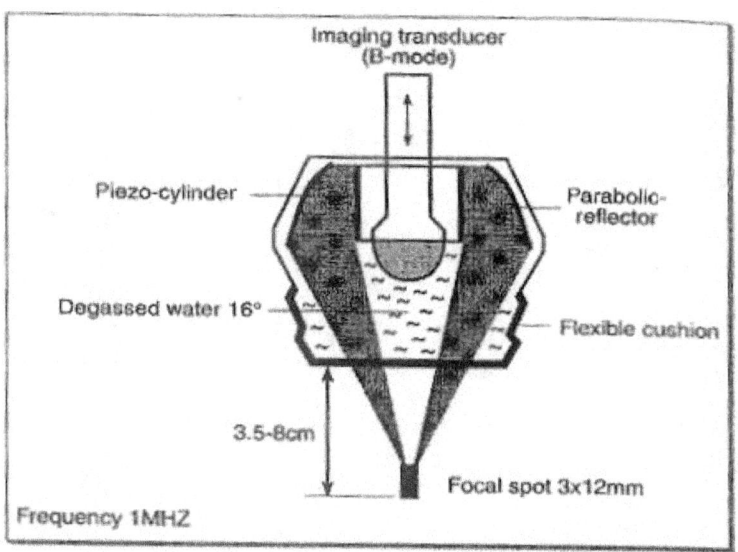

Figure-6: **Treatment Arm Of STORZ ™ For ExtraCorporeal High-Intensity Focussed UltraSound**

A Cylindrical TransDucer Generating UltraSound At $1MHz$ Focussed With An Acoustical Lens To A Focus 3x12mm In Situ;
Degassed Water Filled Flexible Cushion Permitting A Variable Focal Length Of 3.5 – 8 Cm & An Integrated B-Mode Transducer Providing Images Of The Target Zone.

Source – KohrMann KU, Michael MS, Steidler A, MarLingHaus E, Kraut O, Alken P. Technical Characterizations Of An Ultrasound Source For Non Invasive ThermoAblation By High Intensity Focussed UltraSound. BJU Int

Extra- Corporeal High Intensity Foccused UltraSound Tissue LithoTripsy Role In-
Prostatic Diseases (22)
Gelet et al. Pioneered The Use Of High Energy Focussed UltraSound System For The TreatMent Of Localized Prostate Cancer. 2002;90:248-252.

Testis Tumours
A Clinical Phase III Study, In Patients Of Tumours In Solitary Testis(ContraLateral Testis Removed For Malignancy), Demonstrated The Possibility Of Cure With HIFU & PostOperative Irradiation.
Renal Tumors
Widely Employed PerCutaneous Techniques

Reported Study, Curative Attempt In Vivo (24-32)

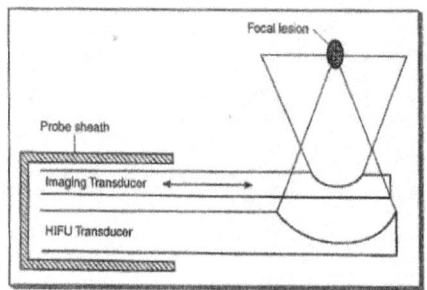 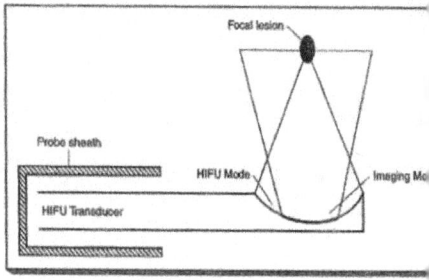

Figure-4:
Transrectal High Energy Focussed UltraSound System:
Separate Transducers For Imaging & Therapy Incorporated Into A 'Joint TransDucer Probe' Are For Intermittent Use.
(AbiaTherm ™ ,EDAP ,Paris, France)

Figure-5:
Trans Rectal HIFU System;
The Same Transducer Operating At 4.0 MHz Is Utilized For Imaging & Therapy.(SonoBlate ™, Focus Surgery, IndianaPolis, Indiana).

<u>Source</u> - MadersBacher S, Marberger M. Therapeutic Applications Of UltraSound In Urology.In Marberger M.edApplication OF Newer Form Of Energy In UroLogy.OxFord:ISIS,1995:115-136

<u>Chongqing HAIFU, Chongqing, China System</u>

In The Chongquing **"High-Intensity Focused Ultrasound" Extracorporeal Device**, Exchangeable Ellipsoidal Therapeutic Transducers Of 12 Or 15 Cm Diameter Are Mounted Around A Centaral 3.5 Mhz Diagnostic Transducer And Positioned Aithin A Basin Filled With Degassed Water Under The Patient Table.
Depending On The Transducer Used, Frequencies Of 0.8, 1.2, And 1.6 Mhz, And Focal Length Of 100 , 130, 135, 150 And 160 Mm Are Available.
In Vivo Focal Region For The 1.6 Mhz Transducers.

In Situ Intensities Are Estimated As Ranging Between 5.000-20.000W/Cm2 (83). Ablation Can Be Achived By Placing Individual Lesions Side By Side As With All Other Systems,
But The Device Also Has The Capacity To Achieve **More Rapid Ablation Through "Painting Out" The Target Area In Sequential Linear Tracks**. Smooth, Three-Dimensional Movement Of The Activated Transducer Enables This Process. And By Exposing The Same Target Are 2-6 Times, The Value Of Ablated Tissue Increase In A Linear Fashion (Fig.7) (35)
At These Energy Levels **Cavitations Processes** Are Clearly Also Involved, But Detailed Experimental And Clinical Studies Provided No Evidence For Tumor Cell Dissemination.

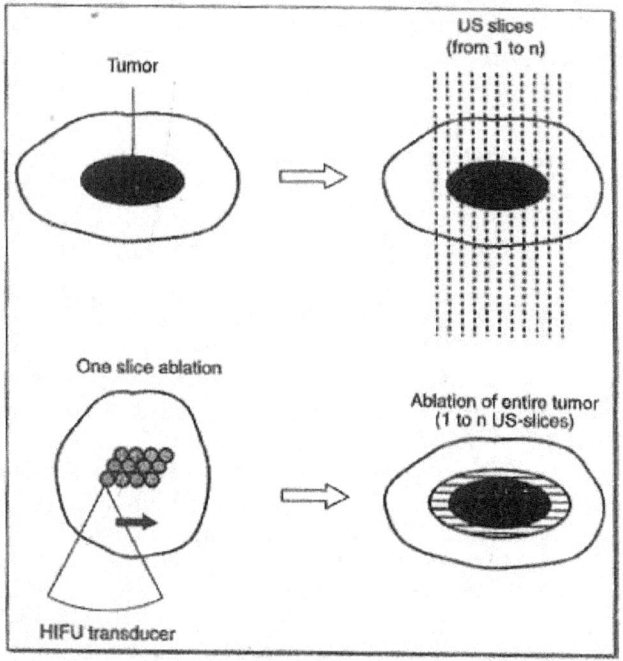

Figure-7: Chongqing HAIFU System:Involved TreatMent Principle Schematic Depiction
The Target Is Dissolved Into Multiple Two Dimensional UltraSound Slices At 5-10 mm Internal, Which In Sum Establish A Three-Dimensional Target Image.With Directional Movement Of Transducer, Each Slice Is Treated & The Effect Monitored By Immediate Reimaging Thereafter.**Source** – Wu F, Chen WZ, Bai J.et al. Pathological Changes In Human Malignant Carcinoma Treated With High Intensity Focussed UltraSound. UltraSound Med Biol 2001;27:1096-1106.

Because Of The **High In Situ Intensites Used**, Treated Tissue Become Hyperechoic On Ultrasonography And This Effect Is Used For On –Line Targeting And Feedback.

Wu Et Al. Have Employed The System For The Treatment Of Patients With **Malignant Tumors, Mainly Of The Liver, Breast, And Soft Tissue**. In Spit Of Large-Volume Ablations And Reportedly Good Tumor Control, Side Effect Were Low, And Mainly Consisted Of Fever In Up To 20% And Skin Burn In 5% Of The Patient.

The Authors Also Mention Treating Patients With Renal Tumor, And In A More Recent Report They Give Details Of A Subgroup Of Patients With Tumors 2-25 Cm In Diameter.

Patients Were Treated **In Anesthesia With A 0.8 Mhz Transducer With A Focal Length Of 135 Mm, At A Median Treatment Time Of 5.4 Hours And Median 1.3 Session Per Patient,** The Tumors Were Completely Ablated In Three Patients And Between 40% And 70 % In The Rest.

A Similar System Was Installed At The Churchill Hospital, Oxford, United Kingdom In May 2002 And Has Been In Use In Phase II Clinical Trials Since November 2002. Sixteen Patients Have Treated In Phase II Clinical Trials, Four With Renal Tumors, And The Remaining 12 With Liver Tumors

All Patients Have Been Treated **Under General Anesthesia, And Respiratory Movement Is Minimized By Selective Intubation**, With Ventilation Of Only The Contralateral Lung.

During Ultrasound Exposures. Acoutics Power Of 180-300 W Have Been Used, And The Most Common Exposure Regime Has Been The Placement Of Single Lesion Adjacent To One Another (With An Overlap Of Half The Transverse Diameter Of The Focus). Maximum Transverse Diameters Of The Target Renal Tumor Have Ranged From 2.5-5.4 Cm, And According To The Trial Protocol, Only A Proportion Of Each Renal Tumor Was Exposed To High-Intensity Focused Ultrasound. Estimated Treated Volumes Range From 4.0-8.0 Cm^3. No Skin Burns Were Seen Despite The High Exposure Powers, And The Most Significant Adverse Event Reported Has Been A Transient Bruising Sensation. Magnetic Resonance And Color Doppler Imaging After Two Weeks Provided An Early Indication Of The Treatment Outcome, And Following An Interval Of Approximately Six Weeks Post-High-Intensity Focused Ultrasound, Three Of The Four Patients With Renal Tumors Progressed To Surgery.(33)

At The Time Of High-Intensity Focused Ultrasound Treatment,
The Hyperechic Change On Ultrasonography , Which Are Characteristic Of Successful Ablation, Were Not Seen In Any Of The Treatment Despite The Very High Acoustic Powers Used. A Small Region Of Reduced Contrast Uptake On Magnetic Resonance Imaging In One Patient, And Reduced Perfusion Color Doppler Sonography In Another Patient Indicated A Possible Volume Of Ablation.

Unfortunately, these regions could not be identified confidently on histological examination, and other than some adherent Gerota's fascia and fat necrosis in the perinephric fat, no conclusive evidence of successful ablation has been found in the other three excised renal tumors. However, the sample size is too small to draw meaningful conclusions and result have been considerably more encouraging in the treated liver tumors. Treatment parameters will be adjusted as the trial progresses, and if consistent ablation continues to prove difficult, the combination approach of embolozation plus high-intensity focused ultrasound as employed in China (34) will be explored.

The process of developing a thermal lesion by high-intensity focused ultrasound in vivo, over sound propagation and absorption to heat generation, conduction and adequate temperature distribution, is subject to a multitude of variables. These are especially difficult to control with high-intensity focused ultrasound of renal tumors.

Source- Extra Corporeal Tissue LithoTripsy In UroLogy
M.Marberger & Y.K.Fong DepartMent Of Urolgy, University Of Vienna, Austria.

REFRENCES

1. Ponsky LE, Crownover RL, Rosen MJ, Et Al. Initial Evaluation Of Cyberknife Technology For Extracorporeal Renal Tissue Ablation. Urology 2003; 61:498-501.
2. Krawitt DR, Addonizio JC. Ultrasonic Aspiration Of Prostate And Bladder Tumors And Stones. Urology 1987; 30:579-742.
3. Papchristou DN, Bartens R. Resection Of The Liver With A Water Jet. Br J Surg 1982; 69:93-94.
4. Higashihara E. Mechanical Energy In Urology For Non-Lithiasis Treatment. In: Marberger M, Ed. Application Of Newer Forms Of Therapeutic Energy In Urology. Oxford: Isis Medical, 1995:1-13.
5. Basting RF, Djakovic N, Widmann P. Use Of Water Jet Resection In Organ-Sparing Kidney Surgery. J Endourol 2000; 14:501-505.
6. Chopp RT, Shah BB, Adonizio JC. Use Of Ultrasonic Surgical Aspirator In Renal Surgery. Urology 1983; 22:157-159.
7. Hodgson WJ, Del Guercio LRM. Preliminary Experience In Liver Surgery Using The Ultrasonic Scalpel. Surgery 1984; 2;230-234.
8. Gill BS, Macfadyen BV Jr. Ultrasonic Dissectors And Minimally Invasive Surgery. Semin Laparosc Surg 1999; 6:229-234.
9. Schmidbauer S, Hallfeldt KK, Sitzmann G, Kantelhardt T, Trupka A. Experience With Ultrasound Scissors And Blades (Ultracision) In Open And Laparoscopic Liver Resection. Ann Surg 2002; 235:27-30.
10. Lingeman JE, Mc Atreer JA, Kempson SA, Et Al. Bioeffects Of Extracorporeal Shock-Wave Lithotripsy. Urol Clin North Am 1988; 15:507-504.
11. Coleman AJ, Saunders JE. A Survey Of The Acoustic Output Of Commercial Extracorporeal Shock-Wave Lithotripsy. Ultrasound Med Biol 1989; 15:213-227.
12. Madersbacher S, Marberge M. Therapeutic Application Of Ultrasound In Urology. In : Marberger M, Ed. Application Of Newer Forms Of Therapeutic Energy In Urology. Oxford:ISIS, 1995:115-136.
13. Crum LA. Cavitations Microjets As A Contributory Mechanisms For Renal Calculi Disintegration In Shock-Wave . J Urol 1988;140:1587-1590
14. Suhr D, Bruemmer F, Huelser DF. Cavitations Generated Free Radicals During Shock-Wave Exposure: Investigators With Cell-Free Solutions And Suspended Cells. Ultrasound Med Biol 1991;17:761-768.
15. Morgan TR, Laudone VP, Heston WDW, Et Al. Free Radical Production By High Energy Shock Wave-Comparison With Ionizing Irradiation. J Urol 1988;139:186-189
16. Randazzo RF, Chaussy CG, Fuchs GJ, Et Al. The In Vitro And In Vivo Effects Of Extracorporeal Shock-Wave On Malignant Cells. Urol Res 1988;16:413-426.
17. Kohri K, Vemura T, Iguchi M, Et Al. Effect Of High Energy Shock-Waves On Tumors Cells. Urol Res 1990;18:101-105.
18. Gambihler S, Delius M, Brendel W. Biological Effect Of Shock Waves: Cell Disruption, Vitality And Proliferation Of LI210 Cells Exposed To Shock Waves In Vitro. Ultrasound Med Boil 1990;16:587-594.
19. Woerle K, Steinbach P, Hofstadter F. The Combined Effects Of High-Energy Shock Waves And Cytostatic Drugs Or Cytokines On Human Bladder Cancer Cells. Br J Cancer 1994;69:58-65.
20. Hoshi S, Orikasa S, Kuwahara M, Et Al. High Energy Underwater Shock Wave Treatment On Implanted Urinary Bladder Cancer In Rabbits. J Urol 1991;146:439-443.
21. Vallancien G, Chartier-Kastler E, Chopin D, Veillon B, Brisset JM, Andre-Bougaran J. Focused Extra-Corporeal Phyrotherapy: Experimental Results. Eur Urol 1991;20:211-219.

22. Gelet A, Chapelon JY, Effects Of High- Intensity Focused Ultrasound On Malignant Cell And Tissues. In : Marberger M Ed. Application Of Newer Forms Of Therapeutic Energy In Urology. Oxford: ISIS, 1995:107-114.
23. Lacoste F, Schlosser J, Vallancien G. The Benefit Of Electronic Scanning In Extracorporeal HIFU. In:Andrew MA, Crum LA, Vaezy S, Eds. Proceedings, 2nd International Symposium On Therapeutic Ultrasound. Seattle: University Of Washington, 2003: 314-322.
24. Kratzik C, Schatzl G, Lackner J, Marberger M. Transculataneous High-Intensity Focused Ultrasound Can Cure Testicular Cancer, Urology 2006; 67:1279-1273
25. Thuroff S, Chaussy C Vallancien G, At Al. High-Intensity Focused Ultrasound And Localized Prostate Cancer. Efficacy Result From The European Multicentric Study. J Endourol 2003; 17:673-677.
26. Kramer G, Steiner GE, Grobl M, Et Al. Response To Sublethal Heat Treatment Of Prostatic Tumor Cells And Of Prostatic Tumor Infiltrating T Cell, Prostate 2004; 58:109-120.
27. Huber PE, Pfistere R. In Vitro And In Vivo Transfiction Of Plasmid DNA In The Dunning Prostate Tumor R3327-ATI Is Enhanced By Focused Ultrasound. Gene Ther 2000:7: 1516-1526.
28. Heidenreich A, Weissbach L, Hotl W, Et Al. Organ Sparing Surgery For Malignant Germ Cell Tumors. Jurol 2001; 166:2161-2165.
29. Madersbacher S, Kratizk C, Susani M, Pedevilla M, Marberger M. Transcutaneous High-Intensity Focused Ultrasound And Irradiation: An Organ-Preserving Treatment Of Cancer In A Solitary Testis. Eur Urol 1998; 33:195-201.
30. Paterson RF, Barret E, Siqueria TM, Et Al. Laparoscopic Partial Kidney Ablation With High Intensity Focused Ultrasound. J Urol 2003; 169:347-351.
31. Adams JB, Moore RG, Anderson JA, Et Al. High Intensity Focused Ultrasound Ablation Of Rabbit Kidney Tumors. J Endourol 1996; 10:71-75.
32. Watkin NA, Morris SB, Rivens H, Ter Harr GR, High Intensity Focused Ultrasound Ablation Of The Kidney In A Large Animal Model. J Endourol 1997; 11:191-196.
33. Kohrmann KU, Michel MS, Steidler A, Marlinghaus E, Kraut O, Aklen P. Technical Characterizations Of An Ultrasound Source For Noninvasive Thermoablation By High-Intensity Focused Ultrasound. BJU Int 2002; 167:2397-2403.
34. Wu F, Chen WZ, Bai J, Et Al. Pathological Change In Human Malignant Carcinoma Treated With High-Intensity Focused Ultrasound. Ultrasound Med Biol 2001; 27:1096-1106.
35. Smith NB, Buchanan MT, Hynynen K. Transrectal Ultrasound Applicator For Prostate Heating Monitored Using MRI Thermometry. Int J Radiat Oncol Biol Phys 1999; 43:217-225

CHAPTER(5.)
(i.)DISCUSSION

With Gradual Successful Availability Of Recent Noninvasive, Minimally Invasive, And Endoscopic Techniques, Classical Open Surgical Removal Of Calculi (OSS): Pyelolithotomy, Nephrolithotomy, Ureterolithotomy, Cystolithotomy, Urethral Stone Extraction Etc.Are Considered Of Decreasing Interest.

ESWL Has Emerged As A Convenient, Practically Safe,Noninvasive OPD Procedure, With Comparative Result Outcomes,
In The Absence/Exclusion Of Nonsupportive Anatomical Parameters, And Associated With Anatomico-Functional Urinary Tract Abnormalities, Such As Outflow Obstruction e.g PUJ Obstruction, Promoting Future Stone Formation By Stasis, The Indications For Surgical Exploration Of Stone, And Simultaneous Correction Of Defect
And/Or Associated Management.

Advantages (Lithotripsy):
(1) Noninvasive,
(2) Usually Done As OPD Procedure,
(3) Patient Resumes Routine Work Within 24 Hrs. And Is Stone Free Within 1-To-2-Month Time,
(4) Avoiding Hazards Of Anesthesia And Surgical Procedures In Patients Not Willing For And/Or Unfit For Such Extensive Procedures.

KEY POINTS FOR BETTER RESULT OUTCOMES

The Discussed Scientific Presentation Study Includes About More Than 500 Patients With Renal And Ureteric Calculi ,
That Were Completely Removed By
ESWL, With An Average Of About Two Sittings And Complete One Sitting Clearance, In Several Cases.
DJS Insertion Was Done In < 10% Cases, Especially In Large Stones >4 Cm, And In Cases Of Repeated Resistant
Urine C And S,Associated Obstructive Lesions Delineation By Radiodiagnosis And Various Scans Indicating
Decreased Renal Function Status Etc.
Proper Forced Diuresis Compliance Was Encouraged And Used In About 15–20% Cases; Improved Results Outcome Was Achieved By Reducing Number Of Sittings In Large Kidney And Ureteric Stones, While Improved Overall Treatment Efficacy
In LPS, Inf. Calyceal, Lower Ureteric, Especially VUJ Stones, Residual Stone Fragments And Also As An Adjunct To Medical Therapy, Achieved In Selected Cases.

Essentials Of Litho-Tripsy

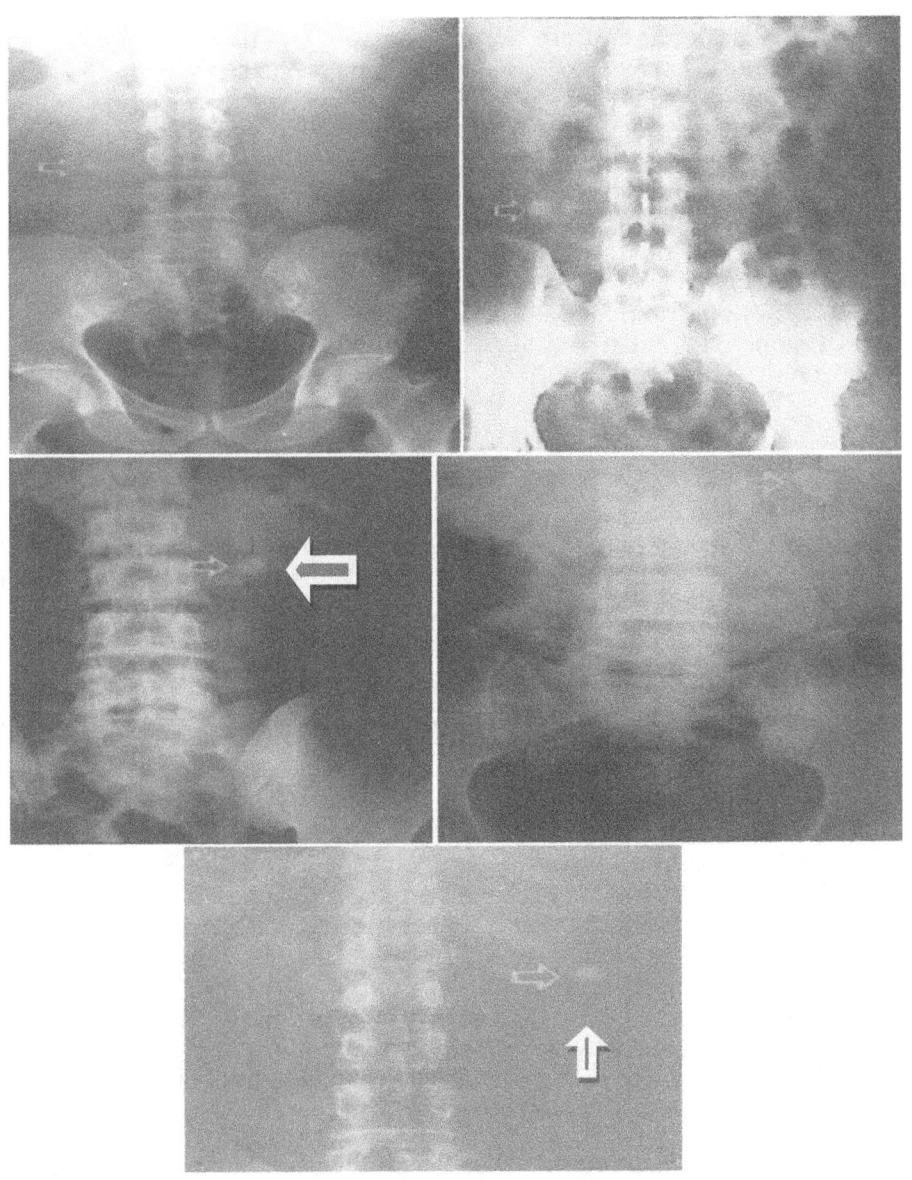

Kidney And Ureteric Stones Of Different Sizes, Locations, Completely Removed

Prophylactic Medical Therapy, In About 10–15% Cases Was Administered, With Crystalluria As Important Therapeutic Parameter.

Special Emphatic Care Compliance, In Regards To Supportive Measures, Especially Gravitational Support Etc In LPS,
 Inf.Calyx, Lower Ureteric, VUJ Stones And
Appropriate Shock Delivery Upon Discretely Contrast Delineated Gall Stone Disease, Choledocholithiasis.

Carefully Conducted Lithotripsy Sittings, With Intensive Radiological Screening For Complete Stone Removal, Supported By Sterile Urine For Urinary Asepsis, Evidence And Diet Regulation In Accordance With Stone Analysis, Stone Composition And Metabolic Evaluators (Indices) Management Formed The Crucial Guidelines To Achieve About >95% Success Rate.

HowEver, The Availble Reports Of Different Studies Regarding **Outcome And Prognosis**, Include-

In **Appropriately Selected Patients**, The Overall Success Rate Of **ESWL** Is >90% For **Stone Clearance**, With Patients Remaining Stone-Free For Up To 2 Years. Compared With **Ureteroscopic Removal** Of Stones, ESWL Leads To Less Complications And Shorter Hospital Stays. (1)

ESWL Is **Safe And Effective**. Small Series Have Shown Successful Treatment Of Stones In **Young Children**, With An Acceptable Short-Term Safety Profile. (2) However, Long-Term Follow-Up Of The **Potential Complications**, Including Hypertension And Decreased Renal Function, Are Not Yet Mature.

As **Stone Burden** Increases And Exceeds 2 Cm, The Stone-Free Rate Drops Significantly. With Stones Sized 2-3 Cm, The Stone-Free Rates With **ESWL Monotherapy** Is Typically 50%, While With Larger Stones (Complete And Incomplete Staghorn Calculi) Are Correspondingly Lower. The **Stone Location** Also Affects The Efficacy Of ESWL. (3)
Studies Suggested That Patients With **Appropriate Renal Collecting System Anatomy, Lower-Pole Stone Location**, Approximately 50% Overall Stone-Free Rate Variations Of 85% In Patients With **Favorable Anatomy** Versus 7% In Those With **Unfavorable Anatomy**.

An Inverse Relationship Was Found Between Stone Size And Stone-Free Rate. In Patients With Stones Or Stone Aggregates Measuring Larger Than 1 Cm, Percutaneous Nephrolithotomy Was The Most Efficacious Modality To Render Patients Stone-Free.

Sheir Et Al (2003) Evaluated The Safety And Efficacy Of ESWL In Patients With An **Anomalous Kidney**, Including 49 Patients With A Horseshoe Kidney, 120 Patients With A Malrotated Kidney,
And 29 Patients With A Duplex Kidney. (4)

Essentials Of Litho-Tripsy

Two Second-Generation Lithotriptors Were Used. Although The Type Of Renal Anomaly And The Type Of Lithotriptor Did Not Affect The Stone-Free Rate, Stone Length And Number (Stone Burden) Significantly Influenced The Stone-Free Rate. The Prone Position Facilitated Treatment In 38% Of The Patients With A Horseshoe Kidney And In 31% Of Patients With A Duplex Kidney. The Overall Retreatment Success Rate Was 64.1%. However, With An Overall Stone-Free Rate Of 72.2%, Sheir Et Al Deemed ESWL To Be Safe And Reliable In Patients With An Anomalous Kidney And To Be Considered The Primary Treatment Option For Stones Smaller Than 20 Mm.

Early-Generation Lithotriptors Required Pushback Of Stones Into The Renal Pelvis For Treatment. With Advancements, Specifically Higher-Amplitude Waveforms With Smaller Focal Zones, Newer Lithotriptors Are Able To Treat Ureteral Stones In Situ. Results Tend To Be Better For Proximal Stones, With Stone-Free Rates Of 65-81%, Versus 58-67% For Distal Ureteral Stones.

ESWL:Future & Controversies

Technical Improvements, Such As **Bidirectional Synchronous Twin-Pulse Technique** With Variable Angles Between The Shockwave Reflectors, Have Been Attempted To Increase The Quality And Rate Of Stone Disintegration.
With This Technique, Shock Waves Are Produced Simultaneously From Separate Reflectors Through Nonopposing Directions To The Same F2 And Appear To Be Particularly Effective With Right Angle Orientation Between The Two.
The Effect Demonstrated In Vitro And Then Demonstrated By **Sheir In A Study Of 50 Patients** With Renal Or Ureteral Stones (Mean Size, 12.3 Mm; Range, 9-18 Mm). Using This Technique, 17 Patients (34%) Were Rendered Stone-Free, 20 Patients (40%) Had Less Than 5 Mm Of Residual Stone, And 13 Patients (26%) Had 6-9 Mm Of Residual Stone At 14 Day Follow-Up. Thirteen Patients (26%) With More Than 5 Mm Of Residual Stone Underwent Repeat ESWL.(5)

The Same Authors Followed This Initial Clinical Study With One That Randomized Patients To **The Twin-Pulse Technique Versus Standard ESWL**. The Study Group Included 240 Patients With Single Radio-Opaque Stones Less Than 2.5 Cm. Stone Disintegration Rates Were Significantly Greater In The Twin-Pulse Group While Stone Free Rates Were High In Both Groups But Not Significantly Different For Stones Less Than 10 Mm (67% And 74%; Standard And Twin-Pulse, Respectively). (6)

An Additional Purpose Of This Study Was To Compare **Collateral Parenchymal Damage** Caused By Each Technique. **N-Acetyl-B-Glucosaminidase (NAG)**, A High-Molecular Weight Enzyme

Not typically filtered by the glomerulus, was measured post-ESWL. The degree to which this enzyme is lost in the urine immediately after ESWL is thought to be reflective of the severity of tubular damage. Both groups in this study had elevated post-ESWL NAG levels, but the levels normalized in the twin-pulse group after 2 days and remained elevated up to 7 days in the control group.

Patients also underwent dynamic MRI post-ESWL to assess changes in renal perfusion. Decreased renal perfusion was demonstrated in the standard ESWL group (control), but not in the twin-pulse group.

The studies concluded that bidirectional synchronous twin-pulse lithotripsy has superior efficacy to standard lithotripsy while possibly decreasing damage to surrounding parenchyma.

Other groups have attempted to improve **the fragmenting capability of the cavitation bubbles created during lithotripsy** by forcing their collapse with a second weaker pulse timed immediately after the initial pulse. Using a porcine model with Begostone phantoms, Young et al (2003) used a 22-Kv shock from an HM3 followed with a 4-Kv shockwave 500-600 ms later from a separate piezoelectric source. Their initial results showed increased stone comminution rates with reduced renal injury.

The **Smaller Focal Zone** and newer lithotripter tabletop designs have increased the indications for treatment and lowered the anesthetic requirements, but some have demonstrated decreased overall efficacy of the treatment. Many newer generators require precise localization, with little margin for error in light of the greatly reduced focal zones. Future studies are necessary to define the preferable anesthetic regimen, localization technique, and shock-wave delivery sequence to optimize outcomes.

A prospective study comparing the **Clinical Effectiveness of the HM3 to the newer MODULITH SLX-F2 Lithotripter** found that the HM3 showed higher stone-free rates for solitary ureteral stones and multiple stones at 3-month follow-up. The HM3 also required fewer shock waves and led to fewer kidney hematomas. (7)

Certainly ESWL has a role in the armamentarium against urolithiasis. Recent trends however, show that its popularity is yielding to endoscopic management of stones. Perhaps this decline can be attributed not to any shortcomings of ESWL, but rather to the rapid improvement of endoscopic instruments used in minimally invasive approaches. (8,9)

Essentials Of Litho-Tripsy

REFERENCES

1. Aboumarzouk OM, Kata SG, Keeley FX, Nabi G. Extracorporeal shock wave lithotripsy (ESWL) versus ureteroscopic management for ureteric calculi. *Cochrane Database Syst Rev*. Dec 7 2011;12:CD006029.[Medline].
2. Fayad A, El-Sheikh MG, El-Fayoumy H, El-Sergany R, Abd El Bary A. Effect of extracorporeal shock wave lithotripsy on kidney growth in children. *J Urol*. Sep 2012;188(3):928-31. [Medline].
3. Lingeman JE, Zafar FS. Lithotripsy systems. In: Smith AD, Badlani GH, Bagley DH, et al. *Smith's Textbook of Endourology*. St Louis, Mo: Quality Medical Publishing; 1996:553-89.
4. Sheir KZ, Madbouly K, Elsobky E, Abdelkhalek M. Extracorporeal shock wave lithotripsy in anomalous kidneys: 11-year experience with two second-generation lithotripters. *Urology*. Jul 2003;62(1):10-5; discussion 15-6. [Medline].
5. Sheir KZ, El-Diasty TA, Ismail AM. Evaluation of a synchronous twin-pulse technique for shock wave lithotripsy: the first prospective clinical study. *BJU Int*. Feb 2005;95(3):389-93. [Medline].
6. Sheir KZ, Elhalwagy SM, Abo-Elghar ME, Ismail AM, Elsawy E, El-Diasty TA. Evaluation of a synchronous twin-pulse technique for shock wave lithotripsy: a prospective randomized study of effectiveness and safety in comparison to standard single-pulse technique. *BJU Int*. Jun 2008;101(11):1420-6. [Medline].
7. Zehnder P, Roth B, Birkhäuser F, Schneider S, Schmutz R, Thalmann GN, et al. A Prospective Randomised Trial Comparing the Modified HM3 with the MODULITH(®) SLX-F2 Lithotripter. *Eur Urol*. Apr 2011;59(4):637-44. [Medline].
8. Miernik A1, Wilhelm K, Ardelt P, Bulla S, Schoenthaler M. Modern urinary stone therapy: is the era of extracorporeal shock wave lithotripsy at an end?. *Urologe A*. Mar 2012;51:372-378. [Medline].
9. García-Galisteo E1, Sánchez-Martínez, Molina-Díaz, López-Rueda, Baena-González. Invasive treatment trends in urinary calculi in a third level hospital. *Actas Urol Esp*. Jul 2014;[Medline].

Source-Extracorporeal Shockwave Lithotripsy Treatment & Management
Author: Michael Grasso III, MD; Chief Editor: Bradley Fields Schwartz, DO, FACS

(ii.)CONCLUSIONS

Being A Well-Established Routine Urological Technique,
Great Majority Of Urolithiasis Patients Can Be Best Managed By ESWL.

However, As With Any Other Type Of Therapy Some Contraindications
And Potential Complications Existence, Needs To Be SafeGuarded
By Proper Precautions & Preventive Measures.

The Discussed Scientific Study Presentation Conclusion,
That For All Practical Purposes,Renal And Ureteric Calculi Can Be
Treated With ESWL, With Almost Cent Percent (Complete) Success
Up To A Solitary Stone Size/Stone Burden Of About 4 – 5 Cms,
With Varying Retreatment And Ancillary Procedures Support,
ReAffirms The Rapid Worldwide Acceptance Of ESWL.

However, Recent Availabilities Of Successful Minimally
Invasive Endourology And Laparoscopic Procedures Are
Debatefully Comparable With Regards To Individual Choice,
Availability Compliance, And Comparative Result Outcome
Variations.[46,47]

The Basic Fundamentals Of **Successful Extraction Of Complete Stone**,
Leaving No **'Nidus'** For Future Stone Formation, With Supportive
Scientific Life Style Diet Regulations Advise, In Accordance
With/Without **Stone Analysis**, **Geographical Considerations** &
Management Of The **Altered Biochemical Indices**, Associated Medical
Problems, Etc., Need Cautious SecureMent,
Irrespective Of Stone Removal Techniques, For
Complete Comprehensive Management Of "Stone Disease".

Scope Of Role For Other Applications-
For **Biliary Diseases & Others**, Along With UpDates Of Gradual
Availabiility Of Comparative Sophisticated Appliances **For
IntraCorporeal Utilizations & Extra-Corporeal Tissue Lithotripsy**,
Have Been Compiled Under Various Chapters,
In Accordance To Scope Of The Present Text.

46. Lehtoranta K, Mankinen P, Taari K, Rannikko S, Lehtonen T, Salo J. Residual stones, after percutaneous nephrolithotomy; sensitivities of different imaging methods in renal stone detection. Ann Chir Gynaecol 1995;84:43-9.

47. Carr LK, D'A Honey J, Jewett MA, Ibanez D, Ryan M, Bombardier C.New stone formation: A comparison of extracorporeal shock wave lithotripsy and percutaneous nephrolithotmy. J Urol 1996;155:1565-7.

ACKNOWLEDGEMENTS

With Gratitudes & Humble Special Thanks To-

- Consulted 'Study Materials'- Books, Literature-
  Print & OnLine Available Resources, With Requested
  Permission AvailAbility, For Compiling The Present Text.

- Senior & Junior Colleagues, ParaMedical,Technical Staff
  Involved For Performing Significantly Large No. Of Complete
  LithoTripsy Sitting Procedures Personally By The Author.

- **The Association Of Surgeons Of India,**
  Urological Society Of India,
  For Selecting The Present Text,
  Amongst Several Papers On "Lithotripsy", By
  'The Scientific Paper Computer Code For
  'Sectional Scientific Session: Urology',
  "New Technology In The Urological Field",
  "The Association Of Genito-Urinary Surgeons Of India",
  ASICON'2002, Science City, Kolkatta, India.&
  Is The First Paper On ESWL (Lithotripsy) Presented,
  At National Level.

- **Scientific Presentations- 'FacultyLectureSeries',**
  MuzaffarNagar Medical College & Hospital,Muzaffarnagar(UP),
  M.A. Medical College, Agroha (Hisar), India.
  Academic Year:2007-08-09,
& Various Other Programmes, Before & AfterWards.
Widely Appreciated For, Comprehensive Summary Including
Various Aspects,Of The Topic, Satisfying 'CME', 'CPD', 'LLL'
Norms Of Medical Education.

- **International Journal of Scientific and Engineering**
  Research (IJSER) (ISSN 2229-5518)
  Paper Number: I019112,
  Paper Title: "Extracorporeal Shock Wave Lithotripsy (ESWL),
  And Its Role In Urolithiasis, With Emphasis On Lower Pole,
  Inferior Calyx Kidney Stones, Lower Ureteric, VUJ Stones,
  And Gall Stone Diseases".
  Paper published in IJSER Volume 3, Issue 11,
  November 2012

  & All Others.

"ABOUT THE AUTHOR"

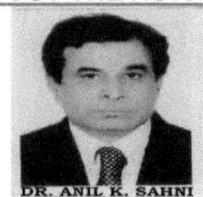

PROF.DR. ANIL K. SAHNI   Address: A-1/F-1 Block-A Dilshad Garden
B.Sc, M.B.B.S, M.S, F.I.C.S, Advanced D.H.A   Delhi-110095 India.
SURGEON, UROLOGIST, ENDOSCOPIST, LITHOTRIPSY SPECIALIST.
LIFE MEMBER :   Mobile : 09873083100
AUSTRIAN MEDICAL SOCIETY   E-mail : dranil_sahni@yahoo.co.in
THE ASSOCIATION OF SURGEONS OF INDIA   dranil_sahni@hotmail.com
DELHI UROLOGICAL SOCIETY   dranilksahni@gmail.com
ASSOCIATION OF MINIMAL ACCESS SURGEONS OF INDIA
INDIAN ASSOCIATION OF GASTRO-INTESTINAL ENDOSURGEONS
MEDICAL COUNCIL OF INDIA REG.No.: 3599(06.01.2005) / 27417(30.05.1983)U.P.
DATE OF BIRTH : **02-06-1958**
"QUALIFICATIONS": **PASSED ALL EXAMS IN FIRST ATTEMPT WITH POSITION.**
B.Sc :1977, Rohilkhand University, Bareilly. Merit Position, National Scholarship
M.B.B.S :1983, G.S.V.M. Medical College, Kanpur.
M.S : 1986, G.S.V.M. Medical College, Kanpur.
F.I.C.S :1995-96, International College of Surgeons, Chicago, Illinois, USA.
ADHA (Advanced Diploma Hospital Administration) : 2006, Institute of Health Care Administration,Chennai.
"EXTRA-CURRICULUM":First Aid Certificate,1968, NSS & NCC Certification,1975-77, Joint Treasurer, Physiology Society,1978: Executive Member, Socio-Cultural Society, G.S.V.M. Medical College,
Kanpur, 1982 Etc., Sports, Music, Print - Live Media & Others.
"EXPERIENCES"   (A)TEACHING EXPERIENCE:
DEMO./TUTOR/REG./RSO/SR:-GSVM Med.Coll.Kanpur (31.05.83 To 31.08.86);
            3 Yrs & 3 Months
              -MCKR Hosp.& Ayur.Res.Inst.Delhi:(10.11.87 To 30.06.89);
            1 Year & 8 Months
              -Yashoda Hospital,Ghaziabad..: (1.1.1993 To 1.12.1994);
            2 Years
ASSISTANT PROFESSOR (SURGERY) :- SantoshMed.Coll.Ghaziabad:
             (06.04.98 To 26.03.2001);2Yrs&11Months
             - SRMS IMS,Bareilly:(1.07.2004 To17.05.2006);
             1Yr & 11 Months
             - M.M.C.H., Muzaffarnagar: (18.05.06 To 31.08.07);
             1Yr & 4 Months
             - M.A.M.C., Agroha (Hisar): (1.09.07 To 31.06.08);
             10 Months
ADDITIONAL :Urology,Lithotripsy,Non-Invasive/Minimal Invasive Surgery, Endoscopy,
       Surgical Teaching, BPT(Physio-Therapy) Courses, G.J Univ.Hisar.
ASSOCIATE PROFESSOR (SURGERY):-M.A.M.C.,Agroha(Hisar):
             (1.07.08 To 15.03.09);9Months
             -VCSG Govt.Med.Sciences & Res.Inst.
             Sri-Nagar,Pauri-Garhwal: 15/16.03.2009 - Till Date.
             HOD (Surgery),Offi.Med.Suptd.
             Co-ChairMan'CME','CPD'...,
             I/C Med.Edu.Unit
PROFESSOR: Forwarded & Recommended Thrice, Confirmed (MCI)
w.e.f 01/07/2011, Complete Experience & Publications Including Books.

Essentials Of Litho-Tripsy

(B) ASSOCIATED ASSIGNMENTS(TRAINING):Esteemed Tertiary Care Hospitals, P.G Teaching, DNB Courses:
  -Sir Ganga Ram Hospital, Delhi: (Dec. 1998 To Dec. 2001); About (3) Year
  -Narendra Mohan Hospital, Ghaziabad: (08.05.1999 To June 2005); About (6) Years
  -Surya Hospital, Delhi:About (4)Years
& Others: In Various Capacities , Including "ADMINISTRATION".

(C) FOREIGN ASSIGNMENTS: -National Iranian Oil Company Hospitals,Iran. - About (1)One Year, 17.12.1991 To 17.12.1992.
  -Aviation & Submarine (Metiga) Hospital, Tripoli, Libya.- About (1) One Year, 26.05.1996 To 25/26. 05. 1997.

Versatile, Wide, Experience in Gen. Surgery, Urology , Lithotripsy & Working Experience Of Other Surgical Super Specialities, Including Intensive Care (Incharge ICU).

"Advanced Diploma In Health Administration" & • Others : Certification In Process.

*(CME),(CPD),(LLL)...: Various National & InterNational Medical Education Programmes,Constant Participation Throughout, Graduation Onwards,
 About(>50) National & International Conferences, Seminars, Symposiums Etc. Participation By Important 'Scientific Studies', Useful Presentations, Discussions,Chairing Session, Publications.

-"3rd AMASI Skill Course", AIIMS, N.Delhi, 29th Nov. - 1st Dec.2006.
-"N.S.V Training Course": PGIMS, Rohtak, March'2008 ; C.S.M Medical University Lucknow, September'2011.
-"Post Graduate Surgical Course", Royal College Of Surgeons Of Edinburgh, U.K, Oct.'2008.
-"MCI CoOrdinatorsOrientationProgr.(1Day):MCIBasicWorkshop (3)Days, (MCINodalCentreCMCLudhina:Sept.2009.
-"AIIMS Ultrasound Trauma LifeSupport (AUTLS) Course",ASITECH,ASICON'2010, AIIMS,N.Delhi,15-20Dec.2010.

*About (50) : Publications, Including Books; 1."Arabic Language. . ."RNI, I & B Ministry,GOI,2003,Several Reprints, 'Supplement',Consideration By UN,ICRC,WHO & Others 2." Students Surgery Manual", Dec.2010...

*About (>25) : 'Scientific Presentations'; Computronics Media Publications,Colloborating Trauma,Filariasis,Breast Care Global Projects ICMR & Others

*About (20): 'Scientific Projects'(In Process); Common Clinical Entities, Useful 'Research Projects' & Or 'Thesis Topics', Including Books; "Surgery For Physio-Therapists" & "Essentials Of Litho-Tripsy".

* Name, Selected, Nominated, Proposed, Published With Other Esteemed Personalities, Of Different Pioneering Magnitudes, By Various National & InterNational Reputed Institutions.

www.ingramcontent.com/pod-product-compliance
Lightning Source LLC
Chambersburg PA
CBHW051801170526
45167CB00005B/1832